FIREARMS AND CLINICAL PRACTICE

Firearms and Clinical Practice

A HANDBOOK FOR MEDICAL AND MENTAL HEALTH PROFESSIONALS

Gianni Pirelli, PhD, ABPP

Sarah DeMarco, PsyD

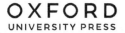

OXFORD
UNIVERSITY PRESS

Oxford University Press is a department of the University of Oxford. It furthers
the University's objective of excellence in research, scholarship, and education
by publishing worldwide. Oxford is a registered trade mark of Oxford University
Press in the UK and certain other countries.

Published in the United States of America by Oxford University Press
198 Madison Avenue, New York, NY 10016, United States of America.

CIP data is on file at the Library of Congress

ISBN 978-0-19-092321-1

DOI: 10.1093/med-psych/9780190923211.001.0001

9 8 7 6 5 4 3 2 1

Printed by Lakeside Book Company, United States of America

This book is dedicated to our colleagues practicing in the medical and mental health professions. Our goal in writing this book was to provide a useful resource that will assist you in providing care and services to those in need, consistent with the contemporary research and best-practice standards in our respective disciplines.

Contents

Disclaimer

———

THIS BOOK IS designed to provide readers with education and information related to firearms and mental health, including but not limited to gun safety and relevant laws and procedures. Our primary goal is to promote awareness and education in this arena and, also, to facilitate clinical decision-making in medical and mental health contexts. Please note: The information presented in this book does not represent the type of professional advice intended to be directly applicable to readers' specific situations, as such should be sought from consulting attorneys and/or mental health experts specifically retained for that purpose.

Preface

꙰ ──

IT IS HARD to believe I have been conducting firearm-specific evaluations in private practice for nearly 10 years. In 2019, I published a book with Drs. Cramer and Wechsler, *The Behavioral Science of Firearms: A Mental Health Perspective on Guns, Suicide, and Violence* (Pirelli et al., 2019). In its preface, I described the genesis and evolution of my expertise in this area—which, like most meaningful things in life, was unplanned, unforeseen, and unconventional.

I am proud that my colleagues and I at Pirelli Clinical and Forensic Psychology, LLC have remained committed to scientist-practitioner principles through and through, whereby our practice informs our research, and our research informs our practice. Through our Center for Research and Training (CRT), our scientific pursuits have also remained organic and completely independent. I have not received any funding since completing my PhD in 2010, and the vast majority of my research and writing has been completed in the early morning hours at my dining room table before work. Fortunately, the pursuit of truth through science has intrinsically motivated me for the last 20 years.

In the guns and mental health arena, staying independent, nonfunded, and objective is uncommon, and staying apolitical is basically unheard of. There are few, if any, more hot-button issues in the United States today. However, it occurred to me at some point in or around 2015 there was a glimmer of hope in bridging certain gaps that divide us as a society. Namely, there was perhaps one non-controversial area of focus that could bring everyone to the table: *education*—specifically, the education of medical and mental health professionals on firearm-related issues. I still have yet to meet anyone who has opposed such and, frankly, I have yet to even think of a cogent argument in this regard. It is difficult to imagine how one could genuinely contend that it is a bad idea to educate doctors, nurses, therapists, and others working in our fields. The so-called "stay in your lane" debate is simply a red herring seemingly fueled by frustrations from those on various sides of gun safety and Second Amendment issues. The truth is this: As medical and mental health professionals, we have not even established a lane yet. When nine out of 10 of us have not received formal training in gun safety and other firearm-related areas, we haven't even left the driveway.

In 2019, Dr. Liza Gold and I published the article *Leaving Lake Wobegon: Firearm-Related Education and Training for Medical and Mental Health Professionals Is an Essential Competence* (Pirelli & Gold, 2019), wherein we wrote that medical and mental health professionals are neither inherently equipped nor professionally trained to help manage firearm-specific suicide and violence risk. This statement remains empirically supported (not to mention having copious amounts of anecdotal support).

As medical and mental health professionals, we must recognize that neither politicians nor media outlets will carve out a viable lane for us. How can we help reduce gun-involved deaths if we are detached from or otherwise alienated by those who own and operate firearms? Physical structures pale in comparison to the proverbial walls that separate so many of us from our patients and examinees. Indeed, communication barriers can be vast and impenetrable.

One salient reason many politicians and media outlets cannot help us overcome these barriers is because, when they are not the primary source of them, they are often fanning the flames. We know what happens when we multiply fractions. Instead, calculations in the guns and mental health arena require a reversal of the typical order of operations, such that addition must precede division.

Typically, politicians who boast about being "tough on guns" are not actually 'taking it to' inanimate objects but, rather, to gun owners. It is also rare to hear that the *reduction of gun deaths* is the actual basis of legislation. Certainly, if such were the case, the foci would largely have to be on preventing such actions as suicide, gang violence, and other primary sources of gun-involved deaths that have essentially nothing to do with "the mentally ill mass shooter armed with an AR-15." Of course, we need to do all in our power to prevent tragedies perpetrated by the latter from ever happening again, but in the process, let us not turn a blind eye to the sources responsible for the other 99.9% of gun deaths occurring in our country every year.

As medical and mental health professionals, we must do our part in our nation's overarching effort to promote gun safety and reduce gun deaths by coming to the consensus that firearm-related competence is one of our essential professional competencies. We can accomplish a lot together, but *we have to decide what we want*. For politicians to continue to be "tough on guns" (owners) while gun death rates remain unchanged for another 20 years? For the media to continue to spearhead firearm-related education? As medical and mental health professionals, we are often the primary gatekeepers in our communities tasked with assessing and managing violence and suicide risk. It is no longer a question of whether we should develop our professional and cultural competence in relation to firearms; we must do so now.

[B]ecause we are all a great deal luckier that we realize, we usually get what we want— or near enough.

Roald Dahl, *Charlie and the Chocolate Factory*
Gianni Pirelli, Ph.D., ABPP

Acknowledgments

WE WOULD LIKE to thank Oxford University Press, particularly the editorial team who worked with us on this project. Special thanks goes to Sarah Harrington—for her unwavering confidence in us and this project, and for the necessary guidance and support to bring it to print. We would also like to thank the proposal reviewers for their feedback and support, which helped improve our conceptualization of this book at the onset. Thanks also to Stephanie Apolo, MA, CASAC-T, our research assistant, for helping to organize and edit references throughout the book.

GIANNI

Thank you to my co-author and colleague, Dr. Sarah DeMarco, for her collaboration on this project and for her seemingly endless positivity and support over the years. I want to also thank my mentor, Dr. Patricia Zapf, for apparently seeing a meaningful spark in a highly motivated, organized, *and naive* 21-year-old two decades ago; Patty, you quite literally opened a door for me that has led to countless others, and I will be forever grateful. My deepest thanks also go to my wife, Dr. Lina Aldana, for always providing me with the love, space, and time needed to complete my writing, and for taking care of our most precious treasures (tqs). Thanks also to Gemma, Ryan, Sandie, and my mother, Susan, for their ongoing love and encouragement. And, to my beautiful children—Miguel, Tiago, and Milena—for filling my heart and mind with never-ending amazement, pride, and love. And to Winston (and Rio) for always knowing just what to say.

SARAH

I must first express my sincere and boundless gratitude to my co-author Dr. Gianni Pirelli, who has shared with me an invaluable wealth of knowledge and expertise in this particularly niche area of practice. Thank you for your mentorship, support, and friendship. I am also deeply thankful for my husband. Your optimism, encouragement, and love have fostered a grounded space in which I can achieve my professional and personal goals. I am extremely fortunate for our partnership. I would also like to thank my mom, whose ever-present love and motivation have carried me throughout my life. And last but certainly not least, thanks to my loving pets, whose unconditional affection supports me in ways they will never quite understand.

About the Authors

⌒

DR. PIRELLI HAS published extensively in the forensic psychology arena, to include but certainly not limited to the application of professional principles to firearm-related issues. Along with colleagues, he developed the Know, Ask, Do (KAD) framework to provide guidance for clinicians addressing gun-related issues in practice (see Pirelli & Gold, 2019). Within this context, Dr. Pirelli et al. have also provided recommendations for developing professional and cultural competence in this area (Pirelli & Witt, 2017), and they have formally addressed particularly important cultural considerations related to conducting gun evaluations, such as the incorporation of local norms (Wechsler et al., 2015). They also developed the Pirelli Firearm-10 (PF-10), a 10-domain structured professional judgment guide for use in firearm-specific evaluations (Pirelli et al., 2015, 2019).

Drs. Pirelli and DeMarco have continued to share their expertise by regularly providing trainings and talks to their colleagues in the medical and mental health professions vis-à-vis navigating firearm-related issues in practice. They have continued to give presentations, teach courses, and provide consultation to a wide range of groups—from Second Amendment groups to community groups focused on gun control and firearm-based violence prevention, as well as many others (e.g., legislatures, state mental health professionals tasked with conducting gun rights restoration evaluations). Their guidance is in line with Pirelli et al.'s KAD model and overarching recommendations to improve gun policy in the United States (see Pirelli et al., 2020).

In addition to their research and publication records, Drs. Pirelli and DeMarco have extensive clinical and clinical-forensic experience, and they regularly testify in court. They are recognized experts in a range of areas within forensic psychology, particularly in the New York/New Jersey/Pennsylvania region, where they conduct forensic mental health assessments in criminal, civil, and administrative matters.

Pirelli Clinical and Forensic Psychology, LLC is distinct from others, as it is an independent practice of doctors with high levels of firearm-specific specialization and expertise—in both practice and research contexts (https://gpirelli.com). Drs. Pirelli and DeMarco have expertise in numerous areas within firearm-related evaluations contexts—administrative, civil, and criminal. Namely, they conduct pretrial and sentencing risk-mitigation evaluations in criminal matters, including but not limited to *Graves Act* matters. They also conduct evaluations in contexts related to gun permit applications and appeals; mental health expungements; gun forfeitures (including restraining orders: Temporary Restrainning Orders [TRO], Final Restraining Orders [FROs], and so-called "red flag" confiscations—Temporary Extreme Risk Protective Orders [TERPO], Final Extreme Risk Protective Orders [FERPO]); carry permits; retired law enforcement officer program (RPO) carry permits; pre-employment and fitness-for-duty evaluations; and evaluations for armed security personnel. Together, Drs. Pirelli and DeMarco have conducted gun-specific evaluations in well over 150 municipalities in New Jersey alone across nearly all 21 counties, and in Pennsylvania and New York as well as in the context of federal matters.

GIANNI PIRELLI, PHD, ABPP

Dr. Pirelli is one of just five people who is Board Certified in Forensic Psychology based out of New Jersey, and one of approximately 300 or so nationally. He received his doctorate in clinical-forensic psychology from the Graduate Center at John Jay College of Criminal Justice, and is a Licensed Psychologist in New Jersey, New York, and Pennsylvania. He currently leads the group practice Pirelli Clinical and Forensic Psychology, LLC.

Dr. Pirelli's primary areas of research pertain to forensic mental health assessment, ethics and standards of practice in forensic psychology, and guns and mental health. He has given many professional conference presentations and invited talks, and he has numerous publications, including being the lead on two books also with Oxford University Press: *The Ethical Practice of Forensic Psychology: A Casebook* (2017) and *The Behavioral Science of Firearms: A Mental Health Perspective on Guns, Suicide, and Violence* (2019), as well as chapters in books such as *Handbook of Forensic Psychology* (4th ed.); *Advances in Psychology and Law* (Vol. 5); *Violent Offenders: Understanding and Assessment*; and *Psychology in the Courtroom*. In addition, his articles have been published in leading practice-oriented journals such as the *Journal of Forensic Psychiatry and Psychology*; the *Journal of Forensic Psychology Practice*; *Professional Psychology: Research and Practice*; and *Psychology, Public Policy and Law*. Of additional note: Dr. Pirelli's research has been cited in amicus briefs to the U.S. Supreme Court and the New York State Court of Appeals, and in the U.S. Department of Justice President's Commission on Law Enforcement and the Administration of Justice Final Report (2020).

Dr. Pirelli is also the former Editor of the New Jersey Psychological Association's (NJPA) journal, the *New Jersey Psychologist*, and served as an editorial board member on the leading forensic psychology journal, *Law and Human Behavior*, for many years. He has also served on the editorial board and routinely reviews for numerous other journals, including but not limited to the *Journal of Aggression, Conflict and Peace Research*; *Psychology, Public Policy, and Law*; *Journal of Forensic Psychology Practice*; and *Journal of Forensic Psychiatry and Psychology*.

SARAH DEMARCO, PSYD

Dr. DeMarco is the Director of Training at the Center for Research and Practice (CRT) at Pirelli Clinical and Forensic Psychology, LLC. She earned her MA in Forensic Psychology from John Jay College of Criminal Justice and her PsyD in Clinical Psychology from the Philadelphia College of Osteopathic Medicine. Dr. DeMarco has worked with adults and adolescents in a variety of clinical-forensic and correctional settings, such as a forensic psychiatric hospital, state prisons, inpatient and outpatient substance abuse treatment centers, and a juvenile detention center. Dr. DeMarco conducts forensic mental health assessments to address various psycholegal issues, and she has extensive experience conducting risk assessments, in particular. Dr. DeMarco is also an Adjunct Professor in the Forensic Psychology graduate program at John Jay College of Criminal Justice and has been designated Adjunct Faculty for the doctoral internship program at Rutgers University. She remains active in research and continuing education efforts, and recently published a chapter in the 2020 book, *Trauma in Forensic Contexts* (Springer).

Introduction

⌒

ACCORDING TO THE Centers for Disease Control and Prevention (CDC, 2021), there were nearly 40,000 gun deaths in the United States in 2019, and 60% (24,000) were suicides. Such is generally consistent with counts from recent preceding years, which have typically totaled approximately 30,000 annual gun deaths, two-thirds of which were from suicide. In 2019, the highest death rate (per 100,000 total population) was Alaska (24.4), followed by Mississippi (24.2) and Wyoming (22.3), and the lowest rate was in Massachusetts (3.4), followed by New York (3.9) and New Jersey (4.1). It has also been noted that the rate of firearm-related deaths in the United States is significantly greater than that of 25 other industrialized countries (CDC, n.d.). Furthermore, the presence of a firearm in the home has been found to be positively correlated with gun-related homicide and suicide risk (Dahlberg et al., 2004; Miller et al., 2013).

All that said, the relationship between mental illness and violence and suicide is nuanced and complex (see American Psychological Association, 2013; Gold & Simon, 2016; Pirelli et al., 2019). These issues have become a part of a national discussion among many people and across various groups, and their saliency rises notably following highly publicized tragic events, such as mass shootings (e.g., Columbine, Sandy Hook, Virginia Tech, Colorado movie theater, Florida's Pulse nightclub, and the relatively more recent ones—the Las Vegas concert, Texas church, Highland Park parade, and Uvalde elementary school shootings). These types of incidents often involve perpetrators using firearms with large-capacity magazines (Barry et al., 2013) and, in some cases, shooters had already been diagnosed with mental health problems (Jenson, 2007). So-called mass shootings, especially school shootings, are the most widely covered and sensationalized sources of gun deaths but, fortunately, one of the least common. In contrast, firearm-involved suicides are the most common, and acts of interpersonal violence closely associated with domestic violence and criminal activity are exponentially greater than those associated with mass shootings.

Firearm-involved violence and suicide is commonly and collectively, yet improperly, referred to as "gun violence." It has been labeled a public health problem of *epidemic* proportions that has led to the involvement of policymakers, community groups, mainstream media outlets, and professional associations (e.g., the American Public Health Association; see Degutis & Spivak, 2021; Greenberg, 2016). For the first time since 1920, the *New York Times* published a page-one editorial in 2015, titled "End the Gun Epidemic in America." President Barack Obama issued an executive order on January 4, 2016, which set forth the following firearm-related initiatives: (1) hiring 230 additional "examiners and other staff" to conduct 24/7 background checks; (2) hiring 200 new Bureau of Alcohol, Tobacco, Firearms and Explosives (ATF) agents and investigators "to help enforce our gun laws"; and (3) a new $500 million investment to increase access to mental health care ("Fact Sheet," 2016). He also indicated that the Social Security Administration would "begin the rulemaking process to include information in the background check system about beneficiaries who are prohibited from possessing a firearm for mental health reasons" (although the administration of President Donald Trump reversed this policy).

Debates regarding the "epidemic" and "public health problem" frequently include the widely held but incorrect assumption that medical and mental health professionals are either inherently equipped or professionally trained to help reduce these types of incidents. As we have previously pointed out, this is inaccurate in both respects (see Pirelli & Gold, 2019). In fact, medical and mental health professionals receive virtually no systematic, formal training on firearm-specific issues—and numerous peer-reviewed studies have empirically documented this lack of training and associated practice-related concerns. This is a problem seen across our disciplines, including but not limited to psychology, psychiatry, and counseling.

For instance, Traylor and colleagues (2010) surveyed a national sample of 339 clinical psychologists and found that the vast majority (79%) believed firearm safety issues were greater among those with mental health problems, but about the same number of psychologists (78%) also reported they did not regularly chart or maintain a record of patients who owned or had access to firearms. Approximately half (52%) of the psychologists indicated they would initiate firearm safety counseling for patients assessed to be at risk for self-harm or harm to others. That said, almost the same number of psychologists (46%) reported that they had not received any information on firearm safety issues. Notably, 20% of those who reported that they had received such information indicated their source was the mass media; only 13% received this information in graduate training and only 7% received it from reading professional journals. These compelling data led Traylor and colleagues to recommend that firearm safety counseling training be integrated into the graduate training of all clinical psychologists and for this to be a priority.

Studies of psychiatric clinical practice with respect to asking about access to firearms and making efforts to eliminate access have also been discouraging (Yip et al., 2012). For example, in one study (Carney et al., 2002), as few as 6% of psychiatric patients in an outpatient setting reported being screened for access to firearms. In a survey of psychiatrists regarding the provision of anticipatory guidance about firearm safety, Price et al. (2007) found that only 27% of psychiatrists had a routine system for identifying patients who owned firearms, even among suicidal patients. One of the most common reasons cited by psychiatrists in this study for not providing firearm safety guidance was "lack of expertise." In a later survey of psychiatric residency training directors, Price and colleagues (2010) found that only 13% reported providing firearm injury prevention training to residents; 79% reported that they had not seriously thought about providing such training. The most significant barriers reported by residency training directors to providing firearm injury prevention training to residents were:

- Lack of standardized teaching material for resident training (50%)
- Lack of faculty expertise on firearm issues (49%)
- Lack of guidelines for training residents on firearm issues (47%)
- Absence of American Psychiatric Association—or American Council on Graduate Medical Education—approved curriculum competencies or guidelines (42%).

Most recently, Nagle et al. (2021) investigated the knowledge and attitudes of approximately 200 psychiatrists in South Carolina with respect to the gun rights of those with mental illnesses. They found that 29% were gun owners, yet only one-third even knew a medical doctor could conduct a mental health evaluation for the purpose of gun rights restoration. Of particular note is that only 4% of psychiatrists correctly answered all five knowledge questions given. Ultimately, Nagle and colleagues noted that firearm-related education in this regard is not required in psychiatry residency or forensic psychiatry fellowship and, based on the results of their study, concluded:

Although state laws may mandate the involvement of a psychiatrist in the evaluation of a patient for the purpose of restoring gun rights, psychiatrists may be ill-prepared to do so . . . Psychiatrists in South Carolina, and perhaps other states, have significant knowledge deficits pertaining to gun laws restricting and restoring gun ownership for persons with mental illness . . . These results show that there is a need for further education regarding this topic during general psychiatry residency and forensic psychiatry fellowship training and with continuing medical education activities for practicing psychiatrists. (p. 34)

In an article published in the same issue of the *Journal of the American Academy of Psychiatry and the Law*, Simpson (2021) reflected on Nagle et al.'s findings, which he indicated "highlight the pressing need for increased training of psychiatrists on this subject" (p. 38). He wrote:

> We should not leave education about this important topic to the vicissitudes of courts and the randomness of referrals. Didactics on the subject should occur in all forensic psychiatry fellowships to provide trainees with a solid framework of knowledge on which to build . . . Nagle et al. make a strong case for the incorporation of training on this topic into the curriculum of all U.S. forensic psychiatry fellowships. (pp. 40–41)

Price and colleagues (2009) also examined college counselors' perceptions and practices regarding anticipatory guidance on firearms for student clients. They surveyed a national sample of 213 counselors and found that very few (6%) were likely to provide anticipatory guidance in this regard and only a somewhat greater number (17%) charted or kept records on client ownership of and access to firearms. As in other disciplines, the majority (54%) of counselors had never received any information on firearm safety and, of those who had, most reported receiving such information from mass media (15%), followed by graduate school training (14%). Less than 10% received firearm safety information from professional meetings, workshops, continuing education classes, or professional journals, respectively. Nevertheless, nearly all of the counselors felt at least moderately confident in their ability to:

- Ask clients about the presence of firearms in their residence (97%)
- Advise clients to remove the firearms from their residence (94%)
- Assess the willingness of clients to remove firearms within the next 30 days (89%).

Furthermore, the majority of counselors felt at least moderately confident in their ability to assist clients in what to do with firearms removed from residences (59%) and arrange follow-up contact within 4 weeks to assess firearm removal (83%). These data are concerning given counselors' self-reported lack of knowledge and training in the specific area of firearm safety.

Slovak et al. (2008) surveyed 697 licensed social workers from Ohio with regard to their attitudes, knowledge, and behaviors associated with client firearm assessment and safety-related counseling. They also found that the vast majority of clinicians (85%) did not routinely counsel on firearm safety and most (66%) did not routinely assess for firearm ownership and access, although the likelihood of routine firearm assessment and counseling increased exponentially in cases wherein clients presented with depression or suicidality.

As medical and mental health professionals, we are taught to engage in general inquiries related to clients' *access to lethal means* related to concerns of dying by suicide or engaging in interpersonal violence, particularly in the context of crisis situations that require assessment of risk of suicide and violence risk. However, even those of us who ask about firearm access are often unsure how to proceed once such access is confirmed. While some of us have learned how to engage in what is referred to as *means restriction counseling*, restricting access to guns is not always clinically indicated or practically possible.

The (incorrect) assumption that addressing mental health issues is "the" answer to reducing firearm-involved violence, particularly violence committed against others, is common. Even President Obama's executive order implicitly connected decreasing gun violence with increasing mental health funding. In addition to allocating an additional half-billion dollars to mental health care access in his 2016 executive order, President Obama also used the terms "mental health" and "mental illness" almost 30 times without ever defining them. Sensationalized mass shootings and their media coverage reinforce the common belief that individuals with serious mental illness are violent and dangerous, especially if they have access to firearms (McGinty et al., 2013), and the axiomatic assumption that mental health professionals should therefore be able to prevent such violence is widespread but, as demonstrated, incorrect. For example, the Las Vegas shooting during President Trump's tenure was the deadliest mass shooting in U.S. history, but he labeled it a "mental health problem at the highest level," not a "guns situation" (Merica, 2017).

Such beliefs are not limited to our political leaders. One survey found that the top perceived cause of gun violence (80% of people polled) is failure of the mental health system to identify individuals who are a danger to others (Saad, 2015). Another survey found that 80% of Americans support laws to prevent individuals with mental illness from purchasing guns (Pew Research Center, 2013) in the belief that this will keep all of us safer from irrational and unpredictable gun violence.

However, along with leading scholars and mental health organizations, we have clearly indicated that firearm prohibitions associated with mental illness should be evidence-based and correspond to the results of an evaluation of people's current risk levels—not simply their mental health diagnoses or histories. As we wrote in a relatively recent chapter on U.S. gun policy:

The association between firearms and mental health is complex and nuanced. Nevertheless, there are certain particularly relevant statistics to consider as a foundation for our understanding of issues related to such: less than 1% of gun deaths have been the result of an active shooter; 2% of murders have been committed with rifles; 3–5% of all acts of interpersonal violence are attributable to even severe mental illness; and two-thirds of gun deaths are suicides. Despite the compelling nature of these numbers, they tend to be disregarded or overshadowed by certain politicians, advocacy groups, and media outlets who often portray the sensationalized image of the "mentally ill mass shooter with an assault weapon"—a stereotype actually drawn from the lowest base rates in each respective area. (Pirelli et el., 2020; p. 404)

Moreover:

A key component of the concept of a moral panic is that the beliefs and percep-tions of the identified topic to be feared are disproportionate to what is occur-ring or has occurred in actuality (Burns & Crawford, 1999). While the connection between mental illness and interpersonal violence, especially gun-involved vio-lence, is steeped in emotion, it lacks empirical support from a statistical stand-point (i.e., with respect to its actual, proportional incidence and prevalence). Thus, the media's focus on mass shootings and associated depiction as a rampant issue particularly linked to mental illness reflects moral panic. (p. 378)

As noted, only 3% to 5% of all acts of violence in the United States are attributable to severe mental illnesses (Swanson et al., 1990, 2015), and even smaller numbers of those with serious mental illness commit acts of violence against others with firearms (Steadman et al., 2015; Swanson et al., 2015; e.g., see also Gold & Simon, 2016; Pirelli et al., 2018; the American Psychiatric Association's resource documents: Pinals et al., 2015a, 2015b; and the American Psychological Association's Panel of Experts Report, 2013). In fact, people with mental illness are more likely to be victims, not perpetra-tors, of violence (Desmarais et al., 2014; Roy et al., 2014).

Indeed, firearm-related violence and suicide is associated with mental health *cri-ses*, not simply mental health problems or diagnoses per se. The Consortium for Risk-Based Firearm Policy, a multidisciplinary group of gun violence prevention and mental health experts, has proposed guiding principles and recommendations to advance an evidence-based policy agenda on the issue of mental illness and firearms (Consortium for Risk-Based Firearm Policy, 2013a, 2013b). The members agreed on a guiding prin-ciple for future policy recommendations: "Restricting firearm access on the basis of certain dangerous behaviors is supported by the evidence; restricting access on the basis of mental illness diagnoses is not" (McGinty et al., 2014, p. e22).

But how do medical and mental health professionals acquire knowledge and guid-ance about firearm-specific issues? Until recently, no comprehensive sources have been available; however, we have previously published a book (Pirelli et al., 2018) as well as various articles and chapters in this arena. We have also developed a frame-work to guide practitioners when conducting firearm-specific evaluations: the Pirelli Firearm-10 (PF-10). In addition, we teach and provide presentations and continuing education seminars on these subjects. However, only particular subsets of medical and mental health professionals will formally be exposed to the literature or other sources of continuing education related to guns and mental health. Therefore, as licensed psy-chologists who have spearheaded some of the contemporary literature and education in this arena, we knew there was a great need for the development of a practical *hand-book* like this—for our colleagues, medical and mental health professionals, to consult when firearm issues arise in clinical practice.

The overarching firearm-related education framework we have developed in this regard is our Know, Ask, Do (KAD) model, which is addressed throughout the book, and in detail in Chapter 4. In this vein, ask yourself:

KNOW: Do I have sufficient information about the issue at hand, generally, as well as in relation to this specific patient? Have I developed sufficient professional and cultural competence to identify, assess, and manage firearm-related issues with patients and examinees? Do I subscribe to a risk assessment and professional decision-making approach grounded in best-practices standards that lends itself to procedural consistency across cases?

ASK: Am I aware of what I need to gather from this patient or examinee to make my next decision in this situation? What might I be asked in the future by a patient, their family member, or an ethics board or a cross-examining attorney? Are my inquiries informed by formal training in the intersecting area of guns and mental health? Are my questions necessary, relevant, appropriate, and (legally and ethically) permissible? Are they focused on addressing proper referral questions?

DO: Am I able to determine the best course of action (or inaction) based on the information I have gathered? Am I able to avoid engaging in black-and-white or biased thinking to ensure my clinical decisions are appropriately nuanced and case-specific? Am I making decisions on an island, or have I consulted as needed? Have I differentiated between crisis situations and those that are serious but not urgent? Have I differentiated between transient and substantive threats? Are my interventions in line with the risk level at hand?

Scope and Format of This Book

FIRST AND FOREMOST, this is a compass, not a cookbook. Our mission throughout this handbook is to facilitate sound clinical decision-making rather than pretend we can prescribe it or somehow point you to "the answer." There are certainly some answers we provide, corresponding with clearly required and prohibited areas of practice—but they are few and far between. What is much more common is our need as medical and mental health professionals to engage in proper procedures and, ultimately, come to a decision that is inherently limited and potentially incorrect. We are not mind readers nor fortune tellers; we are data analysts. As such, our opinions can only be as reliable and strong as the data from which they are derived. We often find ourselves reminding others that *we are psychologists, not psychics*. We have no special ability to predict the future. In fact, we are not at all good at it. So, we can either take our ball and go home or we can remain focused on what we can do quite well: assessing and managing risk.

Risk concerns are at the heart of most if not all firearm-related issues that arise for all of us in our respective practices. Therefore, assessing violence and suicide risk is a necessary yet insufficient component of most of our firearm-related engagement with patients and examinees. Having a handle on contemporary risk assessment principles will likely serve most of us well in many cases wherein gun-related issues arise—but it is not enough. At this point, the professional literature, practice standards, and laws are too wide ranging, and the stakes in each case are too great. As medical and mental health professionals, we must acquire more specialized education and training specific to guns and gun safety. This handbook is intended to serve as your starting and reference point from which you can go on to research the laws and regulations in your respective jurisdictions and apply the concepts and considerations we set forth to your practices.

SCOPE

In this book, we provide our colleagues in the medical and mental health professions with a practical guide on the intersection between mental health and firearms. It is designed to provide readers with a resource that will help them apply firearm-related information and concepts grounded in the empirical literature and best practices in the clinical and forensic treatment and evaluation arenas. As such, our aspiration is that this handbook will be more than solely an informational and educational source, given that its primary goal is to facilitate clinical decision-making for a wide range of medical and mental health professionals practicing across various settings and contexts. Concepts are presented using a best-practices model that encourages and promotes engaging in empirically supported practice and decision-making. This book is distinct from others published in this area due to its inclusion and integration of the following:

1. A focus on the behavioral science aspects of firearm-related matters
2. Review of the professional literature and case law/legal statutes, particularly related to firearm development and use, laws, regulations, violence, suicide, and safety
3. Considerations and information from various relevant areas, including psychology and psychiatry, counseling, sociology, criminal justice, and law
4. Presentation and review of formal frameworks and models for treating and evaluating clinicians to incorporate when firearm-related issues arise in therapeutic contexts, especially when assessing suicide and violence risk is necessary
5. Presentation and review of newly developed and proposed forensic mental health assessment (FMHA) models and applications for evaluating civilians seeking initial firearms permits, gun rights restoration and reinstatement of their firearms subsequent to revocation and forfeiture matters, and for those in related contexts (e.g., mental health expungement evaluations)
6. A focus on how behavioral science principles and our developing empirical knowledge can be applied to clinical practice across settings—to promote and facilitate sound clinical decision-making.

FORMAT

First, please note that we use the words "we" and "us" throughout this handbook because it was primarily written for practicing medical and mental health professionals, and we are licensed psychologists in full-time private practice. Also, as is indicated in the dedication, this book is for you, our colleagues.

We have also worked very hard to write in a scientific yet welcoming and conversational manner. To do so, we have focused on conveying information in a manner akin to presenting at a professional conference, teaching a course, and providing peer consultation and supervision. For instance, we have also included eight case examples and many professional tips throughout. If we were successful in striking the proper tone, this book should be all the more useful to you. In this regard, we use the terms "patients," "clients," and "examinees" somewhat interchangeably throughout—again, to be as inclusive of and useful to such a broad readership across disciplines.

This book consists of six chapters, each of which corresponds to a major area of consideration for clinicians vis-à-vis the intersection of guns and mental health.

In Chapter 1, we provide a primer on guns, including information related to their history and general use, as well as guidance on how to develop cultural competence by recognizing firearm-related subcultures. In addition, we review guns in relation to their types, basic operation, and gun safety principles. Readers are also directed to Appendix A, *Glossary of Firearm-Related Terms*, because, in addition to understanding the mental health–related aspects of the firearm discussion, we must also develop at least a general firearm-related vocabulary (e.g., caliber, semiautomatic, AR-15, bump stock) to be able to put relevant information in context.

In Chapter 2, we review relevant federal and state laws and policies related to guns, including those more specifically associated with mental health. Specifically, we review the Second Amendment; landmark Second Amendment rulings by the U.S. Supreme Court; mental health–related prohibitions; domestic violence–related prohibitions; "red flag" laws (gun violence restraining orders and extreme risk protection orders); gun rights restoration and relief-from-disability considerations; reporting duties of medical and mental health professionals; and gun ownership and safety laws related to magazine capacity, storage, transportation, and right to carry. Readers are also directed to Appendix B, *Glossary of Firearm-Related Law and Legal Cases*.

In Chapter 3, we review the professional literature associated with firearms and mental health, particularly in the context of violence, domestic violence and intimate partner violence, and suicide. We also outline overarching emerging roles for us as medical and mental health professionals, which sets the stage for the second half of the handbook.

Namely, Chapter 4 is devoted to therapeutic contexts—specifically, addressing guns during treatment contacts and the presentation and review of our Know, Ask, Do (KAD) model (see also Appendix C). We also provide guidance on navigating situations such as when patients request gun-specific "clearance," and set forth considerations for treating law enforcement, corrections, military, and related professionals in our practices. Lastly, we address conducting mental health evaluations and comprehensive assessments in both outpatient and inpatient mental health settings.

In Chapter 5, we provide a comprehensive overview of forensic mental health assessment principles as well as those that pertain to firearm-specific evaluations, which represent a specific class of such assessments. In this context, we address considerations for evaluating gun applicants, those seeking mental health expungements, and those involved in gun rights restoration matters (i.e., forfeiture, reinstatement, "red flag," and related scenarios). We also review foundations of violence and suicide risk assessment, in addition to firearm-specific assessment. In addition, we provide a relatively in-depth outline of the Pirelli Firearm-10 (PF-10), a structured professional judgment framework (see also Appendix D).

In Chapter 6, we set forth ethical considerations for medical and mental health professionals. We first review various ethics codes and professional guidelines across disciplines, followed by three ethical decision-making models developed for forensic psychology practice. We then provide guidance on applying such to firearm-related contexts before turning to a discussion on biased decision-making. Specifically, we address the concepts of hired guns, forensic identification, adversarial allegiance, and cognitive bias. Finally, we highlight six areas associated with ethical principles and professional guidelines that are particularly relevant to firearm-related matters: identifying the client; dual roles and relationships, the "therefore" problem, and weapon focus; termination of services; cultural competence and personal beliefs and experiences; breaking confidentiality (reporting requirements, duty to warn and protect, and releasing data); and considerations for internet-based data.

1

A Primer on Guns

GIVEN THAT MANY of us have had relatively little or no exposure to guns on personal or professional levels, this chapter is devoted to providing a general overview of firearms and firearm-related concepts. First, we briefly review the history of guns, including their use by military and law enforcement personnel, as well as civilians. We then address the prevalence of guns in pop culture and public sentiment associated with firearm-related issues. In the second section of this chapter, we discuss the importance of developing professional and cultural competence, including but not limited to being able to identify firearm-related subcultures and related factors that may be relevant to our patients. Lastly, we provide an overview of guns as a matter of hardware and their functionality as such; namely, how they work, various types of guns and ammunition, and gun safety principles. Throughout the chapter, we stress the benefits of becoming familiar with gun-specific concepts, such as to facilitate rapport with certain clients and to improve clinical decision-making across the board. Indeed, this entire book has been designed with these ideals in mind. We also weave in case examples throughout the book to illustrate how various considerations may play out and to demonstrate the applicability of various firearm-related principles in our clinical practices.

THE HISTORY OF GUNS IN A NUTSHELL

Guns, as a type of *arms*, have been used by many civilizations for over 600 years in at least some form, and ancient Chinese alchemists are often credited with creating gun powder as early as the ninth century. Ironically, such seems to have been developed inadvertently in their quest to develop an elixir for eternal life. While they found that combining substances such as saltpeter, sulfur, and charcoal had some healing qualities for skin problems and the like, they also discovered their explosive qualities. This led to the development of the first fireworks as well as a range of explosive weapons, such as bombs, grenades, fire lances, and fire arrows (see McNab, 2009). Guns eventually made their way to the United States in the 17th century via European settlers. They were valued by many for the same types of reasons as they are today; namely, as hunting tools to secure food, for protection, for sporting purposes, and as collector's items. Of course, guns played an essential role in securing independence from Great Britain, and the new U.S. government subsequently began to mass produce guns for military purposes around the turn of the 18th century. As we will illustrate in the *How Guns Work* section below, guns have significantly evolved since that time, particularly because of advancements in their firing mechanisms. Indeed, guns have become a mainstay in many military, law enforcement, civilian, and pop culture contexts in this country.

Gun Use by Military and Law Enforcement Personnel

In the United States, military, law enforcement, and correctional personnel receive training on firearms, and many are required to interact with service weapons at some level during the course of their duties. Military personnel are trained on various types of guns and weaponry very early on, during basic training. Infantry-based personnel and specialists, such as snipers and Special Operations members, receive much more extensive and specialized firearms training. Law enforcement officers in the United States have always carried guns, although such was first standardized by Theodore Roosevelt in 1895 when he became the president of the New York City Board of Police Commissioners. Now, departments throughout the country often have policies identifying which guns are standard issue for service, and other weapons may be used by specialized units (e.g., Special Weapons and Tactics, or SWAT, teams). Correctional and sheriff's officers also receive training and regularly qualify (i.e., demonstrate satisfactory proficiency) in this regard. However, the vast majority of correctional personnel do not carry on the job because guns are not allowed in jails or prisons; they are only used in the most extraordinary circumstances, such as in response to riots or escapes. That said, officers outside security perimeters usually carry guns, including those assisting at the front entrance of correctional facilities, on job details in the community, and in courthouses.

Civilian Gun Use and Ownership

This book primarily addresses firearm-related issues associated with civilians, but the distinction between civilian versus non-civilian gun use was less clear in the early days of this country. American Revolutionary soldiers were essentially armed civilians, Confederate Civil War soldiers used non-regulated arms, and civilians have certainly always used guns for protection, especially during the exploration of new territories throughout the continent. However, as we address in greater detail in Chapter 2, formal gun laws and regulations did not come about for some time. Nevertheless, the Second Amendment (2A) of the U.S. Constitution was ratified in 1791 and acknowledged citizens' inherent right of gun ownership:

> A well regulated Militia, being necessary to the security of a free State, the right of the people to keep and bear Arms, shall not be infringed.[1]

So, how many people in the United States own guns? The easy answer is: We do not know. Because there is no national gun registry, the best we can do is estimate. Most estimates suggest there are approximately 100 million gun owners in the country, which is approximately one-third of the population, and 300 million (legal) guns. These estimates come from what are referred to as *proxy variables*, such as gun death statistics extracted from suicide and homicide databases, as well as from surveys conducted with samples of U.S. households. Two relatively recent polls, for example, indicate that gun ownership is significantly down from the early 1990s. To illustrate, in 2020, Gallup found 32% ownership, which is down from its highest point of 51% in 1993 (https://news.gallup.com/poll/1645/Guns.aspx).

That said, national statistics can be somewhat misleading because states vary greatly in terms of their gun ownership rates. For example, states like Delaware, New York, New Jersey, Rhode Island, and Hawaii have relatively low rates of gun ownership—both in aggregate and per capita—whereas states like Alabama, Arkansas, Virginia, New Mexico, and Wyoming have high rates. For instance, gun ownership in Arkansas is nearly 60%, or 41 guns per every 1,000 residents, and Delaware has only 5% gun ownership, or 4 guns for every 1,000 residents (Capatides, 2015, "49. Delaware section"). As we will emphasize throughout this book, it is important for us as practitioners to pay attention to these types of *local norms* (statistics), in addition to case-specific factors (i.e., noteworthy considerations for a particular client). Furthermore, it is equally important to be aware of laws and regulations in our respective jurisdictions because reliance on national statistics and legislation is unlikely to be particularly helpful insofar as facilitating our clinical decision-making. How might this look in practice? Let us turn to a case example.

---

[1] The landmark U.S. Supreme Court ruling in *District of Columbia v. Heller* (2008) has set the contemporary interpretation of the 2A, including pointing out that it was a preexisting, or inherent, right that "shall not be infringed." The first Supreme Court case on this issue also recognized that this is not a right that is granted (i.e., *United States v. Cruikshank* [1875]). The Court in *Heller* also pointed out that, although some people focus on the use of the term "militia," such is the prefatory and not operative clause in this context. It also addressed the individual versus collective rights issue that is often raised, in part by pointing out that the "right of the people" is used in the Fourth Amendment's search and seizure clause and similarly in the Ninth Amendment—both of which reflect individual and not collective rights. Moreover, the Court cited the founding-era works of William Rawle, Joseph Story, and St. George Tucker (vis-à-vis his version of Blackstone's commentaries) to illustrate the longstanding intention to preserve gun ownership as an individual right.

CASE EXAMPLE 1: MELISSA PORTER (INTEGRATING LOCAL NORMS AND CASE-SPECIFIC FACTORS)

Melissa Porter, a 29-year-old African American female, applied for a firearms purchaser identification card (FPIC) and handgun permit at her local police department in Essex County, New Jersey. She lives alone in an urban area and wants to purchase a five-shot revolver for home defense. However, she was flagged when a 36-hour psychiatric hospitalization from 10 years earlier was discovered during her mental health background check. Melissa did not realize that this would be an issue because she voluntarily went to the hospital at her psychotherapist's recommendation at that time. Specifically, she had been feeling very depressed after her boyfriend of 5 years broke up with her when she was 19 years old. She had no prior mental health problems, but her mother encouraged her to see a licensed professional counselor to help her get through the distress she was experiencing. Melissa did so and, during the third session, she told the therapist she "should just give up" and expressed feeling hopeless. The therapist was concerned, especially because she had only seen Melissa for two sessions to that point and suggested she "get checked" at the hospital. Melissa did so and was released fairly quickly, within a day and a half, as she was not deemed to be at elevated risk to engage in self-harm. The attending psychiatrist diagnosed her with an adjustment disorder associated with the breakup and suggested she continue therapy—without the need for any medication. Indeed, Melissa's low mood and hopelessness resolved within a few months, at which point the therapy ended. She did not experience any notable mental health problems again and she has never had to see a mental health professional since.

Given this information, how can we integrate local norms and case-specific factors to make an informed (clinical) decision about Melissa's appropriateness for firearm ownership? After all, it is not particularly useful and, in fact, can be misleading to simply consider that there are approximately 30,000 gun deaths each year in this country and somehow apply that information to this case. Even knowing that two-thirds are suicides does not get us much further along in our decision-making. Instead, we must delve into New Jersey statistics to get a better handle on the local base rates, particularly those relevant to Melissa. In that vein, it is useful to consider the following based on New Jersey State Health Assessment Data (NJSHAD; https://www-doh.state.nj.us/doh-shad/) and data from the New Jersey Department of Health (Jacquemin, 2016):

- Overall suicide rate: New Jersey's suicide rate is the third lowest in the nation, after D.C. and New York, and it is less than half the national rate (5.4 vs. 11.1 per 100,000).
- Geography: While Essex County has the *highest* death rate due to firearm-related injuries in New Jersey, it has the *lowest* suicide rate in the state (5.6

per 100,000). In direct contrast, the highest suicide rates are in the more rural counties.

- Sex: The male suicide rate in New Jersey is over three times that of females (4.0 vs. 13.0 per 100,000), as nearly 30% of male suicides in the state are with guns as compared to 9% of female suicides.
- Ethnicity: The suicide rate of White persons in New Jersey is nearly three times greater than Black persons (4.2 vs. 11.4 per 100,000), and Black females have an even lower rate (2.5 per 100,000).

It is also worth noting that most suicides in New Jersey are with long guns rather than handguns. Nevertheless, the reality is that female firearm-involved suicides are so exceedingly rare that the 2017 New Jersey Violent Death Reporting System (NJVDRS) report could not even include a line on their graph of suicide weapon trends in the state from 2003 to 2015 because no single year had more than 20 such deaths and, therefore, rates could not even be calculated (Jacquemin, 2017).

As we will illustrate throughout this book, there are certainly a number of clinical considerations relevant to evaluating someone like Melissa that we are not mentioning here, which may either increase or decrease her firearm-related suicide risk. Indeed, there have certainly been some women in New Jersey who have died from suicide with a gun over the years. However, we must use base rates as a starting point and decide how to weigh clinical factors that may elevate, reduce, or have no likely effect on one's risk. Our starting point in Melissa's case might be conceptualized as: An African American female from Essex County, New Jersey, using a handgun to die by suicide would be an anomaly in and of itself. Could it possibly happen? Yes, it is possible, but sound clinical decision-making needs to be based on *probabilities* and not simply possibilities. Many things are possible, but what is likely? In this case, we would still need to conduct a proper suicide (and violence) risk assessment with Melissa, but this is our starting point: an extremely low base rate—in fact, among the lowest we are going to see in the context of gun-involved deaths. This book is devoted to helping medical and mental health professionals think through cases like Melissa's in greater detail, with empirically based confidence.

Guns, Pop Culture, and Public Sentiment

Guns are inextricably linked not only to U.S. history, but also to its ever-evolving pop culture. Guns are present across media, including in our movies, television shows, music, books, theater, and video games. They are omnipresent in Westerns and storylines involving gangs, the Mafia, and other criminal activities. You may also reference Andy Warhol's famous gun art from the early 1980s. In fact, guns are present in so many aspects of our pop culture that we may overlook their presence, particularly when seamlessly woven into our media. For instance, many superheroes and their villainous counterparts use guns regularly, and some heavily rely on them (e.g.,

Deadshot, Punisher, War Machine, Hellboy; see, e.g., Herschberger, 2017; Scole, 2016). Guns are also present in many Looney Tunes cartoons and Disney movies in somewhat subtler ways. For example, in Disney-Pixar's 2007 animated film *Ratatouille*, the main rodent character (Remy) is seen by an elderly woman (Mabel) watching television. She proceeds to wield a loaded, unlocked shotgun and recklessly fires a dozen shots in all directions and, ultimately, through the ceiling. She then dons a gas mask and chases the rodents outdoors near a bridge and fires an additional three shots toward the open waterway. The movie grossed more than half-a-billion dollars and won the Academy Award for Best Animated Feature. At least two of the lead celebrity cast members have publicly addressed guns. Namely, Patton Oswalt has made various tweets mocking gun owners and Janeane Garofalo has participated in at least one gun safety event associated with the Brady Campaign to Prevent Gun Violence—reportedly to raise gun safety awareness (Czajkowski, 2016).

Perhaps more readily known are characters such as Yosemite Sam and Bugs Bunny, who often wielded firearms, as did Davy Crockett, Gaston (*Beauty and the Beast*), and John Smith (*Pocahontas*). References to hunting and shootings have also been used as a main plot point in various stories (e.g., *Bambi* and *Old Yeller)*, and certain types of guns have also become iconic, such as the Model 29 .44 Magnum Smith & Wesson revolver Clint Eastwood used in *Dirty Harry* and the numerous firearms used by John Rambo and James Bond over the years. Undoubtedly, guns are as present in our pop culture today as they always have been ("Hollywood & Guns," 2013).

But how does the American public feel about guns? In short, there are certainly notable divisions in the United States regarding views on guns and gun rights. Indeed, gun-related activities such as hunting and trap and skeet shooting are a significant part of the family heritage and subcultural experience of some, whereas others remain vehemently opposed to any type of civilian firearm ownership. It is accurate to say most Americans, regardless of gun ownership, support a range of gun control measures, such as enhancing certain background check procedures, imposing regulations on gun dealers, and prohibiting certain people from owning guns—including those deemed dangerous, those with domestic violence restraining orders, and those with mental health problems (Barry et al., 2013). Moreover, policies that allow people with mental illnesses to have their gun rights restored even if they are determined not to be dangerous have received the *lowest* support (i.e., 31% to 43% support among gun owners and nonowners). Nonetheless, we will discuss the restoration of gun rights numerous times in this book moving forward because such legal processes are in place in many jurisdictions throughout the country, and they are also the types of issues we, as clinicians, are increasingly more likely to be called upon to address.

What is relevant to point out in this context, though, is that public sentiment regarding gun laws has continued to move in an upward trajectory in recent years, such that most Americans (67%) believe laws pertaining to the sale of guns should be stricter (Jones, 2018). This does cut along party lines, however; namely, there are significant differences among Democrats (90%), Independents (65%), and Republicans (41%) in terms of their support for stricter laws related to gun sales. However, if history repeats itself, we can expect a downward trend in the future given that support for such was at 78% in 1992 and then decreased steadily to 51% by 2008, at which point such support began to rise again. These trends seem to be associated with national violent crime rates as well as the occurrence of high-profile shootings, as the violent crime rate in the United States was at an all-time high in the early 1990s and a number of high-profile mass shootings have been perpetrated since 2008. High-profile shootings tend to keep issues related to firearms and gun control at the forefront of the national discussion, which is reinforced by politicians and media outlets. For example, in 2015, the *New York Times* set forth a page-one editorial for the first time since 1920, entitled "End the Gun Epidemic in America" (www.nytimes.com/2015/12/05/opinion/end-the-gun-epidemic-in-america.html).

The question, though, is: How do mass shootings and media outlets' responses to them affect public opinion related to guns, mental illness, and associated laws and policies? Research has suggested media coverage on mass shootings, for example, increases negative attitudes toward those with serious mental illnesses and heightens support for gun restrictions for them, in addition to imposing general bans on large-capacity magazines (McGinty et al., 2013). This finding is consistent with the aforementioned general lack of support for gun rights restoration procedures. Although we have seen Americans' trust in the media reach its lowest point in decades in recent years, the media's influence on public perceptions and misconceptions associated with guns remains significant.

One particularly concerning issue related to the media's influence in this regard is that "mental health" has become inextricably linked to gun-related legislation and policies. There are a number of reasons for this, not the least of which is sensational media portrayals of the stereotyped "mentally ill mass shooter with an AR-15." The image this term evokes is linked to a heightened emotional response but is actually drawn from essentially the lowest base rate in each respective area: (1) less than 5% of violent acts are attributable to persons with even severe mental illnesses, (2) mass shootings are responsible for much less than 1% of gun deaths, and (3) rifles are used in approximately 2% of homicides in this country (Advanced Law Enforcement Rapid Response Training [ALERRT] Center at Texas State University & FBI, 2018; Blair et al., 2014; Swanson, 1994; U.S. Department of Justice & FBI, 2017).

Some have also pointed out that gun-related violence in low-income areas is largely overlooked and absent from national and political discourse, which corresponds with the belief that the media gravitates toward the "worthy victim" (see Parham-Payne, 2014; Schildkraut & Muschert, 2014).[2] Still, media portrayals often promote emotion over education and, although attention subsequent to high-profile shootings is warranted and understandable, the prosocial and appropriate use of firearms rarely, if ever, gains attention in our media even though the vast majority of those who own or

---

[2] The concept of the "worthy victim" is also apparent in death penalty sentencing; namely, the importance of the race of the victim as opposed to the race of the perpetrator (see, e.g., Kleck, 1981; Klein & Rolph, 1991; Paternoster, 1984; Zeisel, 1981).

otherwise interact with firearms do so safely. Approximately one-third of Americans own guns, or about 100 million people, and many more have potential access to them. It is fortunately the case, then, that the overwhelming majority of people own, handle, and otherwise interface with guns in a responsible and safe manner. However, prosocial activities with guns such as hunting and shooting sports are rarely highlighted by the mainstream media, and they may not be very well understood by many people, including those in our professions—especially in particular regions of the country where firearm ownership and use rates are relatively low. We highlight this issue because one of our primary goals in writing this book is to promote the position that it is important to understand firearms from a perspective broader than solely focusing on gun-involved violence, suicide, and other types of misuse. In no way do we intend to negate or minimize the significance of mass shootings or other situations that involve guns and result in death or injury. However, as medical and mental health professionals, we are trained to work with a wide range of clients and, therefore, developing our competence to work with diverse groups is essential.

DEVELOPING CULTURAL COMPETENCE BY RECOGNIZING FIREARM-RELATED SUBCULTURES

As medical and mental health professionals, it is our ethical obligation to develop and maintain professional competence, which includes *cultural competence*. Although we might have a tendency to conceptualize cultural competence as pertaining to sex, gender, race, religion, ethnicity, and language, it certainly also includes *social contexts*, and this is clearly recognized by our professional organizations. For example, the Association of American Medical Colleges (AAMC) includes social groups along with racial, ethnic, and religious groups in the definition of cultural competence adopted for use in its Cultural Competence Education for Medical Students resource document (https://www.aamc.org/media/20856/download). Moreover, the very first guideline in the American Psychological Association's Multicultural Guidelines recognizes "individual's social contexts" (American Psychological Association [APA], 2017a). Indeed, the *Merriam-Webster Dictionary* (n.d.) defines *culture* as:

a: the customary beliefs, social forms, and material traits of a racial, religious, or social group; *also*: the characteristic features of everyday existence (such as diversions or a way of life) shared by people in a place or time

b: the set of shared attitudes, values, goals, and practices that characterizes an institution or organization

c: the set of values, conventions, or social practices associated with a particular field, activity, or societal characteristic

d: the integrated pattern of human knowledge, belief, and behavior that depends upon the capacity for learning and transmitting knowledge to succeeding generations

As such, cultural influences are those that impact people's languages, thoughts and beliefs, actions, and customs. Moreover, providing clinical services in a culturally competent manner includes recognizing not only potential cultural influences on clients but also those that affect us as providers. It is also important to be aware of how these factors may play out in the client–clinician dyad. In other words, there are three overarching factors to which we should pay attention: (1) the cultural influences clients bring to the relationship, (2) those we bring, and (3) the ways in which our clients' cultural influences interact with ours and the effects of such. Thus, we can envision three entities in any given clinical room: the client, clinician, and client–clinician.

As clinicians, we have been trained to pay attention to the ways in which we interact with clients, but again, our cultural awareness has likely primarily centered around their sex, gender, race, religion, ethnicity, and language, and not necessarily our clients' social contexts. However, it is important to remember that, while people do not choose attributes such as their sex, race, or ethnicity, they typically choose their social activities and groups. As a result, such affiliations may have a greater or special meaning to them, at least in some respects. Later in this book, we explore more involved interactions with clients in both therapeutic and evaluative contexts, but for now, let us look at an example of a relatively benign firearm-related scenario.

CASE EXAMPLE 2: TOM BILLINGS (RECOGNIZING POTENTIAL
CULTURAL INFLUENCES WITH PATIENTS)

Tom Billings is a 42-year-old male who has been seeing Dr. Morrisey, his primary care physician, throughout his adulthood (i.e., for over 20 years). Tom had no particularly notable mental health history, but he has been taking Xanax over the past 3 years, as needed, for social anxiety. Specifically, he was promoted to a new position at work, which required him to start giving monthly group presentations. He always experienced some difficulty presenting in front of larger groups, but it had never been a particularly relevant issue for him because he had not been required to do so since college. Still, he never took psychiatric medication in his life, nor did he ever engage in psychotherapy, because he was able to work through the few presentations he had to give in the past. However, he could not avoid the realities of his new work responsibilities and felt he could use some help to "knock the edge off." Knowing Tom for so long, Dr. Morrisey readily prescribed him a low dose of Xanax to take just before his monthly talks. Tom has done so for the past 3 years, and it has been helpful, as he continues to perform well during his presentations and in the workplace more generally.

Two months ago, Tom decided to apply for a firearms purchaser identification card so he could attend some of the local hunting trips with members of the Elks Lodge he joined last year. As a matter of background, Tom hunted for a brief period as a teenager with his father and paternal grandfather, who hunted for many years, but he did not continue into his adulthood because he became too busy with work and family obligations. Nevertheless, hunting has always been a relatively strong part of his family history and culture, and he has always wanted to find his way back to it. The camaraderie he has developed in the Elks has prompted him to do so. However, the detective in charge of firearm applications at his local police department is requiring Tom to produce a letter from his doctor, in response to the Xanax prescription Tom reported on his application form. Therefore, Tom asked Dr. Morrisey to issue a letter, but Dr. Morrisey feels conflicted because he is "against guns" and feels strongly that "no one needs a gun in their home." He also does not want to speak to the detective or be involved with any administrative, legal, or otherwise forensic matters. As such, he has been avoiding Tom's follow-up calls and Tom is very frustrated, especially because of his lengthy, positive relationship with Dr. Morrisey.

Although this case example may be uncommon in some regions of the country, it undoubtedly occurs in others. In fact, we have seen it happen numerous times in our practices' jurisdictions. There are two main issues at play here: The first is Dr. Morrisey's discomfort interacting with law enforcement, in general, and the second is his more specific problem with being a part of a firearm-related matter. Regarding the initial issue, the reality is that most medical and mental health professionals do not identify as forensic practitioners, they have not been forensically trained, and they do not engage in such work. Therefore, many practitioners are uncomfortable with legally involved matters and most, regardless of their comfort levels, have not received adequate formal education or training to handle them. In fact, even some of the most benign legal issues can present challenges and discomfort for clinicians, such as responding to subpoenas. Of course, there is also the ethical and professional obligation of staying within one's scope and not engaging in problematic dual roles (see Chapter 5).

The second issue here is Dr. Morrisey's aversiveness toward being a part of a firearm-related matter at all. He is clearly opposed to people owning guns and keeping them in their homes, which apparently has prompted him to distance himself from his client and avoid the request for a letter. While it is good that Dr. Morrisey is being open and honest about his personal position on guns, he still has a professional obligation to fulfill. Namely, he has a responsibility to at least provide a clinical treatment summary and, perhaps, even release all of Tom's records to him; after, all, our clients' records are theirs, not ours. Of course, there are ethical considerations related to having the proper releases in place and we may even recommend against the client seeing progress notes if there is a clinical contraindication to such (e.g., if we believe it will potentially cause harm to the client or others if they read what we wrote). Absent such concerns, though, we are obligated to move forward with a client's request in this regard. What is particularly important to recognize in this context is that the presence of a gun-related issue seems to be distracting and, ultimately, impeding Dr. Morrisey from what he has likely done many times: release records to a third party per a client's consent. The fact that a client is seeking a firearm permit really has little significance in this decision because the doctor should not be directly addressing the psycholegal issue anyhow. In other words, Dr. Morrisey should not set forth an opinion about Tom's suitability for firearm ownership because (1) he did not conduct a forensic evaluation to address this specific issue and (2) he is the treating doctor and, therefore, should avoid engaging in such a dual role even if he were qualified to conduct a firearm suitability assessment, just as he would in relation to any other psycholegal question (e.g., parental capacity, proximate cause of psychological injury in a personal injury lawsuit).

Clinicians must often engage in *moral disengagement* when providing treatment or evaluation services. In Betz and Wintemute's 2015 article "Physician Counseling on Firearm Safety: A New Kind of Cultural Competence" published in the *Journal of the American Medical Association (JAMA)*, they noted that various leading medical, legal, and public health organizations have defended the right of physicians to speak freely with patients about gun safety. However, they further noted that health professionals must also know *how* to speak with patients about guns. They too framed the discussion around professionals' cultural competence and contended that firearm owners can be considered a particular type of culture with additional subgroups within it. Ultimately, Betz and Wintemute made four suggestions for physicians with respect to counseling on gun safety:

1. Adopt a respectful counseling approach that is individualized but also routine for high-risk patient groups (e.g., those presenting with suicidality)
2. Maintain a nonjudgmental attitude and present firearm safety information empathetically and collaboratively, without specific instructions to do something
3. Enact policies to encourage this type of counseling on gun safety
4. Act as leaders in educating and advocating for public health and safety associated with firearm injury prevention

Betz and Wintemute emphasized the power of the "white coat" but simultaneously reminded us:

Yet physicians also need to remember that, in individual patient encounters, that same white coat can serve as a barrier to connection and communication. Physicians are entitled to their own perspectives and political opinions, but to serve patients and protect them from disease and injury, it is important to counsel them in ways that are respectful, meaningful, and effective. At times, clinicians may feel uncomfortable or uninformed when discussing certain subjects, and may disagree with a patient's choices or beliefs. However, this discomfort or disagreement cannot justify either offensive condescension or silent inaction. (p. 450)

Let us look at the case example we are considering here from a different angle: What if instead of a firearm permit, Tom and his husband were seeking a mental health clearance in an adoption context and Dr. Morrisey was against same-sex marriage? Or what about clients who are seeking abortions or engaging in essentially any behavior or lifestyle that is in contrast to clinicians' views? Indeed, many of our clients may have different political affiliations than we do, which is often associated with a whole host of worldviews and perspectives on social issues with which we might very well disagree. Certainly, clinicians working in correctional and forensic contexts may be interfacing with clients who more obviously engage in behaviors and lifestyles that run counter to their personal beliefs and morals. However, we cannot dismiss the more ostensibly benign issues in clinical practice, as the potential for bias remains—and, in fact, it may even be greater in the subtler contexts. For example, a correctional psychologist providing therapy to sex offenders may not pass judgment on her clients or focus much at all on the wrongfulness of their offenses (i.e., moral disengagement), whereas the work of others like Dr. Morrisey is impacted by simply finding out that his client of 20-plus years now wants a gun permit. In fairness to Dr. Morrisey and other clinicians with similar reactions, we do have an ethical obligation to recuse ourselves from services when our personal views or problems will likely interfere with performing our work-related duties in a competent manner. However, if Dr. Morrisey's views on gun use and ownership are so strong, he would have to reconsider the types of services he provides and the patients he sees because, as we will illustrate, there are a number of firearm-related situations and subcultures we are likely to encounter in our work.

Firearm-Related Subcultures

Consistent with Betz and Wintemute's (2015) conceptualization, we have also set forth a cultural competence framework associated with firearms (see Pirelli & Witt, 2018). We went one step further, though, and highlighted the fact that there are actually numerous firearm-related subcultures—including those other than gun owners—and that members of each can cross over into others. Specifically, we identified seven such groups to consider in this regard:

1. 2A groups
2. Shooting sport groups
3. Rod and gun clubs, hunting clubs, and shooting ranges
4. Gun control, gun violence prevention, and anti-gun groups
5. Military, law enforcement, and corrections
6. Members of gangs, organized crime, and other criminal organizations
7. Victims of firearm-related suicide, violence, or domestic violence

Of course, it is also important to remember that these groups are certain to be heterogenous in various ways, including their views on guns, gun safety, gun control, and other firearm-related issues. For instance, there are police officers who are particularly interested in tactical training, guns, and marksmanship, whereas others are not and solely interact with their service gun as a required piece of equipment they only carry while on duty. There are also members of gun violence prevention groups who own guns as well as those who have never even seen one in person. Furthermore, there can certainly be overlap across firearm-related subgroups. For example, a police officer may be a member of both 2A and shooting sport groups, whereas another officer may have been a victim of domestic violence and also a member of a gun control group.

Again, we have identified these groups to provide a preliminary outline for practitioners—a starting point intended to prompt clinical and cultural awareness in the same way we recognize a person's sex, gender, race, religion, ethnicity, and language. These are starting points for consideration, although the clients in front of us may have very little in common with their subgroups because of their differing levels of assimilation and perspectives. Of even greater importance is that one's subgroup affiliation may not make much of a difference in relation to a particular question at hand anyhow. For example, a patient may be an avid hunter, but his treatment pertains to work-related stress and, as such, firearm-related issues may never arise. Then again, we can imagine a situation with a patient who has a similar presentation and presenting problem, but for whom gun issues do arise—such as in the context of assessing for suicide or violence risk. Nevertheless, it is our position that it would be beneficial for us to have developed professional and cultural competence in either case. In the first type of situation, doing so gives us an opportunity to get to know and understand our clients better, including their views, activities, and interests. It can damage rapport and even cause a patient to discontinue seeing us if we do not approach gun-related discussions appropriately; thus, conversely, it can lead to a significant increase in the rapport and therapeutic alliance if we do. In the second type of situation, increasing our firearm-related knowledge and competence can improve our risk assessment procedures and associated decision-making across therapeutic and forensic roles, which we illustrate in Chapters 3 through 6 in this book. Let us first outline some of the relevant, albeit preliminary considerations associated with the seven aforementioned firearm-related subgroups we have identified.

Second Amendment Groups

There are many 2A groups in the United States that function at national and state levels. Members of 2A groups believe the Constitution protects citizens' individual rights to own and operate firearms. They are also likely to promote shooting sports in addition to self-defense–related training and education. Of course, many also become involved in political ventures, particularly in light of the ongoing societal climate associated with firearm-related issues. The most recognizable example of a national 2A group is the National Rifle Association (NRA), but there are numerous others, such as the Firearms Policy Coalition (FPC), Jews for the Preservation of Firearm Ownership (JPFO), the Second Amendment Foundation (SAF), Students for Concealed Carry on Campus (SCCC), and Students for the Second Amendment (SF2A).

State-level 2A groups are those such as the Arizona Citizens Defense League (AzCDL), the Connecticut Citizens Defense League (CCDL), the Pennsylvania Firearm Owners Association (PAFOA), and the Second Amendment Coalition of Florida (SACFLA). The interested reader can visit www.allgungroups.org for additional examples. What is important to reiterate, though, is there is often notable heterogeneity in the perspectives across 2A groups. For instance, some groups have adopted a "no compromise" position, such that they will not consider most if not all forms of gun control, whereas others are much more flexible and nuanced in this regard. As clinicians, it may be helpful to know if our patients or clients are members of 2A groups, as it can provide us with an opportunity to discuss their views on gun safety and related issues. It is important to remember the intention is to learn more about our patients and educate ourselves on some of their views and activities relevant to guns, so that we avoid making assumptions about them. The intention is not to engage in political debates with our patients or try to influence their views on anything outside of gun safety and issues associated with their medical and mental health.

Shooting Sport Groups

These groups typically avoid political commentary and focus on providing firearm-related education and training. They also run shooting competitions for those interested in self-defense–related applications and marksmanship, which may include rifles, shotguns, pistols, and even crossbows and bow-and-arrow. Marksmanship-related activities and events have been a significant part of the history of human civilization, well before the United States was even a thought. Activities such as archery date back at least 12,000 years and other shooting sports date back 3,000 years. For example, according to the International Olympic Committee (IOC), the Pentathlon was first held in the ancient Olympic Games in 708 BC and remains a part of the Games (https://olympics.com/ioc/ancient-olympic-games/the-sports-events). It is now known as the Modern Pentathlon and consists of fencing, swimming, and horse riding, followed by a combined running and shooting event (https://olympics.com/ioc/international-modern-pentathlon-union). There are also an additional 15 shooting sport events in our current Olympics (https://olympics.com/ioc/international-shooting-sport-federation). The Paralympic Games also has a number of shooting sport events wherein air pistols, free pistols, and long rifles are used. It is also relevant to remember that students in colleges and universities throughout the country engage in shooting sports. To illustrate, there are approximately 300 colleges and universities that offer shooting programs, including those at universities such as Harvard, Yale, and Fordham (https://competitions.nra.org/competitions/nra-national-matches/collegiate-championships). Furthermore, the National Collegiate Athletic Association (NCAA) has held its Rifle Championship at the Division I, II, and III levels for both men and women since 1980 (https://www.ncaa.com/sports/rifle). There are other shooting sport groups as well, such as the National Shooting Sports Foundation (NSSF), the Youth Shooting Sports Alliance (YSSA), Shoot Like A Girl (SLG²), and the International

Defensive Pistol Association (IDPA). Members of shooting sport groups are likely to be particularly interested in marksmanship and competitive events. As such, they are also likely to be engaged in ongoing firearm-related education and training, formally or informally, and have a good handle on gun safety and related principles. As with some of the other groups identified here, those who engage in shooting sports may have notable variability with respect to their views on gun control and similar political issues. Some may have very little interest in guns per se outside of a piece of equipment used in their sport—akin to a hockey stick or baseball bat. Nevertheless, it can be beneficial for us, as clinicians, to gain a better understanding of our patients' level of interaction with firearms, their views on gun safety, and their practices in that regard (e.g., gun and ammunition storage and transportation).

Rod and Gun Clubs, Hunting Clubs, and Shooting Ranges

There are approximately 500 rod and gun/hunting clubs and over 600 shooting ranges in the United States (www.wheretoshoot.org; https://directory.usacarry.com/places/category/gun-ranges/). Hunting remains an extremely popular activity and such clubs and shooting ranges are also present across regions. Even states with relatively low levels of gun ownership have many (e.g., there are dozens in New Jersey). Many people who join these types of clubs have been exposed to guns throughout their lives, via family and friends. Moreover, they have been using guns since childhood in contexts such as the Boy Scouts of America (now, Scouts BSA), various junior ranger programs, and the like. Of note, people can legally hunt at relatively young ages as well. Some states have no age requirement for most types of supervised hunting (e.g., Alabama, Florida, Arkansas, Indiana), whereas others allow it as early as age 10, such as in Alaska, Arizona, Delaware, Maine, and New Jersey. That said, essentially all states in the United States allow unsupervised hunting by those who are at least 16 years old (Hunts, 2020). Furthermore, there are generally no legal restrictions on children entering shooting ranges, and many allow children as young age 8 years old to participate under supervision (and ages 18 or 21 otherwise). What is important for us to recognize in this context as clinicians is that, while we believe there are approximately 100 million firearm owners in the country, there are many more people who have had some level of interaction or exposure to guns. Indeed, in most jurisdictions, a person can shoot a gun at a range as long as they are at least 18 years old and have proper identification. That said, there are many different reasons why people join clubs or simply go shooting. As noted, some have an extensive family and personal history of hunting, whereas others may go to a range with a friend on a whim. Therefore, it is important for us to ascertain the nature and levels of our patients' acculturation to develop a better understanding of what firearms mean to them, if anything.

Gun Control, Gun Violence Prevention, and Anti-Gun Groups

Just as with 2A groups, there can be significant variability in the perspectives of members in these groups. For instance, there are certainly gun control and gun violence prevention groups that support the 2A and an individual right to own and operate guns, but who may advocate for stricter laws and policies to prevent firearm-involved violence, suicide, and injury. On the other hand, there are groups essentially against all types of civilian firearm ownership and use. Similar to 2A groups, interested readers can easily find local and regional groups, such as North Carolinians Against Gun Violence (www.ncgv.org) and New Yorkers Against Gun Violence (www.nyagv.org); there are many such groups throughout the country. Many national groups are also the product of mergers between and among various groups; therefore, many are considered campaigns and coalitions rather than independent groups per se. In addition, there are various groups that have been developed in response to specific mass shootings and tragic events, such as the Newtown Action Alliance, which was formed after the 2012 Sandy Hook Elementary School shooting. As clinicians, we must be cognizant that members of gun control and gun violence prevention groups may be even more likely to have been impacted by firearm-involved violence or suicide in their lives, which may have shaped their views on guns. There may also be clinical implications in this regard, such as those associated with bereavement or even suicide contagion.

Military, Law Enforcement, and Corrections

Military, law enforcement, and correctional personnel have generally all received some level of formal firearms training, although the depth of such and their subsequent experience with guns varies greatly among and within these groups. Law enforcement officers are likely to have the most consistency in this regard, whereas military personnel can range from soldiers in infantry units with combat exposure to those who have not interacted with a gun since boot camp. Correctional officers are also more likely to have varied gun experience and exposure because it is a job that requires gun training, ownership, and qualification, but does not permit the vast majority of employees to actually interact with firearms during the course of their work. Nevertheless, we should not make any assumptions about law enforcement officers or military personnel with respect to their firearm-related views, experiences, or current use. Some of our patients in these groups will have no interest at all in guns and would never carry off duty, whereas others will be armed at almost all times. What is particularly relevant to us as clinicians, though, is that members of these groups are often at higher suicide risk than their civilian counterparts and such is often completed with guns, more specifically with their service guns. Moreover, the factors associated with completed suicides among this group are often in sharp contrast to those associated with civilian suicides in that civilians are more likely to have documented mental health and substance use–related problems and diagnoses, a history of and current mental health treatment, and disclosed intent. However, among military and law enforcement personnel, there is a greater stigma attached to seeking professional help, particularly related to the potential repercussions of doing so—namely, jeopardizing one's career if placed on restricted duty or leave. In addition, as we will also point out later in this book (Chapter 5), although members of these groups are often issued service weapons, such does not directly translate to their rights as a civilian. For example, both of us (G.P. and S.D.) have evaluated military and law enforcement officers who actively and legally possessed one or more service firearms, but who were still mandated to undergo mental health evaluations to be granted permission to purchase personal firearms within civilian ownership contexts.

Gangs, Organized Crime, and Other Criminal Organizations

Those who engage in illegal acts and who carry or otherwise possess guns are part of a firearm-related subculture perhaps best known to forensic and correctional mental health professionals rather than other clinicians. Still, we may not tend to think of the connection these groups have with guns because it is so relatively commonplace. In fact, it is almost hard to visualize a gang or organized crime member without a gun, although media and Hollywood portrayals of these groups certainly contribute to such. What is relevant to us as clinicians is that these groups represent a primary source of much of the interpersonal gun-involved violence in our society, which is often perpetrated in urban areas. Those engaged in illegal and otherwise nefarious activities are not going to apply for a firearms purchaser license and, therefore, we are very unlikely to evaluate them in that context. Instead, we are likely to provide therapeutic and evaluative services with members of these groups for various reasons and across contexts and settings, including but certainly not limited to correctional institutions. It is important to address gun-related issues with these groups, especially in institutions, as part of discussions associated with their past and anticipated behaviors and lifestyles in the community. These discussions are particularly relevant to have with youth in urban areas because of their vulnerabilities and corresponding risk associated with gun possession and use. There are many reasons those who engage in criminal and otherwise problematic behavior carry and own guns, such as for protection, control, and influence. It can be beneficial to explore these concepts when working with these groups and to specifically address guns in addition to other aspects of their behaviors and lifestyles.

Victims of Firearm-Related Suicide, Violence, or Domestic Violence

Another very relevant firearm-related subculture includes those who have been victims of firearm-involved crimes and those who have been affected by the firearm-involved suicides of people in their lives. Therefore, medical and mental health professionals working with members of these groups should be aware of firearm-related considerations and not make any assumptions about their personal experiences. For example, people within this subculture are likely to have heterogenous views on firearms, and their history with such may or may not influence their beliefs or future involvement with firearms. As such, victims of violence and domestic violence may seek to own firearms at some point (e.g., for self-defense purposes). States vary with regard to restrictions for people with violence and domestic violence histories, and some have even loosened ownership conditions for such people. As with all groups, practitioners should aspire to gain an understanding of patients' motivations and perspectives on gun ownership and related issues, and perhaps for those in this group, how their past experiences have shaped their current views on guns.

Taking Steps to Develop Firearm-Related Cultural Competence

As medical and mental health professionals, cultural competence is an essential aspect of our professional competence. It has been increasingly important to include the development of some level of firearm-related competence, especially now that gun deaths are widely considered a significant public health problem. Expounding on Betz and Wintemute's (2015) recommendations for physicians and other health professionals, we reiterate the stepwise approach we have previously published (Pirelli & Witt, 2018) for practitioners *as well as researchers and educators* to develop and maintain firearm-related cultural competence:

1. Medical and mental health professionals should *familiarize themselves with the firearm literature*, well beyond the gun violence literature and into the full range of firearm-related matters, including prosocial uses of guns and otherwise.

2. Practitioners should *engage in formal continuing education efforts by taking courses in the firearms and mental health arena*. At this point, these types of courses are relatively rare; therefore, professionals may need to initially take more general firearm courses in such settings as local gun ranges or conferences presented by groups who are familiar with firearms (e.g., law enforcement, public safety, 2A groups). In addition, we encourage *taking courses or attending talks from the full range of groups associated with firearms*, including gun violence prevention and even anti-gun groups. It is insufficient to receive information from just one side, and it is important to develop a broader understanding of opinions from both sides. It is equally important to receive education on firearm construction, use, and safety. In other words, appreciating the reasons why some people support particular gun policies will not be useful for the practitioner who is conducting a domestic violence–related risk assessment and becomes aware of gun-specific information during the course of the evaluation. Having an awareness of a 2A debate will lack utility in this context. To this point, though, much of what is available to us as practitioners pertains to gun violence and others' perspectives on guns rather than information specifically about firearms or about those who own and operate them appropriately (i.e., the overwhelming majority).

3. Furthermore, practitioners who would like to conduct firearm-specific evaluations, such as those for initial applicants or in gun forfeiture matters, should *strongly consider visiting environments frequented by firearm owners and operators* (e.g., gun ranges, gun shows, 2A conferences). This recommendation is consistent with clinical training principles, more generally; namely, the many years and thousands of hours of classroom education, independent reading and study, and engagement in experiential practicum placements. Moreover, we must practice within the bounds of our professional competence, which includes not only the types of services we provide *but also* the types of clients for whom we provide them. Of course, we may develop new areas of professional competence, but this requires us to acquire face-to-face, hands-on experience with the new practice areas and populations. In addition, we should seek formal professional supervision, or at least consultation, until we reach a point of independent proficiency in the area.

4. *Those who conduct research and teach in areas related to firearms should also develop and maintain their professional competence* in this regard given that professional ethics codes also pertain to academicians, students, and researchers. For example, the American Psychological Association's Ethical Principles of Psychologists and Code of Conduct (EPPCC; APA, 2017b) sets forth the following:

(a) Psychologists provide services, teach, and conduct research with populations and in areas only within the boundaries of their competence, based on their education, training, supervised experience, consultation, study, or professional experience. (p. 5, Standard 2.01, Boundaries of Competence)

And, more specifically:

(c) Psychologists planning to provide services, teach, or conduct research involving populations, areas, techniques, or technologies new to them undertake relevant education, training, supervised experience, consultation, or study. (p. 5, Standard 2.01, Boundaries of Competence)

Consistent with these principles and the recommendations we have presented for practitioners, *we recommend academics, researchers, and students take a hierarchical approach* to develop and maintain their professional competence associated with firearms and firearm-related subcultures. As such, those who conduct research on or teach about firearm-related issues should become familiar with the literature pertaining to guns, broadly, and not solely gun violence, for example. Furthermore, those who conduct research and teach in areas more closely connected with guns would be well served in seeking formal continuing education on firearm-specific topics, and even consider getting (direct) exposure to certain types of firearm-related subcultures in natural environments, such as at gun ranges or conventions.

That said, to this point we have covered a range of issues *related* to guns, but we have not quite spoken specifically *about* guns as a matter of hardware. Although we do not believe clinicians need to be gun experts or even have a sophisticated understanding of guns per se, it can be helpful to have some working knowledge and an understanding of corresponding language regarding the various types of guns as well as how guns work, and basic gun safety principles. Acquiring such can be helpful in building rapport with certain clients, but also provides us with context and perspective that can inform our decision-making. For example, it is relevant to know the meaning of terms such as *semiautomatic*, *AR-15*, and *magazine*, so our assessments and decisions are not impacted by our assumptions or misinterpretations. We have included a *Glossary of Firearm-Related Terms* in Appendix A to provide you with some basic terms and their definitions; this is not an exhaustive list but is a good starting point for those unfamiliar with guns.

It can also be useful to have a general idea of how firearms operate, as such can provide context in individual cases as well as in relation to gun-related policies and laws. For instance, it is certainly the case that any firearm can potentially cause harm, but there can be significant differences in the likely degree of harm depending on the gun in question. That said, our ultimate opinions may largely be dependent on the type of outcome we are concerned about in a particular case. For example, it theoretically takes only one bullet (of many different calibers and from various types of firearms) to complete a suicide—in contrast to the amount of ammunition involved in certain types of mass shootings. Given that there are different types of firearm-involved risk outcomes that may be in question (e.g., suicide, violence, domestic violence) and likely (or unlikely) scenarios to consider, risk assessments should be context-specific (see Chapter 5 for more detail in this regard). Last, but certainly not least, it is very important for us, as clinicians, to be aware of general gun safety principles and have some perspective on issues related to firearm-related accidents and misuse. After all, how can we know if a patient is being potentially unsafe or otherwise irresponsible with firearms if we do not understand what being safe and responsible with guns actually looks like?

GUN TYPES, OPERATION, AND SAFETY

Many of us have been concerned about our patients engaging in certain activities, such as driving, working particular jobs, or even raising their children—and even though we might not be motor vehicle, vocational, or parenting experts, we have still been able to appropriately and professionally address our concerns. Why? Because most of us have at least a general sense of the language and contexts associated with vehicles, working, and child-rearing from personal if not professional experiences. Of course, we may refer a patient to a specialist when the situation at hand exceeds the parameters of our professional competence or our identified role in a certain case (e.g., evaluations of fitness to drive, for duty, and to parent). However, most of us are likely comfortable enough to at least broach the subjects. We do not make this same assumption about guns, however. As we noted in the Introduction to this handbook, relatively few medical and mental health professionals receive formal education and training on firearm-specific issues, including gun safety, despite the fact that one in three Americans own guns, and even more have potential access, and at times we are expected (and sometimes required) to inquire about guns.

Therefore, it is important for us to have a basic understanding of various gun types, general components and functions, and safety principles. How else can we be informed commentators and consumers of information related to guns? Otherwise, we run the risk of fostering miscommunication and misunderstanding, and we may also adopt ill-informed thresholds for important clinical decisions—such as those associated with suicide and violence risk (e.g., breaking confidentiality when a duty to warn or protect is incurred). Terms such as *semiautomatic, assault rifle, large-capacity magazine*, and even *gun control* are commonly used, yet misunderstood. While we certainly do not claim to be gun experts in this specific regard and we also acknowledge there may be disagreement even among those who are, we provide an overview of firearm-related foundational concepts and key terms to help inform clinical decision-making and encourage continued education in the following three areas: (1) how guns work; (2) types of guns and ammunition; and (3) gun safety.

How Guns Work

Cannons were developed hundreds of years after the Chinese first created gunpowder and early explosive weaponry. These advancements led to the development of the first guns in or around 1350, which are often referred to as "hand cannons" because they were basically miniature, handheld cannons. The firing mechanism was based on the basic premise of having a tube with a closed end (breech) and an open end (muzzle), loading it with gunpowder and a projectile, and then lighting the gunpowder to create an explosion that would expel the projectile. Modern-day guns still operate from this basic concept; however, their ignition systems have evolved, thereby making them more efficient and capable of more rapid and accurate firing (Supica, n.d.).

All guns basically have four components that define their classification and abilities: *muzzle, breech, hammer*, and *trigger*. The muzzle is the opening on the front from where the bullet is projected, and the breech is the back. The hammer initiates contact with the ammunition primer to ignite the gun powder, which results in projecting the bullet out of the muzzle. The hammer is the component that you may have seen someone pull or click back with his or her thumb, although it is internal on some handguns and on many rifles and shotguns. On some guns, a *firing pin* is used to contact the primer instead. Lastly, the trigger is the part that is pulled by one's finger to release the hammer and fire the bullet ("Guns 101," n.d.). Other common components include but are certainly not limited to *sights, action, frame, barrel, bore, chamber, cylinder release*, and *receiver*.

The ways in which guns specifically work vary to some extent because they can have different types of firing mechanisms. Early firearms, such as matchlock and flintlock guns, functioned by one lighting a match or producing a spark that would ignite the gunpowder. While modern firearms operate from the same general

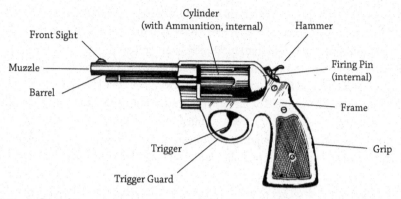

FIGURE 1.1 Basic firing components of a modern firearm (revolver)

premise, there are additional steps: the ammunition, or bullets, sit in the barrel; the operator pulls the trigger, causing the hammer to snap forward; the firing pin strikes the primer, which creates a spark and ignites the gunpowder, thereby creating an explosion that projects the bullet out of the gun. Again, there are various types of firing mechanisms, but these are the basic steps involved in shooting a modern-day gun (Figure 1.1).

Types of Guns and Ammunition

The most basic distinction between guns is that of handguns versus long guns. There are other relevant classifications, such as automatic and semiautomatic weapons, which we will generally address in this section as well.

Long Guns

Most of us can readily visualize long guns in the form of hunting rifles and shotguns (see Figure 1.2). Long guns have longer barrels than handguns, although laws differ across jurisdictions with respect to their definitions of what constitutes a long gun (based on barrel length). Furthermore, short-barreled shotguns (those less than 18 inches and often referred to as "sawed-off shotguns") and rifles (less than 16 inches) are regulated under the National Firearms Act (NFA) unless a taxed permit (stamp) has been obtained from the Bureau of Alcohol, Tobacco, Firearms (2009). The issue, in large part, pertains to their concealability. They are classified as Title II Weapons, or NFA firearms—and although they are not per se illegal under federal law, they are more heavily regulated than other guns. That said, they are illegal in some states, such as New Jersey and New York, along with certain types of silencers and items classified as destructive devices. This is another example of the importance of being apprised of specific state laws and the inter- and intrastate nuances that exist. In New Jersey, for instance, one must apply for a handgun permit for each handgun purchase, whereas there is no specific permit required for long guns.

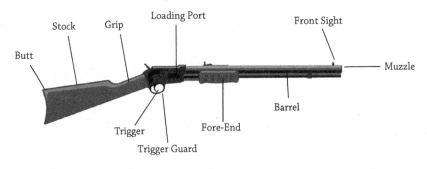

Butt Stock Grip Loading Port Front Sight Muzzle Trigger Trigger Guard Fore-End Barrel

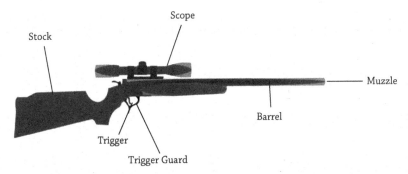

Stock Scope Muzzle Trigger Trigger Guard Barrel

FIGURE 1.2 Shotgun (top) and rifle (bottom)

Typical long guns, however, are designed to be held against one's shoulder and are much more difficult to conceal than handguns or their short-barreled counterparts. There are many reasons people buy and use long guns, ranging from hunting to home defense to engaging in shooting sports and related competitions. What is the difference between a shotgun and a rifle, though?

Shotguns are long guns that project shells packed with one of three types of ammunition: *bird shot*, *buck shot*, or *slugs*. Bird shot shells contain the smallest pellets and buck shot shells have the largest, whereas slugs contain pieces of metal and not pellets. Shotguns will fire a (circular) pattern of these many small projectiles, which is useful for hunting certain types of game (e.g., birds), as well as trap and skeet shooting involving moving targets. Shotguns are also a very popular self-defense choice as compared to guns that expel single bullets, particularly because they require somewhat less aim and accuracy due to the fact that they release multiple projectiles within a single shot. The loud sound a shotgun makes when it is "racked," or when a shell is loaded and chambered, is also rather loud and identifiable—which is thought to be a potential deterrent to would-be burglars or the like. There are many types of shotguns, but perhaps the most commonly known are pump-action and double-barreled. A pump-action shotgun works as it sounds, such that the user loads it manually and then literally pulls the pump forward and back to prepare for firing, whereas double-barreled shotguns essentially fold in half and are prepared for firing once loaded. Some double-barreled shotguns also have a hammer that must be pulled back, like a revolver (handgun).

Rifles are long guns that have grooved barrels, or what are called "rifled bores." This causes the bullet to spin upon firing, which significantly improves the shot accuracy. As such, it is not surprising that rifles are the choice weapon of snipers, hunters, and marksmen aspiring for high levels of accuracy, especially from long distances. Theoretically, a rifle can shoot over 4 miles, albeit with limited accuracy at that distance. Record sniper shots have generally been recorded at distances between 0.5 and 1.5 miles, or 800 to 2,600 yards. However, most (amateur) shooters practice at 50-, 100-, and 200-yard ranges, which reflect typical hunting distances. There is also significant variability in the types of ammunition used in rifles, as these guns range from .22 caliber to much higher-level calibers, with the largest being .950. The smaller calibers, such as .22s, are the types used for small game hunting and "plinking" (i.e., shooting targets such as cans and metal discs) and are popular for use by youth (e.g., in the Scouts BSA).

Civilian rifles are usually either *bolt-action* or *semiautomatic*, which refer to the firing mechanism and, more specifically, the way in which a cartridge/bullet is loaded into the barrel chamber and prepared for firing. For instance, a bolt-action rifle comprises a manually operated bolt, wherein the operator (manually) manipulates the bolt to eject the previous cartridge (i.e., round) and prepares the next for firing. A semiautomatic rifle works like a semiautomatic handgun in that, upon each pull of the trigger, the cartridges, or rounds that are loaded into a magazine, automatically cycle into the barrel *without* the need for an additional step by the operator (e.g., manipulating a bolt or pulling back a hammer).

Simply put: A semiautomatic weapon is one that requires a trigger pull for each shot, as compared to an automatic weapon, which continues to fire so long as the trigger is held back.

We frequently hear the term *assault rifle*, although it does not have a clear definition and is often used incorrectly. An assault rifle is generally considered to be a fully automatic rifle (rather than semiautomatic) that uses a detachable magazine. Automatic, in this context, means that you can hold the trigger down and bullets will continue to fire. These firearms are illegal for civilian use but are used by the military. That said, many of us would not be able to tell the difference between an automatic and semiautomatic rifle just by looking at them, which can lead some to erroneously group assault-style weapons with actual assault weapons.

In Figure 1.3, for example, two rifles are presented. While they *look* similar, they are actually very different in terms of their firepower and capabilities (i.e., functionality). To be clear, every gun can potentially harm someone, but the degree of impact can vary greatly. For instance, the firearm first presented is an AR-15-style semiautomatic rifle. These types of firearms can be made to fire a wide range of ammunition sizes, but one cannot know this simply by looking at a photo. Namely, the one depicted here is for civilian use and can be made to fire .22LR ammunition—to hunt such animals as squirrels and rabbits, or to engage in plinking. Of course, there are rifles that *look* like this one but use much more powerful ammunition. Again, we cannot know this by looking at an image. The firearm below it, on the other hand, is an M4-style automatic

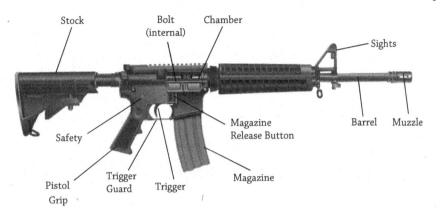

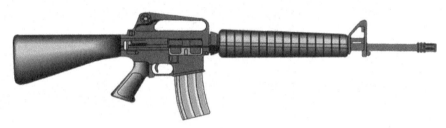

FIGURE 1.3 Semiautomatic (AR-15; top) and automatic (M4; bottom) rifles

rifle used by the military that can shoot .223 ammunition ("ammo"). To reiterate, even ballistics experts would not be able to tell the firepower of these guns, much less laypersons in this context, including clinicians like us. It is likely that these guns appear effectively identical to most of us.

As Figure 1.4 illustrates, bullet sizes can vary tremendously. This particular image contains bullets for both rifles and handguns and demonstrates the significant variability in available bullet sizes. As we will outline in the *Ammunition and Bullet Calibers* section below, bullet size corresponds to what is referred to as the caliber of a firearm (e.g., 9mm, .22LR, .223). To revisit the example corresponding to Figure 1.3, the firing mechanisms (semiautomatic vs. automatic) and ammunition used by these guns are extremely different, unlike their look.

Of additional note is the label *AR-15*, which is a term that is often misused and misunderstood. It stands for ArmaLite Rifle, named after the company that developed it in the 1950s. The AR-15 is a semiautomatic modern rifle, and it is simply one type of design within this category of firearms. It is not a fully automatic rifle (like the M4) and, despite the negative attention they often receive, they are commonly owned and operated by many civilians in the hunting and shooting sports communities. As such, it is certainly possible for the AR-15 depicted in Figure 1.3 to fire the smallest bullet shown in Figure 1.4, whereas the automatic weapon below it can fire the largest (and

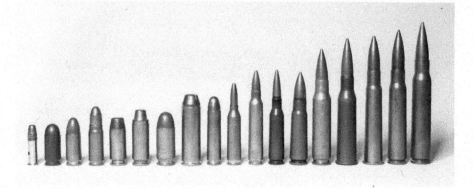

FIGURE 1.4 Bullet sizes: examples of rifle and handgun ammunition

even larger). In other words, an AR-15 like the one shown in Figure 1.3 can theoretically fire any size bullet depicted in Figure 1.4, as well as many other variations. Again, simply looking at an image gives us essentially no information as to the gun's functional capacity in this regard.

Handguns

Handguns are usually designed and used for marksmanship-related activities, such as target and competitive shooting, as well as for self-defense because their size lends to easier handling, carrying, and concealability. There are basically three types of handguns: *single-shot pistols*, *revolvers*, and *semiautomatic pistols*.

Single-shot pistols use one bullet at a time—a mechanism also available for rifles and shotguns. Once the gun is fired, another bullet must be loaded. As such, single-shot firearms are much less efficient than revolvers and semiautomatic pistols and, therefore, are more likely to be owned and operated by collectors and gun enthusiasts today.[3] There are exceptions, however, such as *The Palm Pistol*®, which is a single-shot firearm "intended for seniors, disabled or others with grip limitations due to hand strength, manual dexterity or phalangeal amputations," as it can be fired using the thumb or combinations of other fingers (http://constitutionarms.com/palm-pistol/).

Many of us can recognize revolvers, as they are commonly seen in Westerns. Although police have used them in the past, they are generally not currently used by on-duty law enforcement any longer because civilians have much greater levels of firepower readily available to them, particularly those who engage in criminal activity, which necessitate the use of semiautomatic firearms. Nevertheless, revolvers remain popular among our citizenry. They also continue to be used by off-duty officers as well as armed security guards and those in related professions. Revolvers were

---

[3] Single-shot firearms should not be confused with single-*action* revolvers, which is a term that corresponds to a certain type of firing mechanism.

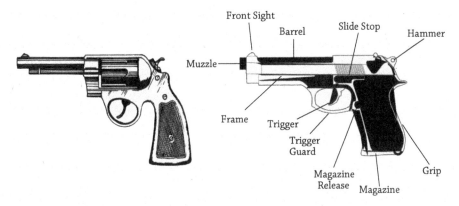

FIGURE 1.5 Revolver (left) and semiautomatic handgun (right)

initially called *revolving guns* because they have a cylinder containing bullets and they are considered repeating firearms, as multiple rounds can be fired without reloading. Each bullet is loaded into the cylinder, which rotates when fired, thereby lining up the next round for fire. Revolvers may be single-action or double-action, and some guns allow for both types of use. Single-action revolvers require the hammer to be manually pulled back, whereas double-action revolvers automatically rotate when the trigger is pulled. If you have ever heard the term *six-shooter*, it is because most revolvers hold six bullets.

Although the term *semiautomatic* may have a negative connotation for some, essentially every modern handgun that is not a single-shot pistol or revolver is semiautomatic (see Figure 1.5). It is the type of handgun we are most likely to see presented by media outlets or even in our everyday lives, particularly given their widespread use by law enforcement personnel. A defining feature of a semiautomatic handgun is the magazine, or clip, that holds the bullets and is inserted into the handle area of the firearm. Whereas revolvers rotate, semiautomatic handguns use the energy of a shot to (automatically) reload the next bullet into the chamber. This occurs at each pull of the trigger, until all of the bullets are used and the magazine is empty. This is why semiautomatic guns can be rapidly fired and reloaded with a backup magazine. In other words, someone can shoot 15 bullets quickly and then, with the push of a button, replace the empty magazine with another, full, 15-round magazine—and continue to fire. As such, they are often used in shooting sports competitions, particularly when speed is desirable, but also by law enforcement as well as those who commit violent crimes. The amount of bullets that can fit in a single magazine varies, ranging from 5 to 30, and includes essentially everything in between. That said, some states have restrictions on magazine capacity, such as New Jersey's relatively recent change to a maximum of 10 for civilians—decreased from 15 (see Ciyou, 2018; Kappas, 2021; Supica, n.d.). That said, some may argue there is not much of a practical difference between having four 15-round magazines and six 10-round magazines for someone seeking to do harm, such as perpetrating a mass shooting.

Ammunition and Bullet Calibers

Ammunition is often thought of as the bullets a gun fires, but it is somewhat more involved than that because ammunition actually consists of a case, primer, gunpowder, and a projectile. The case holds all of the components together and is usually made of brass, steel, or copper. The primer is an explosive chemical compound that ignites the gunpowder when struck by the firing pin. The two types of primer, rimfire and centerfire, correspond to where the primer is located in the case—either in its rim or in the center of its base. Gunpowder is also a chemical mixture but serves as a propellant because it burns rapidly and converts to an expanding gas when ignited. The projectile is the object expelled from the barrel (i.e., the actual bullet). Another important concept to know is caliber, which refers to the internal diameter of a gun's barrel, or the diameter of the projectile it fires. Therefore, it corresponds to the size of the bullet a gun can fire, and it is measured in hundredths and even thousandths of an inch. There are literally hundreds of ammunition and gun calibers available, but some of the most common are .380, .22LR, .40 S&W, 9mm, .45ACP, .38 Special, and .357 Mag. In Figure 1.6, just some of the available rifle and handgun ammunition is shown; note the significant variability in size and type. Also note that the term *gauge* is used to refer to the diameter of shotgun barrels, such as 12- or 20-gauge. A shotgun shell is presented in Figure 1.7 along with ammunition used in a rifle and handgun, and this illustration contains the basic component locations. Please note that some components are internal and cannot be seen in the images presented here; namely, gunpowder, primer, and propellant are internal.

Lastly, it is important for us to know that the typical box of handgun ammo contains 50 rounds, 25 for shotguns, and 20 for rifles. There are exceptions, though, and many gun owners will often store numerous boxes of ammunition. Ammo is relatively inexpensive and can be purchased online fairly easily. While costs certainly vary based on brand and caliber, most can be purchased between 2 and 50 cents per round. For example, one can buy 5,000 rounds of .22LR for about $200 and 1,000 rounds of 9mm ammo for $150. Moreover, it is fairly compact, so it is possible to carry 1,000 rounds in a handheld ammo can, which will weigh about 30 pounds. Figure 1.8 depicts examples of the box contents of both rifle and handgun ammunition.

Gun Safety

Although it is not typically presented to us in our professional literatures, firearm safety is obviously one of the most, if not the most, important issues for us to consider. After all, we are often called upon to assess and opine upon our patients' risk levels, including their suitability for firearm ownership and use. But as we have asked in the previous section: How can we know if a patient is being potentially unsafe or otherwise irresponsible with firearms if we do not understand what being safe and responsible with guns actually looks like? Now that we have provided you with an overview of gun types and their general operating mechanisms, let us specifically address gun safety principles.

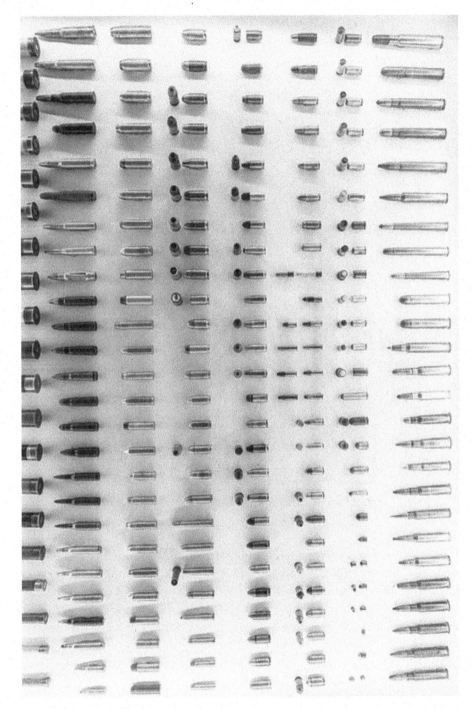

FIGURE 1.6 Additional examples of rifle and handgun ammunition

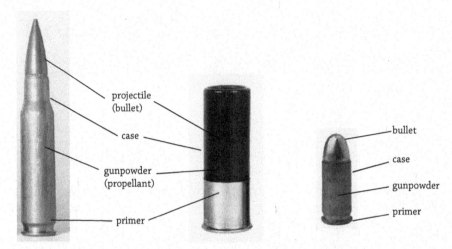

FIGURE 1.7 Basic component locations of rifle (left), shotgun (middle), and handgun (right) ammunition

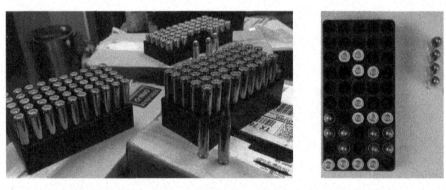

FIGURE 1.8 Examples of box contents of rifle (left) and handgun (right) ammunition

There are many gun safety resources available to us, and they include in-person education and instruction as well as that which is online and in print (e.g., see Luciano, 2015). While health-related organizations may present some general concepts of relevance, it is advisable to go directly to firearm-specific authoritative sources for this information. The NSF and the NRA are two examples of such authorities that have set forth basic safety rules that we should all know.

Specifically, the NSSF has set forth the following 10 rules for safe firearm handling, which we have paraphrased ("Firearms Safety," n.d.):

1. *Always keep the muzzle pointed in a safe direction.* This rule is paramount and underlies all others; specifically, do not aim at something you do not intend to shoot. This rule applies *at all times*, even when loading, unloading, and cleaning a gun. Following this rule would likely eliminate most, if not all, accidental injuries and deaths.

2. *Firearms should be unloaded when not actually in use.* A firearm should only be loaded when it is being prepared for use. In addition, guns and ammo should be stored separately and in safe places, in areas inaccessible to children and unauthorized adults. When a gun is being handled or given to another person, its chamber, receiver, and magazine should immediately be checked to determine if it is loaded and safe. *Assume all firearms are loaded* until they are determined not to be.

3. *Don't rely on your gun's "safety."* Many firearms have what is referred to as a *safety*, a component that is intended to prevent unintended firing. Some firearms do not have safeties, though, and some have fairly ineffective ones. Therefore, a handler can mistakenly assume a safety is engaged, which reinforces the principle that we should assume that all firearms are loaded until otherwise determined. Furthermore, a gun's safety should be in the "on" or engaged position until the user is ready to fire. It is also important to note that a gun can fire even in certain instances when the trigger is *not* manually pulled by an operator, such as if it is dropped or otherwise struck hard enough to engage the firing mechanism.

4. *Be sure of your target and what's beyond it.* Do not fire a gun unless you determine what you believe the bullet will strike, including beyond the intended target, because, once a gun is fired, the operator has no more control over where the projectile might go. Therefore, it is critical that the operator consider the target and beyond it and also estimate where the projectile may travel if the shot is missed or ricochets. Similar to the spirit of Rule #1, firearm operators should only point a gun at something they intend to shoot or otherwise destroy.

5. *Use correct ammunition.* Some guns allow for the use of various sizes of ammunition. It is critical that the operator only use the proper ammunition intended for a firearm, which will be indicated in its instruction manual. Ammo boxes also include relevant information in this regard. A gun can be damaged and injury can be caused by using improper ammo. Guns are designed, produced, and safety tested based on the use of proper ammo. Of additional note is that those who *handload* or *reload* ammo need to ensure that they adhere to the proper specifications as well. Furthermore, ammo should never be submerged in water, lubricated, or modified otherwise.

6. *If your gun fails to fire when the trigger is pulled, handle with care!* There are times when a gun jams or simply does not fire when the trigger is pulled. When that happens, the gun should be properly unloaded and the cartridge should be disposed of. Please note that the gun remains loaded until the cartridge and all ammo are removed.

7. *Always wear eye and ear protection when shooting.* Eye and ear protection is necessary for obvious reasons related to the expelled bullets and associated noise. However, it is also important to note that there are various other materials that could lead to eye injury when firing and even cleaning guns, and noise exposure can certainly lead to hearing damage.

8. *Be sure the barrel is clear of obstructions before shooting.* Any obstruction in the barrel of a gun, regardless of how seemingly small, can impact its pressures and cause injury.

9. *Don't alter or modify your gun, and have guns serviced regularly.* There are approved accessories for guns, such as sights and tactical apparatuses, but only experts who design them should modify firearms otherwise. Moreover, guns should undergo periodic inspection, adjustment, and service, just like other mechanical devices.

10. *Learn the mechanical and handling characteristics of the firearm you are using.* There is an extensive range of guns available for civilian use, varying by brand, type, style, size, and functionality, and many other classifications and specifications. However, people should only handle and operate fire-arms with which they have or gain familiarity, including but not limited to learning their particular loading and unloading, carrying, safety, and firing mechanisms.

These safety principles are consistent with the NRA's fundamental rules as well, and the NRA adds two rules to this list: (1) never use alcohol or over-the-counter, prescription, or other drugs before or while shooting, and (2) be aware that certain types of guns and many shooting activities require additional safety precautions ("NRA Gun Safety Rules," n.d.).

In addition, both the NSSF and the NRA have also developed firearm safety programs: *Project ChildSafe* and *Eddie Eagle GunSafe®*, respectively. The NSSF developed Project ChildSafe in or around 2003 as part of *Project Safe Neighborhoods*, which is a federal gun violence–prevention initiative (www.projectchildsafe.org). Project ChildSafe has partnered with thousands of law enforcement agencies—mostly police departments—who have distributed millions of safety kits, including gun locks and safety materials, to gun owners in every state and five U.S. territories to help reduce firearms misuse. According to the group, this initiative is "an industry-wide commitment to raise the public's consciousness on the issue of firearm safety and responsibility and encourage firearms owners to embrace the importance of proper storage" and to set forth the following message to gun owners: "Store your firearms responsibly when not in use." The group also has an "Own it? Respect it. Secure it." initiative toolkit available for people to "get involved in promoting responsible firearms ownership to your customers and in your community." They also ask gun owners to sign and adhere to the following pledge:

I choose to own a firearm and therefore accept responsibility for using and storing it safely. I commit to securing my firearm when not in use, being aware of who can access it at all times and educating others to do the same.

In 1988 the NRA developed the *Eddie Eagle GunSafe®* program, which they refer to as a "gun accident prevention program that seeks to help parents, law enforcement, community groups and educators navigate a topic paramount to our children's safety." Primarily, it was designed to teach pre-K through fourth graders what to do if they ever come across a firearm (https://eddieeagle.nra.org). They set forth the mantra "Stop, don't touch, run away, and tell a grown-up." According to the group, they provide grant funding for schools, law enforcement agencies, hospitals, daycare centers, and libraries interested in bringing Eddie Eagle to children in the area.

We present these programs for informational purposes, as their ultimate effectiveness remains somewhat unclear and has been contested, as some have found that gun safety programs do not reduce the likelihood children will handle firearms when unsupervised (see, e.g., Holly et al., 2019). Still, while these types of programs cannot and should not replace responsible gun storage and handling practices, they certainly include a number of positive messages about firearm safety and should be included in gun safety planning. In other words, education is necessary but insufficient alone to ensure gun safety for children and adults alike.

RECOMMENDED FURTHER READING

Crites, M. (2020, January 12). Who invented the first gun? A brief history of firearms. American Firearms. www.americanfirearms.org/gun-history/

Luciano, J. (2015). *Guns the right way: Introducing kids to firearm safety and shooting*. Gun Digest Books.

McNab, C. (2009). *Guns: A visual history*. DK Publishing.

National Rifle Association. (n.d.). Gun safety rules.https://gunsafetyrules.nra.org/

National Shooting Sports Foundation. (n.d.). Firearms safety—10 rules of safe gun handling. https://www.nssf.org/safety/rules-firearms-safety/

Pirelli, G., & Witt, P. H. (2018). Firearms and cultural competence: Considerations for mental health practitioners. *Journal of Aggression, Conflict and Peace Research*, 10(1), 61–70.

Supica, J. (n.d.). A brief history of firearms. National Rifle Association.https://www.nramuseum.org/gun-info-research/a-brief-history-of-firearms.aspx

2

Guns and the Law

WHY DO WE, as clinicians, need to know about gun laws? As one of the core components of the Know, Ask, Do (KAD) framework that we detail in Chapter 4, it is important for practicing medical and mental health professionals to have at least a general working knowledge with respect to gun culture, safety, and laws—among other relevant areas. If we can agree that an essential feature of conducting violence and suicide risk assessments is attending to potential firearm-related issues, then the need to understand at least some level of gun safety and laws goes without saying. Indeed, we cannot know if a patient is being unsafe if we do not know what safety looks like. This applies not only to gun handling and operation, but also other areas, such as firearm storage and transportation. Certainly, it is not our role to screen for the legality of our patients' behaviors in most cases, but it is our obligation to develop and maintain a working general knowledge of certain federal and state gun laws if we are going to address gun safety and the like with patients. Given that overlooking firearm-related concerns is not an option when conducting violence and suicide risk assessments (and in other professional pursuits), we must develop sufficient competency to inquire about gun-related issues.

All that said, this chapter will demonstrate not only the differences between federal and state law, in general, but also the high levels of heterogeneity for gun laws across the 50 states. Of course, a whole other layer is that of the procedural differences within each state, as such greatly impacts the way in which laws and policies are carried out for the general citizen. In our practice, we often tell people to think of certain gun policies and procedures within the state as they would motor vehicle violations, as there is a fair amount of discretion embedded in the process. For instance, New Jersey has over 500 municipalities and there is significant variability in the processing of firearms purchaser identification card applications, including but certainly not limited to the ultimate decisions that are made. This can also be true *within* the same town, as screening officers and police chiefs can change over time. Moreover, when someone is denied, there is also great variability across judges at the appellate level in the state superior courts across New Jersey's 21 counties. Perhaps the concept of "think globally, act locally" suits the reality of the situation on the ground—in our day-to-day practices.

> Ψ It is important to develop not only a *global* but also a *local* understanding of state-specific laws and even local policies, where much discretion may lie.

Nevertheless, it is important to have context by providing an overview of the legal landscape, historically and at present. Such an overview will help build a foundation of working knowledge related to guns for clinicians (i.e., a *global* understanding), thereby serving as a jumping-off point to then learn about state-specific laws and even more local policies, such as how particular police departments in our respective areas manage firearm-related matters and laws (i.e., a *local* understanding).

The reality is there are seemingly countless gun laws in many states, and they can be very complex. Whole books can be written on gun laws alone and, indeed, they have (see the *Recommended Further Reading* section at the end of this chapter). There are also a number of online resources that provide synopses of gun laws across the states and in particular areas of interest; for example, the interested reader may search such websites as the Giffords Law Center (https://giffords.org/lawcenter/gun-laws/) and the National Rifle Association's Institute for Legislative Action (https://www.nraila.org/gun-laws/). These types of resources can be helpful in pinpointing certain laws, and also in comparing and contrasting them throughout the country.

In this chapter, we highlight key legal areas relevant for a wide range of clinicians. Namely, we first provide a brief, historical overview of these laws and particularly highlight several landmark U.S. Supreme Court (SCOTUS) cases related to the Second Amendment (2A). Then, we focus more specifically on the history of mental health–related prohibitions at both the federal and state levels, to include an examination of how "mental illness" is defined. In addition, we provide an overview of prohibitions related to domestic violence (DV) and associated restraining orders, while also addressing so-called red flag laws, which are designed to prohibit access to guns during times of crisis. Additionally, we address how individuals can have their gun rights restored, such as by way of pursuing "relief from disability" (RFD) legal avenues. Finally, we explore laws relevant to gun safety, such as firearm storage and transportation laws.

THE SECOND AMENDMENT

Federal law and SCOTUS rulings essentially dictate what is minimally constitutionally required (or prohibited) in the country; however, states can generally go above and beyond these authorities in many respects—and they often do, as we will outline in this chapter. It can be helpful to go through the timeline of gun laws in the United States to provide context before moving into a more detailed discussion.

Gun laws were generally nonexistent in the United States until the mid-19th century. Since then, however, they have expanded significantly at both the federal and state levels. Robert Longley, a U.S. government expert, provided a useful outline of landmark legislation related to firearms. To provide some context, the 2A gained final ratification in 1791. It reads:

> A well regulated Militia, being necessary to the security of a free State, the right of the people to keep and bear Arms, shall not be infringed.

While it is just one sentence with 27 words, the interpretation of the 2A continues to be hotly debated. Throughout the 1800s and the early 1900s very few gun-related laws were set forth and, in fact, it was not until the late 1800s when SCOTUS even began to hear any such cases. Although not directly related to the mental health–related considerations with which we are focused in this handbook, it can be helpful to provide additional context by noting a few early SCOTUS cases that addressed the 2A at some level.

LANDMARK 2A RULINGS BY SCOTUS
Cruikshank (1875), Presser (1886), and Miller (1939)

The first case in this early SCOTUS–2A trilogy was that of *United States v. Cruikshank* (1875). This case involved an armed White militia attack that killed over 100 Black Republican freedman who gathered outside a Louisiana courthouse to prevent a Democratic takeover. Some of the White militia were charged and indicted for alleged conspiracy to prevent Blacks from exercising their civil rights, including to bear arms lawfully per the 2A. SCOTUS ultimately held that the 2A only restricts the federal government from infringing upon the right to bear arms and does not restrict citizens from denying other citizens from their right to do so (or any other constitutional right in the Bill of Rights).

The second early case was that of *Presser v. Illinois* (1886). Presser was part of an armed citizen militia group comprising over 400 German workers associated with the Socialist Labor Party. The group, including Presser, was charged with parading in the streets of Chicago on horseback without a license to do so, or within the context of a recognized organization permitted to engage in such by the government. As a result, Presser contended that his 2A rights were violated, but SCOTUS ultimately held that forbidding armed bodies of people to gather, drill, or parade did not violate an individual right to keep and bear arms.

The third case in this conceptual series is that of *United States v. Miller* (1939). Before addressing the case directly, some additional context is warranted. Despite two earlier SCOTUS cases that touched upon 2A rights, it was really not until 143 years following the ratification of the 2A that any significant regulations were actually put forth. Namely, in 1934, the National Firearms Act was passed, thereby approving the regulation of the manufacturing, sale, and possession of fully automatic guns. Then, four years later, the Federal Firearms Act of 1938 placed the first limitation on firearms sales: Sellers were required to obtain a federal firearms license (FFL), to create a general record of firearm purchases throughout the country. This Act also prohibited the sale of firearms to those who were convicted of violent felonies. The third notable early SCOTUS case followed shortly thereafter: *United States v. Miller* (1930). This case involved a criminal prosecution under the National Firearms Act of 1934, which passed subsequent to the so-called St. Valentine's Day Massacre (i.e., the murder of seven members of Chicago's North Side Gang perpetrated by the South Side Gang associated with Mafia leader Al Capone). The 1934 law, in part, banned fully automatic guns as well as short-barreled rifles and shotguns, which are also referred to as "sawed-off" shotguns. Miller and a co-defendant were charged with violating the Act by transporting a sawed-off double-barreled 12-gauge shotgun across state lines. In response, Miller challenged aspects of the Act, contending there was a violation of his 2A rights. However, SCOTUS ultimately held that banning a shotgun having a barrel less than 18 inches was not a 2A violation because it did not have any relation to either a well-regulated militia or ordinary military equipment. Therefore, the 2A would not guarantee a civilian's right to keep and bear such a firearm.

While the early SCOTUS cases and federal laws were notable insofar as they got the 2A ball rolling in a legal sense, many believe that the gun control debate as we now know it did not truly begin until the 1960s—largely in response to the assassinations of President John F. Kennedy and Dr. Martin Luther King, Jr. In fact, prior to 1968, firearms and ammunition were easily available to adults. Then, a pivotal federal law was passed in the United States: the Gun Control Act (GCA) of 1968. The GCA regulated interstate and foreign commerce of firearms via imposing stricter licensing requirements and regulations, and it also required all newly manufactured guns to have a serial number. We will take another look at the GCA later in this chapter (see the *Mental Health–Related Prohibitions* section). Subsequent to the passage of the GCA of 1968, the Bureau of Alcohol, Tobacco, and Firearms (ATF) was created in 1972 to control illegal use and sale of firearms as well as to enforce federal firearm laws. The ATF has become a household name, but it is important to realize it has only been in existence for 50 years as we write this book and over 60 years *after* the creation of the Federal Bureau of Investigation (FBI). Numerous laws and initiatives followed the ATF's creation, some of which we address throughout this chapter and others that are outside the scope of this book.

That said, before turning to a review of firearm law–related areas most relevant for clinicians, it is important to highlight three additional landmark 2A cases ruled upon by SCOTUS: *District of Columbia v. Heller* (2008); *McDonald v. Chicago* (2010); and *New York State Rifle & Pistol Association, Inc. v. Bruen (2022)*. Perhaps what is most notable is the recency of these highly consequential rulings by the Court, given that they came about over 225 years *after* the ratification of the 2A.

Heller (2008), McDonald (2010), and Bruen (2022)

In *District of Columbia v. Heller* (2008), SCOTUS addressed the question of whether the 2A protects an individual's right to keep and bear (functional) arms in the home for self-defense. This case was prompted by Washington D.C.'s handgun possession ban, which stated that those who legally owned firearms were to keep them disassembled or bound by a locking device (e.g., trigger lock) in the home. The respondent was Dick Heller, a D.C. special police officer who applied to register his handgun to keep at his residence; permission was denied. In a 5–4 decision, SCOTUS held that the 2A applies to federal enclaves and protects an individual's right to possess a firearm for traditionally lawful purposes, such as self-defense within the home. Justice Antonin Scalia wrote the majority opinion, wherein he provided a thorough historical context to the development of the 2A as well as an analysis of the prefatory and operative clauses (and terms used) within it.

Despite the landmark ruling, general uncertainty remained regarding the scope of gun rights with respect to their application at the state level. Therefore, SCOTUS heard *McDonald v. Chicago* in 2010 to address that very question. Namely, in *McDonald*, it was argued that the Court's analysis and interpretation of the 2A in *Heller* should also apply to state and local governments. Ultimately, SCOTUS arrived at a 5–4 decision once again, with Justice Samuel Alito writing for the majority. They decided that the due process clause of the Fourteenth Amendment included the 2A right the Court recognized in *Heller* and, therefore, applied it to the states (i.e., thereby finding Chicago's firearm ban to be unconstitutional). A discussion of the debate between individual and so-called collective rights is well outside of the scope of this book, but the main take-home message for our purposes here is that the individual right to bear arms is the prevailing view substantiated by the higher courts, particularly SCOTUS, at this time.

In June 2022, the U.S. Supreme Court set forth another major 2A ruling in *New York State Rifle & Pistol Association Inc. v. Bruen*. In November 2021, the Court heard arguments proposing a challenge to New York State's law that currently requires those applying for a license to carry a concealed, loaded firearm outside the home to demonstrate "proper cause." This was based on the assertion that carrying a gun outside the home is a constitutional right and not a situation that should require demonstration of need. Via a 6–3 vote, Justice Clarence Thomas wrote the majority opinion:

"New York's proper-cause requirement violates the Fourteenth Amendment by preventing law-abiding citizens with ordinary self-defense needs from exercising their Second Amendment right to keep and bear arms in public for self-defense" (p. 2)

The impact of this landmark ruling was seen within days, particularly in the seven so-called "may-issue" jurisdictions; namely, New York, California, Hawaii, Maryland, Massachusetts, New Jersey, and the District of Columbia (D.C.). For instance, the Attorney General of New Jersey issued a directive literally the next day (June 24, 2022) highlighting the removal of the state's "justifiable need" provision for applicants moving forward. Given the recency of the ruling, time will tell its practical effects otherwise. It is likely the case that we will have a much clearer picture of such by the time you are reading this book.

MENTAL HEALTH–RELATED PROHIBITIONS

Certain people are prohibited from owning firearms per both federal and state laws, which are ostensibly intended to prevent firearm-involved violence and suicide. While researchers over the years have found that there is a strong link between mental illness and suicide (e.g., Price & Norris, 2010), the link between mental illness and (interpersonal) violence is weak. In fact, only a small percentage of people with even serious mental illnesses engage in violence. Namely, research demonstrates that only 3% to 5% of all violence, which includes violence involving firearms, is even attributable to serious mental illness (Swanson et al., 1990, 2015). Moreover, this typically occurs only during a specific period of time in the context of psychiatric crises, or acute phases of the respective illnesses. As we discuss at various points in this book and particularly in Chapter 5, a comprehensive, *clinical* risk assessment can help identify a particular person's risk levels at a given time. Yet, most laws prohibiting firearm ownership identify mental health diagnoses and treatment as a concern in an overgeneralized, blanket fashion: Essentially any diagnosis and sometimes any type of mental health treatment at any point in one's life can potentially prevent one from exercising one's 2A right to gun ownership.

For instance, while federal law requires someone to have been (involuntarily) committed to a hospital and adjudicated mentally defective, police chiefs in states such as New Jersey can flag and deny applications for a firearms purchaser identification card for essentially any mental health-related reason, regardless of how benign. Indeed, we regularly receive calls from people whose applications have been flagged or denied by a police department simply because they engage in weekly psychotherapy on an outpatient basis for relatively minor levels of distress, as well as from those who may have engaged in treatment for a brief period as a child decades ago. Examples are wide-ranging and have included those who engaged in therapy in the context of their parents' divorce, sexual abuse victimization, gender issues, and academic challenges and distress. Another memorable example is a person who contacted us for a forensic psychological evaluation after the police department required his firearm ownership suitability to be assessed because he was taking anxiolytic medication for irritable bowel syndrome (IBS). In some states, like New Jersey, there is a seemingly endless range of discretion by the issuing police department, coupled with a broad-strokes approach to reviewing applications. As such, applications often function as crude screening documents.

Denying a person's 2A right to gun ownership because they took part in therapy *at any point* in their life for *any given reason* is a rather extreme form of prohibition. Yet, it is not uncommon in a state like ours, New Jersey, despite the clear empirical evidence that most people with a diagnosable mental illness do not engage in violence toward others and mental illness is a poor predictor of violence, to include firearm-related violence (McGinty & Webster, 2016). Information on the link between mental illness and firearm-related violence is discussed in more depth in Chapter 3. But for now, let us take a look at the laws that have been passed that prohibit individuals from possessing firearms based on mental health–related factors.

Federal Law

Earlier, we touched upon the GCA, a 1968 federal law that not only established provisions related to the importation of firearms and minimum age requirements for purchasers but also expanded on the categories of persons prohibited from possessing or purchasing firearms (18 USC. § 922). The GCA specifically pertains to mental health insofar as it prohibits the sale of firearms to anyone who has been "adjudicated as a mental defective" or has been "committed to a mental institution," or has been involuntarily psychiatrically committed. The ATF later defined "mental defectives," which was not defined within the original GCA bill, as those who are a danger to themselves or others, who lack the mental capacity to manage their own affairs, who are found not guilty by reason of insanity (NGRI), and who are found incompetent to stand trial (IST) (Protection of Human Subjects, 2009).

Twenty-five years later, in 1993, the Brady Handgun Violence Prevention Act was signed into law. In addition to mandating a 5-day wait period before the purchase of a handgun, it also expanded the GCA by requiring dealers to conduct background checks on those purchasing firearms via a search of the FBI's National Instant Criminal Background Check System (NICS). NICS comprises three national databases (those from the National Crime Information Center, the Interstate Identification Index, and the NICS Index) as well as purchasers' criminal and mental health histories, including any civil orders (e.g., domestic violence–related protective or restraining orders) that may affect their eligibility to purchase a firearm. The NICS can theoretically produce a check in minutes and is valid for 30 days. Essentially, the system provides dealers with instructions on whether to proceed, deny, or delay purchases based on results associated with any (federal) prohibitions. In a "delay" situation, in which more investigation is needed to determine the accuracy of a particular "hit," the FBI has 3 business days to provide such information before a sale proceeds.

Per the Brady Act, however, states were not required to report information to federal databases, which led to incomplete background checks. However, the NICS Improvement Amendments Act (NIAA) of 2007 was enacted in the wake of the Virginia Tech shooting, setting forth provisions for financial penalties as well as incentives to push states to provide relevant information. Currently, 47 states are now either authorized or required to report mental health records to NICS, five of which are authorized but not required. Arkansas, Michigan, and Ohio collect mental health records within an in-state database but do not disclose to NICS. All of the 47 states noted must report records of those involuntarily committed as inpatients. Furthermore, 22 states also require the reporting of records pertaining to those who received outpatient mental health therapy, and 16 require the reporting of those who have been appointed a guardian (i.e., lack the capacity to manage their own affairs). About half of the states are required to report those found NGRI or IST—that is, criminal insanity or incompetence.

NICS firearm checks have increased in numbers over the years and, in Chapter 3, we detail how they have increased exponentially in 2020. For instance, in the year 2000, there were approximately 8.5 million NICS checks. This number remained relatively steady until 2006, at which point we began seeing checks well above 10 million annually and to nearly 30 million—specifically, in 2009, there were 14 million checks; in 2012, 19 million; in 2016, 27 million; in 2019, 28 million; and in 2020, 39 million. As of December 31, 2021, there were approximately 38.8 million checks (https://www.fbi.gov/file-repository/nics_firearm_checks_-_month_year.pdf/view).

State Law

In addition to adhering to federal prohibitions, 34 states as well as the District of Columbia have their own laws that restrict access to firearms based on mental health–related reasons. While a full outline for each state would be too cumbersome here, we strongly encourage readers to familiarize themselves with their respective state laws in this regard. A useful source in this regard is the Giffords Law Center website, which has a section on state-specific restrictions (https://giffords.org/lawcenter/gun-laws/). We also presented a timeline of various types of firearm-related legislation in certain states in Chapter 2 of our previous book (Pirelli et al., 2019). As with much of what we present throughout this handbook, it is incumbent upon the readers to take the extra steps to research their respective laws and regulations and apply them to their respective practices.

Consistent with our KAD model, it is important to familiarize ourselves with relevant gun laws that affect our patients and even our practices, directly or indirectly; however, it is critical to highlight the distinction between the letter of the law and its application. Put differently, just like ethics codes and similar types of procedural documents, laws are often intentionally, sufficiently vague and, therefore, inherently subject to interpretation. Therefore, the resulting discretion is typically wide-ranging. This is not unique to the firearm arena, though, as forensic practitioners can readily acknowledge the differences among prosecutors and other state attorneys vis-à-vis their interpretations and application of the law—as well as, of course, among judges. What will be unique to many practitioners like us in relation to gun laws and regulations is the administrative process handled through police departments at various points.

It is safe to assume that the vast majority of medical or mental health professionals will not interface with law enforcement agencies in their professional lives. However, it is common in certain jurisdictions for departments to contact treatment providers once they are identified by gun permit applicants and, of course, those of us who conduct forensic evaluations to address firearm ownership suitability will be frequently authoring reports intended to be provided to the respective law enforcement agencies in given cases. Just as with prosecutors and judges, law enforcement officers have fairly wide discretion in their decision-making, and such can play out very differently even from one town to the next. As a practitioner conducting forensic firearm evaluations, it lacks utility to think of gun laws on a state-by-state basis per se. Knowledge of certain federal regulations is imperative and we must also have a relatively strong handle on the laws in the state in which we practice; however, it is not particularly useful to be able to compare to another state—outside of certain considerations related to adjoining states.

For example, New Jersey and Pennsylvania have significantly different gun laws, including but not limited to those associated with licensing processes, carry rights, and transportation. Therefore, it is important for practitioners in New Jersey to have at least a general sense of the differences because a fair amount of Pennsylvania citizens travel through the state at any given time. Indeed, there have been a number of people who have received very serious weapons charges for passing through New Jersey with a Pennsylvania-legal gun and carry permit (i.e., that was illegal in New Jersey). It is for these reasons and more that we encourage people to think of gun-related procedures within a given state as they would motor vehicle violations and the like, as we noted in the introductory paragraph of this chapter. Issuing authorities, such as police chiefs, are certainly bound by federal and state

> Ψ Local agencies have wide discretion in decision-making about firearm applications, even within the same state. Such may vary among towns and even among decision-makers within the same department.

laws, but their procedural applications can wildly vary from town to town and across counties within the same state. Moreover, given this discretion, there can be heterogeneity even within the same town over time, as screening officers and police chiefs can change, as can political climates.

There is no way to reasonably and effectively provide summaries and corresponding guidance for each state in the country. Rather, we provide general overviews along with some examples of state laws to give readers a sense of the types of considerations of which clinicians would want to gain an understanding in their respective states. It is important to keep in mind that states have different definitions of "mental illness." Therefore, it is important to ascertain if a given state defines "mental illness" based on DSM-5-TR diagnoses, type of treatment received, or some combination. Moreover, some states can flag and deny people who have engaged in outpatient mental health treatment, despite the federal prohibitor necessitating involuntary psychiatric commitments.

> Ψ It is important to keep in mind that states have different definitions of "mental illness." Therefore, it is important to ascertain if a given state defines "mental illness" based on DSM-5-TR diagnoses, type of treatment received, or some combination.

Some application forms are rather vague in this regard—once again, leaving much discretion to the decision-maker (i.e., law enforcement officer or judge). Despite the fact that we, as clinicians, will operationalize mental illness consistent with our fields' practice standards, it is necessary to be able to apply our (clinical) concepts to the legal standards at hand in order to be most helpful to decision-makers.

As indicated, the characterization of mental illness has been expanded in some jurisdictions to include those who were *voluntarily* admitted to hospitals (i.e., Connecticut, Illinois, Maryland, Washington D.C.). Others use a broader definition of mental illness, whereas some are more specific in their criteria. To illustrate, Illinois expanded prohibitions to those who are developmentally disabled and intellectually disabled. The former was defined as a disability that results in "significant functional limitations" in three or more of the following domains of functioning: "self-care, receptive and expressive language, learning, mobility, or self-direction." Intellectual disability was defined as "significantly subaverage general intellectual functioning which exists concurrently with impairment in adaptive behavior, and which originates before 18 years" (430 Ill. Comp. Stat. 65/1.1, n.d.). Additionally, Illinois prohibits those who are impaired by a mental condition "of such a nature that it poses a clear and present danger to the applicant, any other person or persons or the community" (430 Ill. Comp. Stat. 65/8, n.d.). Maryland prohibits those who "suffer from a mental disorder" and a history of violence against others (Md. Code Ann., Pub. Safety § 5-1330, 2003). Hawaii extended prohibitions to those who have been "diagnosed with a significant behavioral, emotional, or mental disorder" as well as prohibiting those who have received "treatment for organic brain syndromes" (Haw. Rev. Stat. § 134-7, 2019). Again, it is incumbent upon us as evaluating clinicians to address these nuances within the context of our overarching assessment procedures. These examples further support the need to incorporate a flexible framework, like the Pirelli Firearm-10 (PF-10), which covers the range of clinically relevant areas to address in a firearm-specific evaluation while allowing for consideration of state-by-state nuances.

> Ψ It is best to incorporate a flexible framework when assessing risk. The Pirelli Firearm-10 (PF-10) covers a range of clinically relevant areas to address in firearm-specific evaluations and allows for state-level nuances.

It may not be surprising that there are more mental health prohibitions in so-called blue states than red states. For instance, California prohibits those who have had inpatient admissions for dangerousness,[1] but since the beginning of 2020, the state has also permanently prohibited access to firearms by those who have been involuntarily

---

[1] We use the term, 'dangerousness,' throughout this chapter because it a relevant legal term here. However, clinically, we have been using the terms 'violence risk assessment' and 'suicide risk assessment' for decades at this point—a move away from the commonly used term previously: prediction of dangerousness. Such reflects more than simply a semantic difference; rather, it is consistent with contemporary standards advocating for a prevention and management- rather than prediction-based approach to risk assessment.

committed to a psychiatric facility related to dangerousness more than once within a 1-year time period. Furthermore, California prohibits those who were court-ordered/ mandated to receive intensive inpatient treatment related to a mental health disorder or "chronic alcoholism," which specifically prohibits them from firearm access for 5 years, and potentially permanently without a petition to the court for gun rights restoration. Other prohibitions in California include persons who have been adjudicated dangerous to others due to their mental illnesses, those adjudicated a "mentally disordered sex offender," those who have been under a court-ordered conservatorship due to significant disability as a result of their mental illness or chronic alcoholism, and those found IST or NGRI, or anyone who has disclosed to a psychotherapist a serious threat of physical violence against an identifiable victim (for 5 years) (Cal. Welf. & Inst. Code §§ 8100(a), 8103(a), (b), (d), (e), (d), (g) (2016). Conversely, many states have not expanded what constitutes mental illness beyond what has been set forth by federal law; namely, the more conservative states (e.g., Alaska, Mississippi, Montana). Taken together, we hope the importance of having a general handle on certain state laws and definitions is clear, especially in the rather diverse area of firearm laws.

DV-RELATED PROHIBITIONS

Another area of prohibition that is essential to explore for the purposes of this handbook's utility is that of DV, or what may also be referred to as intimate partner violence (IPV).[2] Medical and mental health professionals alike may work with patients who are in DV-related situations. Of course, we may not even know if such is taking place. Before discussing some of the specifics of gun-related prohibitions in this context, we highlight a couple of key points related to the relationship between DV and firearms. That said, please note that we cover this in greater detail in Chapter 3.

Most DV situations do not involve weapons of any kind, particularly firearms (Truman et al., 2014). For example, in New Jersey in 2016, there were approximately 63,000 offenses reported (up from 62,000 in 2015), 31% of which resulted in arrests (Thirty-Fourth Annual Domestic Violence Offense Report: https://www.njsp.org/ucr/pdf/domesticviolence/2016_domestic_violence.pdf). Moreover, approximately 2,500 arrests involved restraining orders and there were 52 murders in this context in New Jersey that year. Of particular note:

- Of the 63,000 offenses in New Jersey, 145 involved a firearm (i.e., 99.8% did not involve a gun).
- In fact, the majority of offenses reported involved no weapon at all (54%), followed by "hands, fists, feet, etc." (42%), "other dangerous weapon" (2%), and knife (1.5%).

---

[2] For our purposes, we will refer to domestic violence (DV) and intimate partner violence (IPV) under the overarching abbreviation, DV.

- Furthermore, the vast majority (76%) of those involving a firearm resulted in no injuries at all.

Yet, firearm-related legislation is often driven based on the premise of concerns in this regard. As with all other types of gun deaths, all must be taken seriously, and we must seek to prevent all of them. The reason for the notable attention to guns in these scenarios despite consisting of such relatively low numbers, overall, is similar to that of suicides—the increased likelihood of fatality when guns are used (e.g., Bailey et al., 1997; Campbell et al., 2003; Kellermann et al., 1993). Indeed, firearms can be used to intimidate or threaten, even if never used to cause physical harm. Notably, however, there is no evidence to suggest that the presence of firearms leads to the onset of interpersonal violence (Sorenson, 2006) nor does it increase already-present interpersonal violence, more generally (e.g., Vest et al., 2002). As clinicians, we must go beyond identifying general DV-related risk factors and assess firearm-specific risk in these situations. Namely, we must identify and assess *lethal* risk factors in DV situations. Although we will cover this in greater detail in Chapter 3, some such factors include child custody situations, the victim having left or threatened that she (usually female) was going to leave, a recent physical assault against the victim, the abuser having substance use problems, protection orders, acute perceptions of betrayal, or stalking (Farr, 2002; Johnson et al., 1999). Based on these data, the presence of a firearm in the home is a potentially exacerbating variable, rather than a high-risk factor in its own right. Thus, noting the presence of a firearm, in and of itself, is insufficient, and thus, other risk factors need to be considered.

Federal Law

Federal law prohibits those who have been convicted of a "misdemeanor crime of domestic violence" from purchasing or possessing firearms or ammunition. In 1996, the Lautenberg Amendment to the 1968 GCA was set forth (18 USC. § 922(g)(9), 1996). It was named after its sponsor, Frank Lautenberg, the late New Jersey U.S. senator. The Amendment defined a "misdemeanor crime of domestic violence" as an offense wherein a person has used or attempted to use physical force or threatened use of a deadly weapon within a domestic relationship—a current or former spouse, cohabitant, parent/guardian, or where they share a child/be similarly situated to a spouse or parent/guardian (42 USC. § 3796gg-4, 2012). However, most of what may be important in the context of DV is the state laws as such pertain not only to prohibitions based on DV history, but also with respect to restraining orders. Restraining or protective orders, according to federal law, can be filed against a current or former spouse, cohabitant, or a person with whom the applicant shares a child (Violence Against Women Act, 42 USC. § 13981, 1994). We provide more context in the next subsection; nevertheless, federal as well as many state laws prohibit a person with a protection order to own, ship, or receive a firearm or ammunition. Such was also expanded in 1994 to those who are subject to a final DV restraining order by the Violent Crime Control and Law Enforcement Act (18 USC § 922[g][8]).

State Law

States have passed additional firearm-related laws prohibiting certain DV abusers who are not covered by federal law, such as restricting them from buying or possessing firearms and/or ammunition, surrendering of such, and reporting identities to databases used in background checks. Because federal law broadly defines a "misdemeanor crime of domestic violence," 30 states, along with Washington D.C., have broadened either the definition of DV or what constitutes a misdemeanor regardless of whether the victim resides with the offender. For example, states such as California, Hawaii, Connecticut, and New York prohibit gun ownership to those convicted of assault, battery, or stalking regardless of the victim's relationship to the offender. While the details of DV statutes may not have significant clinical implications for most of us in the majority of our work, certain aspects may be more relevant to some of us in certain contexts. For instance, forensic practitioners conducting firearm-specific evaluations will likely need to know what constitutes a DV relationship and even a misdemeanor offense. If nothing else, such would help inform our record review in certain instances. As should be readily apparent, one the running themes of this chapter pertains to the importance of having a working knowledge of relevant certain federal and state laws related to firearms, but with a particular emphasis on the way in which particular operative terms are defined (e.g., domestic violence, domestic relationship, mental illness).

All states allow alleged DV victims to seek protective orders, also known as restraining orders, which place certain restrictions on the alleged abusers. There are two types of orders that can be produced: ex parte and final orders. Ex parte orders are temporary orders in an emergency situation (i.e., temporary restraining order). For a final order, the petitioner bears the burden of providing enough evidence to demonstrate that the alleged abuser poses a danger to self or others; however, the standard of proof needed in this context varies somewhat across states. For a final order, a hearing will be held in which both the victim and the alleged abuser appear, so a judge can make an ultimate determination based on the evidence. The time frame during which each of these orders may remain in effect can also vary. For instance, in California, ex parte orders may remain in effect for up to 21 days, whereas a final order may remain in effect for up to 5 years (Cal Fam. Code § D.10, Pt. 4. Refs. & Annos. [West]). Furthermore, 15 states require those subjected to DV restraining orders to surrender their firearms for the period outlined in the respective court order. In many states, this is true even for an ex parte, or temporary, restraining order (18 USC. § 922g).

"RED FLAG" LAWS: GUN VIOLENCE RESTRAINING ORDERS AND EXTREME RISK PROTECTION ORDERS

Numerous states have enacted legislation providing for what are referred to as gun violence restraining orders (GVROs) or extreme risk protection orders (ERPOs), colloquially referred to as "red flag" laws. These laws restrict gun rights by leading to forfeitures of guns, ammunition, and permits, thereby prohibiting individuals in question from accessing their firearms and related items during times of crisis or concern. The name "red flag" relates to observed warning signs that are sufficient evidence for the petition, such as risky and dangerous behaviors like increased alcohol abuse, suicidality, or concerning psychiatric decompensation otherwise (e.g., Elbogen & Johnson, 2009, McGinty et al., 2014; Swanson et al., 2013). GVROs are distinct in that they allow law enforcement to petition for the restraining order.

California was the first state to enact a GVRO law (CA Penal Code § 18100, 2018), which took effect in 2016. Currently, 19 states and Washington D.C. have such laws, and each state with a red flag law has its own parameters such as who can petition, the standard of proof to obtain the order, how long the order lasts, and the firearm relinquishment process. Of the 19 states, 12 (in addition to Washington D.C.) allow household or family members to petition the court. It is particularly important to note that Maryland and Washington D.C. allow mental health providers to petition, New York allows school administrators, and Hawaii allows medical professionals, coworkers, and educators. Once the petition is filed, a judge will decide if the respondent is at risk of engaging in dangerous behavior, thereby warranting the limiting of access to firearms. The factors that judges consider in making this decision are not necessarily clearly delineated and, therefore, are likely to differ across jurisdictions. That said, historical factors such as history of violence, recent threats of violence, or substance use are presumably considered (Wintemute et al., 2001). Some states do provide specific guidance with respect to the evidence showing extreme risk. For instance, California specifies that the court must consider threats or acts of violence toward self or others within the past month, a violation of a DV protective order at the time of petition, any conviction for any crime that prohibits the purchase and possession of firearms, and a pattern of violent acts or threats within the past 12 months.

Formal risk assessments conducted by licensed mental health clinicians are typically not required at this stage even though the standard of proof is usually based on "reasonable grounds" that the respondent poses imminent danger. Nevertheless, if a judge makes this determination, then an ex parte restraining order is granted without prior notice to the respondent. Persons subject to a GVRO are required to relinquish their firearms, and in some states their licenses to possess or carry them. They will then be prohibited from either possessing or purchasing guns for a period of time. Generally, the ex parte order lasts between 14 and 21 days, depending on the state. A final order may be issued that typically lasts up to 1 year. However, a higher standard of proof must be met to obtain this order, which is either a preponderance of or clear and convincing evidence, depending on the state, that the person poses a risk of danger.

With regard to the relinquishing of firearms, no federal laws exist that provide procedures for the removal of firearms in gun forfeiture situations, but some states have specific removal or confiscation procedures. Nevertheless, states generally allow law enforcement to do so. In most cases, however, the respondent typically has a certain amount of time (e.g., 24 to 48 hours) to obtain a receipt, filed with law enforcement and the court, that they surrendered their guns, or a search warrant is typically ordered to authorize a search and seizure of their firearms. In some states, the respondent can decide what happens with their firearms. For instance, in California, the owner can transfer their firearms to a law enforcement agency or licensed firearms dealer or sell them. Given that some states require a license to own a firearm, each state has its own procedure as to its revocation (https://lawcenter.giffords.org/gun-laws/policy-areas/who-can-have-a-gun/extreme-risk-protection-orders/).

There are other instances in which police may be called to a location and thus become involved, in the absence of a GVRO. Although this may include riskier DV, mental health crisis, or threats to self or others, such may also be more benign situations, or ones involving transient threats, or ones in which there is a more general concern with regard to someone's behavior. Upon inquiry about firearms in the house, police may request that the firearms be taken by them for "safekeeping" even if a GVRO or ERPO has not been sought. We see this to some extent, at least in New Jersey, where we primarily conduct our work.

When a GVRO runs out, the respondent does not always get their guns returned to them automatically. In many cases, even those wherein guns have been taken for "safekeeping," the respondent must petition to have their rights restored through a court hearing, at which time the burden of proof rests on the petitioner to demonstrate that they no longer pose a risk. In fact, in some states, they are required to petition the courts to restore their rights to be able to again be in possession of firearms.

GUN RIGHTS RESTORATION AND RELIEF FROM DISABILITY

Up to this point, we have explored various firearm-related prohibitions, including those pertaining to mental health, DV, and the recently enacted GVROs and ERPOs. As we alluded to, when the respondent seeks to have their rights restored and firearms returned, the onus is on said respondent to demonstrate to the court that they no longer pose a risk, regardless of the reason for the forfeiture. The federal government and most states have a process through which a prohibited person must go to restore their rights to possess and purchase firearms, or to have their guns returned to them, regardless of the reason for the prohibition or confiscation (e.g., initial applicant denial, restraining order, GVRO/ERPO). These laws and processes are often referred to as "relief from disability" (RFD) statutes and procedures.

Federal Law

The term "disability" within the RFD context encompasses the federal mental health prohibitor areas covered previously in this chapter, including those who have been involuntarily committed to a psychiatric hospital, and those adjudicated IST or NGRI. As noted, additional state-level prohibitors can come into play, such as having a developmental disability. In 1986, the Firearms Owners Protection Act (FOPA) revised many provisions of the GCA of 1968, such as those pertaining to restrictions on gun and ammunition sales, as well as establishing penalties for those in possession of a firearm during the commission of a crime. Moreover, it expanded on the GCA by including RFD for prohibited persons. Two decades later, the NICS Improvement Amendments Act (NIAA) of 2007 included provisions for states to develop programs allowing prohibited persons to seek RFD, which was added to address the concern that persons with a "mental defective" adjudication were prohibited from gun ownership for life. Of note is that grants are provided to states to create RFD programs. For these programs to become federally certified by the ATF, under the NIAA, certain provisions are required: an application for relief from the federal prohibition on buying or owning a gun through state procedure, a judicial appeal of a denial of the initial relief petition, and updated records removing the name of the person from both federal and state databases if the relief is granted (Gold & Vanderpool, 2018a).

In a 2016 landmark case, *Tyler v. Hillsdale County*, Tyler was involuntarily committed for 30 days and was unable to restore his firearm rights in Michigan, where he resided, because there was not an established program to grant him relief. This case was initially dismissed in the federal district court before it was heard by the Sixth Circuit in September 2016, who held that a lifetime ban based on an adjudicated intellectual disability or a commitment to a "mental institution" infringes on 2A rights, and thus such persons are not permanently barred from owning a firearm. The court also noted that prior psychiatric commitment does not necessarily indicate a current mental illness, nor dangerousness to others. Tyler's suit relied on the opinion in *District of Columbia v. Heller* (2008) that, although the 2A secures an individual right to bear arms, it does not forbid "presumptively lawful" bans on firearms possession, such as mental illness.

State Law

Although most states have some form of RFD programs at this point, approximately a dozen of these programs do not meet the federal criteria (e.g., Maine, California, Connecticut, Mississippi). States without such programs include Arkansas, Michigan, Montana, New Hampshire, New Mexico, Wyoming, and Washington D.C. (Gold & Vanderpool, 2018a). That said, this list also includes states that do not have mental health–related prohibitors (e.g., Wyoming, Montana). Nevertheless, even many states that meet federal criteria do not have clearly delineated gun rights restoration procedures, including but not limited to the process of obtaining relief, such as the corresponding evidence required. Moreover, the burden of proof required varies across states (Gold & Vanderpool, 2018a).

It may stand to reason that if someone is prohibited from owning firearms, based on dangerousness or mental illness, a mental health evaluation to include a risk assessment would be necessary. However, neither the federal government nor most states require such. Although most states with RFD statutes certainly have some process that consists of the review of medical records and the like by the court or some agency, it is unclear what type of records are required for review (Gold & Vanderpool, 2018b). In fact, only 15 states require that evidence be presented regarding dangerousness and that specific documentation be reviewed; namely, that which is related to the prohibitor issue in question. Moreover, only eight of these states require risk assessments. Examples include New York and Oregon, where petitioners must provide their mental health records related to the prohibitor and criminal histories. Oregon further requires a recent violence and suicide risk assessment evaluation conducted by either a licensed psychiatrist or psychologist. In New York, the gun relief authority is the Commissioner of the Office of Mental Health (OMH), wherein a violence and suicide risk assessment evaluation is required. New York also requires additional letters speaking to the petitioner's reputation written by those close to them. In other states, the requirements vary considerably, such as the qualifications of the professional providing evidence, the proximity of time evidence is presented in relation to the petition, and the information to be addressed (Gold & Vanderpool, 2018b).

According to an American Psychiatric Association's Resource Document on Access to firearms by People with Mental Disorders (Pinals et al., 2015), however, "psychiatric evaluations and testimony should be required when persons seek restoration of their firearm-related rights because psychiatrists can describe and interpret the individual's mental health history and current mental health status, and the effects of treatment and other factors on improvement or exacerbation of the person's condition" (p. 191). It is also suggested, though, that the ultimate gun rights restoration decision should be made by an administrative, judicial body. The Consortium for Risk-Based Firearm Policy, comprising legal, medical, and mental health professionals, similarly proposed that, while the court or other such authority makes the ultimate decision in RFD hearings, such should include the consideration of a mental health evaluation, inclusive of an opinion of a psychiatrist or psychologist (Consortium for Risk-Based Firearm Policy, 2013). More specifically, the mental health professional should attest to the following: (1) the individual no longer exhibits symptoms related to the disorder that was related to their involuntary commitment, or that they are no longer at risk of harm to self or others; (2) that they have and will continue to be compliant with recommended treatment; and (3) that ongoing treatment compliance will likely reduce risk for that person to be a danger to self or others in the foreseeable future. However, because this is a relatively new area, there is little information known about how RFD hearings are actually conducted, the frequency with which the court requests a psychiatric or psychological evaluation or risk assessment, and the extent to which mental health evidence might affect decisions (Gold & Vanderpool, 2018b).

REPORTING DUTIES OF MEDICAL AND MENTAL HEALTH PROFESSIONALS

As we have illustrated, medical and mental health professionals alike may play an integral role in the restoration of firearms. However, such evaluations will likely be conducted by a small subgroup of clinicians familiar with the legal and clinical concepts necessary to complete such evaluations. Most medical and mental health professionals are more likely to encounter more acute concerns related to client safety, wherein an assessment of risk is necessary for reporting such safety risks. In Chapter 6, we explore in much greater detail the ethical considerations of professionals in the context of breaking confidentiality when a duty to warn and/or protect is enacted. Here, we will provide a brief overview of the laws associated with such to provide a legal foundation for our mandated reporting requirements as clinicians.

In many clinical roles, we are serving on the frontline of assessing patients' violence and suicide risk, which is legally and colloquially often referred to as their "dangerousness to self and others" (and even property). Of course, assessing risk and reporting our concerns when it is elevated is the responsibility of most clinicians across roles and contexts, well beyond frontline work roles. In this section, we will review some particularly relevant considerations, which are useful reminders for medical and mental health professionals like us. Certain concepts, such as confidentiality in the context of the Health Insurance Portability and Accountability Act of 1996 (HIPAA) get tremendous attention over our many years of academic and clinical training for good reason, but such extraordinary attention can lead to at least some level of desensitization—or, at the very least, cause us to overlook particularly important details. Indeed, anecdotally, it is not uncommon to hear the term "HIPAA" being spoken in clinical contexts to reference essentially everything related to confidentiality, even if HIPAA requirements do not actually apply. That said, the HIPAA Administrative Simplification Regulation Text issued by the U.S. Department of Health and Human Services (Office for Civil Rights, 2013) is 115 pages long, so there is quite a lot covered—not to mention additional requirements set forth in our respective state regulations and ethics codes (see Chapter 6). Suffice to say that the importance of maintaining patients' confidentiality has been instilled in us, many times over, as both an ethical and legal obligation.

Most of the time, maintaining confidentiality is a relatively easy concept to follow, such as protecting personal health information (PHI) through computer and filing systems, and not disclosing PHI to those who are not privy to such. By and large, fairly black-and-white decisions can be made in this regard, and made quickly. However, there are times when we are obligated to break confidentiality to ensure the safety of our patients and others, and these can be rather gray types of decisions—namely, scenarios in which we believe our patients are at imminent threat of harming themselves or other people. Some of us will never be in this situation, perhaps as a result of some combination of our work setting, our caseload, and a little luck. On the other hand, some of us work in crisis centers, emergency rooms, and similar settings where assessing high-risk patients and situations is literally our job. And, of course, many of us work, have worked, or will work in roles that expose us to the full continuum in between—from very benign to extremely high-risk clinical situations. Regardless of the role or

Ψ Professional liability is correlated with clinical thresholds. Clinical thresholds that are too high are associated with potential *external* risk to clients, whereas thresholds that are too low are associated with *internal* risk to practitioners in the form of increased professional liability concerns (e.g., ethics complaints, lawsuits).

setting in which we find ourselves at any given time, the decision to break confidentiality is one that must be taken seriously at all times. As we will address in greater detail in Chapter 6, developing and maintaining rapport and a therapeutic alliance with our patients is an extremely important aspect of engaging in effective clinical work, and it can become significantly impaired and even destroyed if we improperly manage processes related to informed consent and risk assessment.

The inception of our mandated reporting duties came about following the case of *Tarasoff v. Regents of the University of California* (1976). This landmark case is based on the murder of Tatiana Tarasoff by her boyfriend, Prosenjit Poddar, a graduate student in naval architecture at the University of California at Berkeley. Poddar became obsessed with Tarasoff and expressed his intent to kill her to his college counselor, psychologist Dr. Lawrence Moore. Despite disclosing this information to the counselor, neither Tarasoff nor her parents were ever warned, and Poddar ultimately murdered Tarasoff. Her parents subsequently sued the counselor and various employees of UC Berkeley for not warning their daughter and, eventually, the California Supreme Court found that such professionals have a duty to both their patients and (identifiable) individuals who may be in danger. This ruling triggered the enactment of *duty to warn* laws that are currently mandated in 46 states, whereby healthcare professionals are permitted to break confidentiality requirements when there is a risk of imminent danger, to include incurring a legal duty to warn potential, identifiable victims. Many states have established *Tarasoff*-related warnings or duty to warn reporting (see Gorshkalova & Munakomi, 2020). Namely, 23 have statutorily mandated so-called duty to warn laws (e.g., Arizona, California, Maryland, New Jersey, Nebraska, Virginia, Montana), 10 states have duty to warn as a common law (e.g., Alabama, Delaware, Hawaii, Vermont, South Carolina, Pennsylvania), and 11 states are permissive with respect to duty to warn (e.g., Alaska, Connecticut, Florida, New York, Texas). In the permissive states, clinicians are not liable for breaching confidentiality and are not required to do so. Six states have no established legal requirements in this regard (i.e., Arkansas, Kansas, Maine, Nevada, New Mexico, North Dakota).

In any case, the decision of whether a duty to warn has been incurred should be preceded by a formal violence and/or suicide risk assessment, in line with case-specific questions and issues. While we address this in greater detail in Chapter 5, some points are worth highlighting here first. A primary consideration is that our professional decision-making thresholds are critically important to establish, such that they should generally not be too low or too high. Of course, some of us working in screening roles may very well have a low threshold for risk-related concerns, as such would prompt further evaluation. Indeed, this is the point of screening. For others, our thresholds may be largely dependent on our roles and the referral questions at hand in given circumstances. Simply put: The decision of whether or not the scale has been sufficiently tipped to warrant breaching confidentiality and reporting a client of concern is one of the most serious and consequential decisions we can make as medical and mental health professionals. There is inherent subjectivity in this clinical decision-making process, but that is not necessarily a bad thing. To the contrary, clinical experience

Ψ The decision of whether or not the scale has been sufficiently tipped to warrant breaching confidentiality and reporting a client of concern is one of the most serious and consequential decisions we can make as medical and mental health professionals.

Ψ Decisions must be well grounded in risk assessment principles, consistent with the standards of practice in our respective disciplines. They must also reflect consistency in the way in which we assess risk across cases in our respective practices.

and associated expertise is usually highly valued in our fields (e.g., think of the value placed on curriculum vitaes). As we discuss in Chapter 5, a problem can arise when a clinician engages in *unstructured* clinical judgment rather than a structured professional judgment (SPJ) approach, which we endorse. As to the main point here pertaining to breaking confidentiality, what is important to remember is there will usually be bidirectional implications for doing so (and not doing so). Therefore, our decisions must be well grounded in risk assessment principles, consistent with the standards of practice in our respective disciplines as well, reflecting consistency in the way in which we assess risk across cases in our own practices.

Some states have expanded on the duty to warn laws by adding a *duty to protect* element, which includes reporting confidential client information to a third party, typically law enforcement. For example, New York passed the Secure Ammunition and Firearms Enforcement Act of 2013 (i.e., NY SAFE Act) in response to the Sandy Hook school shooting in Newtown, Connecticut. The SAFE Act amended the preexisting reporting requirements, further requiring all mental health professionals, physicians, and nurses to make a report to law enforcement "if they conclude, using reasonable professional judgment, that the individual is likely to engage in conduct that would result in serious harm to self or others." If county officials "agree with the assessments," they will proceed to put the individual's name into the state database, where it will remain for 5 years. During this process, if law enforcement determines the individual has a gun permit, they are required to revoke the license and seize the person's firearms. Furthermore, the person in question is then restricted from obtaining a permit to obtain/possess firearms until the person's name is "purged."

A similar amendment was added to New Jersey's duty to warn law in recent years. Namely, in 2018, Governor Murphy signed a bill into law mandating treating medical and mental health professionals to contact police departments in clients' towns of residence when their duty to warn is incurred. This law pertains to licensed practitioners of psychology, psychiatry, medicine, nursing, clinical social work, and marriage counseling. In addition to engaging in other actions based on options that were already part of the law, such as contacting local law enforcement and arranging for a psychiatric hospitalization, this amendment requires that a treating professional in New Jersey must also contact the chief law enforcement officer of the patient's residential municipality and provide "the patient's name and other non-clinical identifying information." This information will be then used to "ascertain whether the patient has been issued a firearms purchaser identification card, permit to purchase a handgun, or any other permit or license authorizing possession of a firearm," thereby allowing law enforcement to confiscate the patient's firearms purchaser identification card, firearms, ammunition, and related items (NJ Rev. Stat. § 2A:62A-16, 2020). This was an amendment to the existing law, which provided immunity to practitioners for breaking confidentiality in certain instances. A number of other states, such as California and Illinois, have similar reporting requirements.

These state regulations demonstrate the types of nuances often seen in reporting laws throughout the country and highlight the importance of becoming very familiar with the specific reporting laws in our respective states of practice. Clients may have a general familiarity with our obligation to report substantive threats but may not be aware of the additional steps we may decide or even be required to take. It is for this reason that we emphasize the importance of the informed consent process. Not only is it an ethical requirement and the right thing to do, but formally providing informed consent in a comprehensive, thoughtful, and interactive manner facilitates rapport-building with patients. In the context of the discussion at hand, it is also an essential reference point we may need to refer back to when risk-related concerns arise. Indeed, people can become very upset when their expectations are violated; therefore, managing

> Ψ The informed consent process if important not only substantively but also in terms of rapport-building and managing expectations. As a result, there are notable professional liability implications in this regard.

expectations in this way is important for additional reasons, including but not limited to those related to our professional liability. In the context of firearm-related considerations, it is important that our clients understand our reporting requirements as well as the potential, associated repercussions, which may have long-lasting implications for them, personally and professionally.

All that said, some states have considered and brought forth legislation in recent years in an attempt to prohibit physicians from asking patients certain questions about their gun ownership, known as "gag orders." The first gag law introduced was Florida's 2011 Privacy of Firearm Owners Act (FOPA)—also known as the "Docs v. Glocks" law, which sought to block doctors from asking patients about gun ownership or recording it in the file. In 2012, the U.S. Southern District of Florida Court issued a permanent injunction against these provisions (i.e., inquiry, recordkeeping, discrimination, harassment) in this matter the following year, on the basis that such infringed upon doctors' freedom of speech. This matter was then sent to the 11th Circuit of the U.S. Court of Appeals, in the case of *Wollschlaeger v. Governor of Florida* (2014), where medical professionals and organizations sued the governor of Florida and the state (officials) for setting forth the FOPA. It was similarly argued by the petitioners that the Act violated the First Amendment by preventing "open and free exchanges of information and advice with their patients about ways to reduce the safety risks posed by firearms" (p. 2). The 11th Circuit vacated the injunction in 2014 and upheld the Act, however; according to the court, the law only restricted speech uttered in doctors' examination rooms. As such, the Act was exempt from First Amendment scrutiny, which otherwise allowed freedom of speech. However, *Wollschlaeger v. Governor of Florida* was heard again in 2015, and in 2017, in a 10–1 ruling, it was determined that such violated the First Amendment and not the 2A. An additional provision in this ruling barred physicians from discriminating against patients who were gun owners. Florida state officials never filed an appeal to SCOTUS and this law is no longer in effect as of 2019. Numerous other states, since 2011, have introduced gag order laws such as these, but none have been successful to our knowledge.

ADDITIONAL GUN OWNERSHIP AND SAFETY LAWS: MAGAZINE CAPACITY, STORAGE, TRANSPORTATION, AND RIGHT TO CARRY

Consistent with our KAD model, as clinicians, it is imperative to have a working knowledge of what constitutes safe and legal practices in order to gauge such concerns for our patients. We have emphasized the importance of going beyond simply asking whether or not someone has access to guns, which may be too cursory or even misleading. Additional questions are often necessary to form more complete and informed opinions about risk, such as those pertaining to storage and transportation practices, including but certainly not limited to child access. In this section, we provide a brief set of considerations related to magazine capacity limits as well as storage, transportation, and carry laws. While it certainly is not our job to investigate or enforce laws, this type of information can be important for us to know if we need to opine as to our patients' risk levels. Forensic evaluators in gun-related matters often need to know this information even more so to inform their decision-making process.

Magazine Capacity Limits

If we recall back to Chapter 1, a magazine is the detachable part of a gun that holds the ammunition. In recent years, much has been discussed in media and political outlets about what are referred to as *large-capacity magazines.* Namely, policymakers throughout the country have drafted legislation setting increased limits on the number of rounds (i.e., cartridges that contain bullets) that can be loaded into a single magazine to be considered legal in their respective jurisdictions. These large-capacity magazine bans have generally followed high-profile "mass" shootings. The number of rounds that can be held in a given magazine varies, often based on the type of firearm in question. Although high-capacity magazines are typically associated with rifles in media and political presentations, handguns can certainly hold magazines that exceed state minimums. In fact, the magazine capacity for semiautomatic pistols ranges widely, from six to 18 rounds. Certain rifles, including the oft-spoken-about AR-15-style rifle, typically come with a 30-round-capacity magazine, however. The point remains that magazine capacities vary greatly and are largely dependent on the size of the firearm, its manufacturer, and its intended purpose.

All that said, most states do not have any capacity restrictions on magazines. However, the following states have either 10- or 15-round restrictions: California, Colorado, Connecticut, Hawaii, Maryland, Massachusetts, New York, New Jersey, and Vermont (https://giffords.org/lawcenter/gun-laws/policy-areas/hardware-ammunit ion/large-capacity-magazines/). Given that legislation in this regard has increasingly arisen in recent years, many existing gun owners have been faced with surrendering their magazines or even their firearms. In some cases, they have been allowed to possess modified magazines, or those that have them "pinned." In New Jersey, for example, this has happened multiple times; namely, there have been two laws passed regarding capacity limits, including a previous 15-round and a more recent 10-round capacity minimum. At both time points, once the law was passed, it was unlawful to own magazines that did not meet the requirement.

It is important to note, however, that magazines can be unloaded and reloaded in a matter of seconds. In other words, there is little practical difference between someone having four 15-round magazines and six 10-round magazines, particularly in the hands of those intending to do harm—especially when they are among unarmed persons. Legislators who set forth hardware laws like this typically cite their rationale as the prevention of "mass" shootings; however, such is largely predicated on the curious assumption that would-be mass shooters follow gun laws. This, coupled with the (fortunate) rarity of active-shooter events, makes these hardware laws more political than practical—and, in actuality, more of an impediment to lawful gun owners than to impending mass shooters.

Storage

The importance of safe gun storage cannot be overstated. Such not only prevents theft, but also prevents minors and other unintended persons from gaining access to firearms. Safe storage may include such practices as maintaining guns in locked safes or cabinets, in addition to using trigger locks. As always, states have their own nuances, but proper firearm storage is reflective of safe, responsible gun ownership regardless of the letter of the law in a given state. A disproportionate number of unintentional firearm-related fatalities have occurred in states where gun owners are more likely to store their firearms loaded or unlocked (Miller et al., 2005). While accidental shootings are relatively rare in relation to the overarching number of total gun deaths, it has been suggested by researchers that keeping a gun locked and unloaded, with ammunition locked in a separate location, appears to be a good strategy to reduce injuries in homes with minors (Grossman et al., 2005). These are not necessarily legal requirements across the country, and people may even be advised by some to keep home defense firearms loaded and unlocked in residences without minors. Therefore, as clinicians, we need to know the laws in this regard in our states of practice and, in most cases, seek to understand the practices of our patients as opposed to passing (personal) judgment upon them. Indeed, we become aware of many improper and even illegal behaviors of patients that we do not usually act upon (e.g., drug use)—unless, of course, such is linked to concerns of imminent or, at least, foreseeable and specific risk.

Locking Devices

Most contemporary firearms have safeties and locking devices installed; however, they have begun to be shipped to owners with external locking devices in recent years (e.g., trigger locks, cables). Although there are no federal laws requiring locking devices, 11 states do have such laws on the books. Massachusetts is the only state requiring all firearms to be stored with a lock in place, such as with a tamper-resistant mechanical lock. California, Connecticut, and New York require this if the owner resides with a prohibited person. As with many of California's gun laws, the laws regarding firearm locking devices are comprehensive in that all firearms manufactured, sold, or transferred in the state must include a firearm safety device approved by the Department of Justice (DOJ). States such as New York, Michigan, and Ohio prohibit the sales of firearms without a locking device or trigger lock, and some states, such as Connecticut and New Jersey, require locking devices on all handguns sold (e.g., Mich. Comp. Laws § 28.435, 1927; N.J. Stat. Ann. § 2C:58-2a(5)(d),(e), 2009). Illinois and Maryland have similar laws that include not only external safety devices, but also integrated mechanical safety devices (i.e., one that is built into the handgun). Some states, such as California and New York, have actually set specific standards for external locking devices. Maryland and Massachusetts have gone a step farther and have a list of approved external locking devices.

There are also local laws, in certain cities, regarding locking devices and safe storage to be aware of beyond state-specific laws. For instance, New York City mandates a safety locking device with the transfer of a firearm both to and from individuals (i.e., through purchasing or obtaining). San Francisco and Sunnyvale, California, both require that all handguns within a residence must either be in a locked container or have a trigger lock, unless the gun is on their person.

Child Access Prevention

Child access prevention (CAP) laws are targeted at reducing rates of unintentional deaths among minors as well as youth suicides and school shootings, by encouraging the safe storage of firearms. Thus, gun owners face legal problems when they allow children to have unsupervised access to their guns or are otherwise negligent in this regard. Although federal law does not outline gun storage requirements, the 30 state laws that do vary considerably, with some imposing criminal liability when a minor has access to firearms—intentionally or negligently. The definition of a "minor" under CAP laws also varies across states, ranging from 14 to 18. Once again, the nuances in gun laws throughout the country are seemingly countless. For instance, there are states that impose criminal liability when a child "may" or "is likely to" gain access (i.e., California, Washington D.C., Massachusetts, Minnesota, Nevada, New York); for allowing a child to gain access regardless of injury (i.e., California, Washington D.C., Delaware, Hawaii, Maryland, Massachusetts, Minnesota, Nevada, New Jersey, Texas); and if a child uses or carries a gun (i.e., Connecticut, Florida, Illinois, Iowa, New Hampshire, North Carolina, Rhode Island, Washington State). There are also states that impose criminal liability for the negligent storage of unloaded firearms (i.e., California, Connecticut, Washington D.C., Hawaii, Massachusetts, Nevada). However, there are exceptions to CAP laws, such as when the firearm is used for hunting or if the minor uses the gun in self-defense, or to aid law enforcement. Consistent with our KAD model, we cannot overemphasize the importance of taking a close look at the laws in the states in which we practice, to be able to recognize safety concerns among patients.

Although researchers have asserted that safe storage laws are effective in lowering suicide risk among adolescents (Price & Norris, 2010), such findings tend to be more nuanced. For instance, although state-level CAP laws have been ineffective in appreciably reducing unintentional deaths, states with CAP laws had lower rates of youth suicide (Gius, 2015). Furthermore, although state-level minimum age laws have had no effect in reducing youth suicides, after the enactment of a federal minimum age limit, both unintentional death and youth suicide decreased (Gius, 2015). However, it has been found that families living in states with stronger firearm legislation and CAP laws reportedly engage in safer storage practices (Prickett et al., 2014).

Another notable area pertains to programs that have been developed that teach children about gun safety. For instance, *Project ChildSafe* was developed by the National Shooting Sports Foundation (NSSF) in 2003 and is a federally funded, nonprofit charitable organization that partners with law enforcement. They have distributed millions of gun safety kits to owners throughout the country, which include a cable-style gun-locking device and a brochure that discusses safe handling and secure storage guidelines to help deter access by unauthorized users. A primary tenet of the group is "Own it? Respect it. Secure it." Another program, the *Eddie Eagle GunSafe®* program, was developed by the National Rifle Association (NRA) in 1988 and is characterized as a "gun accident prevention program." This program focuses on teaching pre-K through fourth graders what to do if they ever come across a firearm. The basic instructional steps are "stop, don't touch, run away, and tell a grown-up." There are many resources on the program's website, including videos and activities. These programs highlight the importance of gun safety promoted by firearm subcultures alike. However, there have been some concerns raised regarding the effectiveness of these programs, as well as methodological limitations.

Transportation

With regard to federal gun transportation laws, the FOPA protects individuals transporting firearms at some level. Specifically, a person is entitled to transport a firearm from any place where they lawfully possess/carry to another place where they may lawfully do the same, as long as the firearm is unloaded, locked, and out of reach. In a car without a trunk, the gun must be unloaded and locked in a container—not in a glove box or in the console—and ammunition is locked either in the trunk or likewise in a similar container. As we elaborated upon earlier in this chapter (*Mental Health-Related Prohibitions: State Law*), laws pertaining to transporting firearms vary among states. As such, it is imperative that the traveler has copies of any licenses or permits, and it would behoove the person to have printouts of official publications that outline the jurisdiction's provisions in the event of an encounter with law enforcement.

If someone wishes to carry a loaded and readily accessible gun in their car, then state and local carry laws apply. Because carry laws vary greatly among states, crossing state lines with a loaded firearm can lead to significant legal problems. Nevertheless, in many if not most states, guns may be legally transported if done so in the manner we described: unloaded, in a container, and locked in the trunk—essentially not accessible to the people in the car. In any case, there are some states that are especially strict and have numerous, complex gun laws; therefore, travelers must be mindful and consult the relevant laws in states they are traveling to (or through) in advance (e.g., California, Hawaii, Massachusetts, New Jersey, New York, Washington D.C.). Moreover, certain jurisdictions within these states may have their own additional requirements. For example, in New York City, a New York license is not valid on its own; one must have one that is specific to New York City.

When traveling by plane, the Transportation Security Administration (TSA) dictates that both guns and ammunition can be transported if they are unloaded and secured in a hard-sided container. However, this must be checked; in other words, they are not allowed in carry-on luggage. The ammunition may be transported in the same hard-sided case as the unloaded firearm (see www.TSA.gov for additional restrictions). Prior to travel, both must be declared in the manner the airline specifies. Gun owners who do not intend on traveling with their firearms would benefit from double-checking their bags before heading to the airports, as there will likely be not only delays but also potential sanctions for accidentally having them in their bags. Bringing even an unloaded firearm with accessible ammunition to the security checkpoint has penalties. Some airports, such as those near New York City (i.e., Newark, JFK, LaGuardia) have been known to enforce state and local firearm laws against travelers despite federal laws. Therefore, those traveling to or through these airports may want to consider shipping their firearms. In addition, travelers must also be mindful (and planful), more generally, in case an unexpected diversion occurs that requires them to spend time in a city where they did not intend on staying. There may be storage options available, but identifying the laws and related options at hand is incumbent upon gun owners.

Right to Carry

In Chapter 1, we discussed issues of cultural competency as it pertains to firearm-related subcultures, exploring the vast differences that exist across the United States in this regard. For instance, in many states, it would not be out of the ordinary to see someone walking with a gun holstered on their hip, or visible in a motor vehicle. To the contrary, there are numerous states where this would be particularly alarming and would likely lead to the police being called. Some gun owners assert that the 2A affords them not only the right to own firearms, but also to carry them (i.e., "bear" arms), which is consistent with the recent *Bruen* ruling by SCOTUS.

Nevertheless, there are very specific and nuanced laws pertaining to a gun owner's right to carry. In states where such is allowed, these fall under the umbrella terms *open carry* and *concealed carry laws*. These may also be different for those who must carry for work as compared to general gun laws pertaining to civilians. For example, federal law allows certain law enforcement officers to carry concealed firearms. As the names imply, *open carry* refers to carrying a firearm in public that is visible to others, whereas *concealed carry* refers to publicly carrying a firearm that is not visible to others.

Open Carry

Even in states that allow for open carry, such may be prohibited in certain locations (e.g., schools, public transportation). States like California, Florida, Illinois, and Washington D.C. prohibit open carry of any gun in public, while New York and South Carolina prohibit openly carrying handguns but not long guns. Massachusetts, Minnesota, and New Jersey prohibit openly carrying long guns but not handguns; however, in Minnesota, handguns must be unloaded. The remaining states generally allow open carry, with some requiring a permit or license to do so (e.g., Connecticut, Georgia, Massachusetts, Minnesota, New Jersey), which in some states may be very difficult to obtain. Laws do become even more nuanced with open carry of long guns, for instance. In most states, openly carrying a long gun is legal, although Iowa, Tennessee, and Utah require the gun to be unloaded. In certain cities in Virginia and Pennsylvania, there are limitations with regard to the open carry of long guns. Of course, carry permits are a prerequisite in states that allow this type of firearm possession, which were historically essentially impossible for civilians to attain in what were referred to as "may issue" rather than "shall issue" states (e.g., New Jersey). Again, the recent SCOTUS ruling in *Bruen* has changed the trajectory of carrying guns in the United States.

Concealed Carry

Thirty-five states require a permit to carry a concealed firearm in public, and 15 generally allow concealed carry in public without such a permit (e.g., Maine, Alaska, Vermont, Missouri). Of the 35 states requiring a permit, eight of them, as well as Washington D.C., have the aforementioned "may issue" laws. These bestow significant discretion upon the issuing state, such that state officials can simply deny permits based on reasons such as lacking good character (e.g., New Jersey, New York, California). Seven states require that the applicant demonstrate good cause, or justification as to why they are seeking the permit for concealed carry. For instance, in California, this exists when there is a clear and present danger to the applicant or their family, spouse, or employees, particularly when this credible threat cannot be managed through other legal means. In Massachusetts, applicants must demonstrate a "good reason" to fear injury to their person or property, similar to other states, such as Hawaii. Ten states require that the person be of good character, and approximately half of the states require some level of knowledge of firearm use and safety. Moreover, before *Bruen*, in New Jersey, carry applicants had to demonstrate what was referred to as a *justifiable need* to carry, which proved to be a nearly impossible feat in the state. In fact, both New Jersey and Massachusetts have had the second-lowest carry rates in the country (New Jersey: approximately 1,200 people as of 2013), just above Hawaii, which had no people who carried. Time will tell how these numbers change as a result of the SCOTUS ruling in *Bruen*. Nevertheless, for context, Florida, Georgia, Pennsylvania, and Texas each have more than a million permit holders for concealed carry. Fourteen states have limited-discretion "shall issue" laws and 13 states have no-discretion "shall issue" laws. Still, nearly all states place restrictions on where concealed firearms can be carried.

RECOMMENDED FURTHER READING

Ciyou, B. L. (2018). *2018 edition: Gun laws by state: Reciprocity and gun laws quick reference guide*. Peritus Holdings.

Consortium for Risk-Based Firearm Policy. (2013). *Guns, public health, and mental illness: An evidence-based approach for state policy*. Educational Fund to Stop Gun Violence. https://efsgv.org/wp-content/uploads/2014/10/Final-State-Report.pdf

District of Columbia v. Heller, *554 US 570 (2008)*.

Gold, L. H., & Vanderpool, D. (2018a). Legal regulation of restoration of firearms rights after mental health prohibition. *Journal of the American Academy of Psychiatry and the Law, 46*(3), 298–308.

Gold, L. H., & Vanderpool, D. (2018b). Psychiatric evidence and due process in firearms rights restoration. *Journal of the American Academy of Psychiatry and the Law, 46*(3), 309–321.

Kappas, J. S. (2021). *2021 traveler's guide to the firearm laws of the fifty states*. Traveler's Guide.

McGinty, E. E., Webster, D. W., & Barry, C. L. (2014). Gun policy and serious mental illness: Priorities for future research and policy. *Psychiatric Services, 65*(1), 50–58. https://doi.org/10.1176/appi.ps.201300141

Pirelli, G., Schrantz, K., & Wechsler, H. (2020). The emerging role of psychology in shaping gun policy in the United States. In M. K. Miller & B. H. Bornstein (Eds.), *Advances in psychology and law* (vol. 5, pp. 373–411). Springer.

Swanson, J. W., Robertson, A. G., Frisman, L. K., Norko, M., Lin, H. J., Swartz, M. S., & Cook, P. J. (2013). Preventing gun violence involving people with serious mental illness. In D. W. Webster & J. S. Vernick (Eds.), *Reducing gun violence in America* (pp. 33–51). Johns Hopkins University Press.

3

Firearms and Mental Health

A REVIEW OF THE PROFESSIONAL LITERATURE AND EMERGING ROLES FOR MEDICAL AND MENTAL HEALTH PROFESSIONALS

AN IMPORTANT ASPECT of developing competency in any area is having at least a general understanding of the state of the respective literature. Although research examining the relationship between firearms and mental health is ever-growing, there is a solid foundation of empirical studies that have addressed the nature of the connection and the lack thereof in certain respects. That is, while certain media outlets, politicians, and other groups may try to portray what appears to be a rather strong link between mental illness and gun deaths across the board, the research clearly indicates that, in actuality, the relationship is complex and nuanced. Indeed, such nuances are very important for us as clinicians to understand when firearm-related issues arise in clinical practice. Therefore, in this chapter, we provide an overview of the current literature addressing the relationship between mental illness and violence, domestic violence, and suicide—both generally and firearm-involved, more specifically. We cover these areas in their own respective sections, as they warrant distinct sets of considerations in many respects. Then, we review the emerging roles for us, as medical and mental health professionals, in both clinical and policy contexts related to guns.

MENTAL ILLNESS AND VIOLENCE

Before diving into the more specific relationship between firearms and interpersonal violence, it is important to address the broader connection between violence and

Ψ Although mental illness can be a moderating factor in some instances and, therefore, weighted accordingly on a case-by-case basis, the reality is the vast majority of people diagnosed with even severe mental illnesses do not commit acts of interpersonal violence—with or without a gun.

Ψ Throughout this chapter, and in various parts of this book, we refer to *moderating* variables, or factors. The term *moderation*, statistically speaking, means that the relationship between two variables depends on another—a *moderating variable*. To illustrate, we might consider the relationship between having a family history of heart disease and a person's risk of heart attack. The risk often largely depends on the impact of various *moderators*, such as nutrition and exercise as well as other habits (e.g., smoking). These are all factors that *moderate* the relationship between family history of heart disease and one's potential to suffer a heart attack. Thus, in our context here, it is important to consider factors that may *moderate* the relationship between firearm ownership, possession, or easy access otherwise, and various types of gun-involved deaths.

mental illness. This is a critically important starting point because many people endorse the faulty assumption that there is a strong link between mental illness and (interpersonal) violence. Although mental illness can be a moderating factor in some instances and, therefore, weighted accordingly on a case-by-case basis, the reality is the vast majority of people diagnosed with even severe mental illnesses do not commit acts of interpersonal violence—with or without a gun (Swanson et al., 1990, 2015). Still, various politicians, media outlets, and other groups have played a large role in propagating this misconception, especially in the context of tragic events that become sensationalized, such as active shooter incidents and "mass shootings."

Of course, the language often used by many feeds this misconception—for example, collectively referring to all gun deaths as "gun violence" when, in fact, the majority are suicides and relatively few are the result of active shooter-driven mass shootings, which have become the face of the so-called gun debate. However, politicians and media outlets are not solely responsible. Despite working diligently for decades to destigmatize mental illness, some medical and mental health professionals have continued to foster stigma by literally grouping the most heinous school shooters with those who have died by suicide via a firearm. While suicide has been technically considered self-directed violence, particularly in academic circles, there are a whole host of concerns with characterizing all gun deaths as gun violence, which is by no stretch of the imagination a unitary construct. Given those who die by suicide are typically thought of as victims rather than perpetrators, the precise method used during the act should be inconsequential in terms of how we view the deceased. Yet, many promote the message that all deaths resulting from a gunshot are the result of someone who has perpetrated "gun violence," be it via suicide, accidental discharge, or an active shooter situation. All are entered into the same databases and analyzed in the aggregate. However, when conceptualizations are faulty, so will be everything that follows (i.e., data collection, analyses, interpretations, and recommendations). As it is said in the world of meta-analysis, *garbage in, garbage out*. Fortunately, by developing our professional competence in this arena, we have the ability to provide clarity and increased accuracy in our work as clinicians.

The connection between mental illness and violence is complex and nuanced. First and foremost, we must identify how the constructs of mental illness and violence are being operationally defined. Then, we need to avoid black-and-white thinking; rather than asking if mental illness is associated with (interpersonal) violence, there is greater utility in conceptualizing violence risk in a contextualized manner—for instance, asking *when* and *how* the manifestations of a given mental illness lead to certain *types* of interpersonal violence acts, by *particular* people in *specific* contexts. We outline risk assessment principles and concepts in greater detail in Chapters 4 and 5, but let us take a moment here to address the issue of operationally defining important terms, such as violence.

A primary tenet of science is the need to operationalize constructs, or to define the variables examined in a particular study. This may simply include providing a clear definition or explaining how we measure a given construct, such as using a particular assessment instrument to measure intellectual functioning (e.g., an IQ test). The oft-cited gap between research and practice is real but can be significantly narrowed if we embrace a scientist-practitioner model, whereby our research informs our practice and vice versa. A central step in doing so is to recognize that variables can (and usually should) translate from research studies to practice, just as many questions that arise in practice provide excellent fodder for empirical study. Indeed, applied research with strong ecological, or external, validity would be reflective of such. If we can agree on the relative importance of these ideals, then it follows that the frameworks and inherent concepts used in both practice and research should be symmetrical if not precisely the same.

In the gun context at hand, it is important to more closely look at the ways in which researchers operationalize or otherwise define the terms "violence" and "gun violence," more specifically, particularly in studies designed to examine their associations with mental illness. For instance, the construct of violence employed in one study may include acts that do not include physical contact (e.g., verbal threats, certain types of robberies), whereas another study may only include acts comprising physical contact. This seemingly minor difference among studies can have a rather significant impact when the time comes to aggregate data for the purpose of drawing conclusions about the relationship between these variables (e.g., in meta-analyses or even qualitative literature reviews). There are various types of violence that may be accounted for in a research study, such as physical, verbal, and sexual violence, in addition to subtypes within each of these constructs (e.g., contact vs. non-contact violence). Thus, we must look carefully at others' use of various constructs and be transparent about our own use, in both research and practice, to ensure consistency across sources. Otherwise, our terms essentially boil down to jargon, which can be misinterpreted or, worse, misleading.

Again, this is why we avoid using the term "gun violence," which is typically defined by the inclusion of all types of gun deaths regardless of the actual cause—via suicides, homicides, and accidental discharges. Instead, it is much more transparent and, therefore, useful to speak of particular types of gun deaths separately (e.g., firearm-involved suicide). Another example is the term "mass shooting," which is typically defined by the number of deaths resulting from a shooting (historically, three or four), whereas the term "active shooter" has greater utility, as it pertains to the behavior and even *motivation* behind the act rather than the outcome. Indeed, there are active shooter scenarios that do not result in any gun deaths. As a result, they do not wind up in databases with similar shooting events. It comes as no surprise then that our collective knowledge and associated interventions remain relatively limited in this arena, given that most databases are driven by the amount of gun deaths rather than the reason behind the shootings.

Ψ We avoid using the term "gun violence," which is typically defined by the inclusion of all types of gun deaths regardless of the actual cause—via suicide, homicide, and accidental discharges. Instead, it is much more transparent and, therefore, useful to speak of particular types of gun deaths separately (e.g., firearm-involved suicide).

In the past few decades, much research has been conducted examining the link between mental illness and violence. Although a full review is outside of our scope here, a number of seminal studies have set the groundwork for future research in this area. Namely, the National Institute of Mental Health (NIMH) Epidemiologic Catchment Area (ECA) study was the first of its kind. Published in the 1990s, it was a survey-based study of a community sample of about 10,000 participants from numerous U.S. cities (e.g., Baltimore, Los Angeles, New Haven). Violence was operationally defined as consisting of physically assaultive behaviors, such as hitting, pushing, shoving, kicking, or throwing objects at someone, and multiple researchers analyzed these data. Over a 12-month period, just about 12% of those with a serious mental illness (i.e., to include schizophrenia, bipolar disorder, or major depression) committed any type of violence, as compared to a 2% prevalence rate of violence by those without a mental illness or substance use disorder (Swanson et al., 1990, 2015). However, it was estimated that just 3% to 5% of all acts of interpersonal violence, with or without guns, were attributable to even these serious mental illnesses. In other words, based on these findings, over 95% of violent acts are not attributable to even severe mental illnesses.

Ψ Just 3% to 5% of all violence, which includes violence involving firearms, is attributable to even serious mental illness.

Another study of note is the MacArthur Violence Risk Assessment Study, wherein Steadman et al. (1998) examined the link between mental illness and violence over a 1-year period among those discharged from inpatient psychiatric units as compared to their community counterparts. Violence was operationalized as falling into one of two categories: (1) acts resulting in physical injuries and, also, sexual assaults, threats with a weapon, and acts involving the use of a weapon otherwise, or (2) other aggressive acts that did not result in physical injuries. It was found those diagnosed with a mental illness alone (i.e., not with a comorbid substance use disorder) were no more likely to commit violence than their community counterparts. Of additional note is that, in 2015, Steadman et al. again examined the MacArthur data to determine the prevalence of firearm involvement. They found that just 2% of patients committed a violent act involving a gun.

While both the ECA and the MacArthur studies found a weak link between violence and mental illness per se, both sets of findings indicated that having a substance (both alcohol and drug) use disorder (either alone or comorbid with another psychiatric condition) significantly increased violence risk. Namely, Steadman et al. (1998) found that the prevalence rate of violence for those with a major mental illness alone was approximately 18% as compared to 31% for those with a comorbid substance use-related diagnosis. Thus, the presence of a substance use disorder was found to be a particularly salient concern in the context of violence risk in these samples, which is consistent with other research in this area (e.g., Elbogen & Johnson, 2009; Moberg et al., 2014). That said, subsequent research has shown that alcohol use alone is a particularly salient concern with respect to violence even in the absence of other types of substance use. For example, alcohol is a factor in 40% of all violent crimes (National Council on Alcoholism and Drug Dependence). The link between alcohol use and violence and aggression has been well established in the literature (e.g., Chermack & Giancola, 1997; Kachadourian et al., 2012).

While the empirical research has demonstrated most people with mental health–related problems, even severe illnesses, rarely perpetrate violence toward others, there is undoubtedly a subgroup of people who do—albeit a relatively small one. Nevertheless, identifying who they are and when they will act violently is perhaps one of the most consequential tasks for us as clinicians. Because we cannot and should not simply draw a line from mental health diagnosis to violence risk, assessment is a critical component of our work. In Chapters 4 and 5, we address the ways in which we can effectively conduct risk assessments in clinical and forensic contexts. As we will continue to emphasize throughout this book, we should avoid the temptation to engage in prediction-based assessments and subscribe to a risk management and prevention approach. It is also generally more useful to conceptualize a mental health symptom or diagnosis as being more or less *associated* with violence risk as opposed to being the *cause* of a specific violent act (i.e., it is serving as a potential moderator variable). Hence, we need to seek to conduct context-specific risk assessments that account for mental illnesses and their manifestations but that do not overvalue their presence in a given case.

Although the presence of a mental illness alone is a relatively weak predictor of violence in general (see also Corrigan & Watson, 2005), there are specific disorders and symptoms of disorders that may be more closely *associated* with acts of interpersonal violence than others. Thus, it may be more useful to focus our attention on symptoms and related functional manifestations rather than on diagnostic labels per se. Still, some of the more closely associated syndromes observed in the context of interpersonal violence are personality disorders and substance use disorders—as compared to suicidality, which is more closely related to mood and anxiety disorders (Harford et al., 2013).

Other important considerations relate to the experience of psychotic symptoms associated with severe mental illnesses. Although there is a modest relationship between psychosis and violence (e.g., Douglas et al., 2009), certain features of psychosis associated with severe mental illness, when active, may increase the risk of someone engaging in interpersonal violence. Psychosis can be a feature of serious mental illnesses, such as schizophrenia, schizoaffective disorder, bipolar disorder, and even major depressive disorder (American Psychiatric Association, 2013). So-called positive symptoms (i.e., hallucinations, delusions) and disorganized presentations have been found to be more strongly related to violence than negative symptoms, which are more depressogenic in nature (Douglas et al., 2009). Delusional beliefs and hallucinations with violent themes can be particularly problematic. For instance, command hallucinations, or voices that direct people to do certain things (e.g., harm others), or persecutory delusional beliefs may motivate violence (Douglas et al., 2009). Psychosis can cause anxiety, impair one's judgment, and negatively impact the ability to make sound decisions and even experience remorse.

Mental Illness and Firearm-Involved Violence

Now that we have provided some foundational understanding related to the link between mental illness and violence, we can move on to addressing the more nuanced link between mental illness and firearm-related violence. First, let us take a look at the statistics associated with firearm-involved homicide, which accounts for approximately one-third of all gun-related deaths in the United States—a rate that has remained stable for over two decades. Of additional note is that firearms, predominantly handguns, are involved in two-thirds of all homicides.

Ψ In the context of concerns related to firearm-involved violence (and suicide), we must be very vigilant when working with clients who misuse substances, particularly alcohol. While a history of alcohol abuse alone is not dispositive, clients with more chronic, severe, and recent histories should certainly heighten our awareness when considering firearm misuse.

With regard to mental health considerations, it is worth reiterating that just 3% to 5% of all acts of interpersonal violence, including but not limited to acts with firearms, are attributable to serious mental illnesses (Swanson et al., 1990). As such, the number of those with serious mental illness engaging in interpersonal violence with a firearm is even lower (Knoll & Annas, 2016). However, it is also important to restate that chronic alcohol misuse is strongly associated with violence, in general, and with engaging in risky behaviors involving a firearm, specifically (Wintemute, 2015). Therefore, in the context of concerns related to firearm-involved violence (and suicide), we must be very vigilant when working with clients who misuse substances, particularly alcohol. While a history of alcohol abuse alone is not dispositive, clients with presentations of more chronic, severe, and ongoing usage should certainly heighten our awareness when considering firearm misuse.

As for active shooter situations, according to FBI data, they contribute to less than 1% of all firearm deaths each year. Such a relatively low base rate makes these types of events challenging to empirically study (Trestman et al., 2016). Yet, many gun laws passed in the wake of these tragedies are typically centered on mental illness, such as calling for increased mental health screenings during background checks, even though most of the guns used in active shooter incidents have been legally obtained (i.e., shooters were subject to and passed background checks; Buchanan et al., 2018). In fact, the organization Everytown for Gun Safety (2019) found this to be the case two-thirds of the time, whereas illegally obtained firearms were more likely to be used in the commission of violent crimes, such as robbery, murder, and rape (https://www.everytown.org). Of course, there have been exceptions. For instance, the tragedies at Columbine and Sandy Hook Elementary involved the use of guns that were legally owned but stolen by the perpetrators.

As we have discussed, the link between firearm-related violence and most mental illnesses is not particularly strong. In fact, those diagnosed with a serious mental illness are more likely to be victims of violence rather than perpetrators (McGinty & Webster, 2016). The stereotype of the "mentally ill mass shooter armed with a semiautomatic rifle" is quite literally derived from drawing from the lowest base rates in each respective area, as most acts of violence are not attributable to even severe mental illnesses, and active shooter/mass shootings are responsible for a very small proportion of gun deaths, as are rifles. Once again, media and political attention fuels much of the misperception here: Even according to FBI data, active shooter incidents lead to less than 1% of firearm-related deaths in the United States.

> Ψ The stereotype of the "mentally ill mass shooter armed with a semiautomatic rifle" is quite literally derived from drawing from the lowest base rates in each respective area, as most acts of violence are not attributable to even severe mental illnesses, and active shooter/mass shootings are responsible for a very small proportion of gun deaths, as are rifles.

We are still left with a primary issue of particular importance to us, as clinicians; namely, the motivation behind active shooter incidents. Although there are numerous misconceptions in this context as well, Fox and DeLateur (2014) provided five potential themes thought to occur either independently or in combination with one another:

1. Revenge (e.g., a deeply disgruntled individual seeks payback for a host of failures in career, school, or personal life)
2. Power (e.g., a "pseudo-commando"-style massacre perpetrated by some marginalized individual attempting to wage a personal war against society)
3. Loyalty (e.g., a devoted husband/father kills his entire family and then himself to spare them all from a miserable existence on earth and to reunite them in the hereafter)
4. Terror (e.g., a political dissident destroys government property, with several victims killed as "collateral damage," to send a strong message to those in power)
5. Profit (e.g., a gunman executes the customers and employees at a retail store to eliminate all witnesses to a robbery). (p. 3)

Of these, revenge was the most common due to active shooters perceiving themselves as victims of injustice. That said, school shootings are thought to be a distinct type of active shooter situation, as they tend to occur in low-crime suburban or rural settings, lack specifically targeted victims, and result in higher fatalities, and the shooter is typically a middle- to lower-class white male (Rocque, 2012). Some researchers have examined mental health–related variables associated with high-profile school shootings. Namely, violent ideation has been found to be related to perceptions of inadequacy, low self-esteem, depressive affect, hopelessness, anger-induced aggression, lack of peer and parental support, and impaired or otherwise damaged masculine identity, as well as considered attempting suicide prior to the shooting (Harter et al., 2003; Rocque, 2012).

Another commonly held, albeit erroneous, belief is that school shooters are "loners." However, this is not supported by the literature by and large. Although they may have ended up isolated, they have tended to be "boys with a history of trying to join peer groups, but find themselves socially marginalized" (Bushman et al., 2016, p. 19). Many have lacked in both their social skills and the physical characteristics typically valued within their peer group (Langman, 2009). These findings highlight the importance of identifying social concerns when assessing firearm-related risk, particularly with youth. Of course, many teenagers experience these types of issues but do not go on to become school shooters (Bushman et al., 2016; Vossekuil et al., 2004). There is no way to predict who will engage in such extreme, low–base-rate actions, which is precisely why employing an approach based on risk management and prevention is essential.

Ψ There is a general misconception that school shooters are "loners," whereas they have tended to actually have made attempts to join peer groups and found themselves socially marginalized and isolated. Still, there is no way to predict who will engage in such extreme, low–base-rate actions, which is precisely why employing an approach based on risk management and prevention is essential.

MENTAL ILLNESS AND DOMESTIC VIOLENCE AND
INTIMATE PARTNER VIOLENCE

We use the terms "domestic violence" (DV) and "intimate partner violence" (IPV) interchangeably for our purposes here, but they are distinguishable. For instance, IPV is typically thought to involve either a current or former partner (e.g., boyfriend, girlfriend, spouse), whereas DV can include others such as parents, siblings, or other relatives. With respect to the prevalence of DV in the United States, a Department of Justice (DOJ) investigation of data from 2003 to 2012 revealed that nonfatal DV accounted for approximately 21% of all violent crime within that period of time (Truman & Morgan, 2014). IPV, in particular, accounted for a greater number of these victimizations (15%) versus those incidents committed by immediate family members (4%) or other relatives (2%). IPV incidents also resulted in injury more often. Moreover, the World Health Organization (WHO) published the World Report on Violence and Health in 2002 and found consistency across both industrialized and developing countries in terms of the factors associated with IPV perpetrated by males. They include heavy drinking, depression, personality disorders, witnessing or experiencing violence as a child, low income, low academic achievement, and young age. Dysfunction within the relationship, including marital conflict and instability, poor family functioning, and economic stress, have also been found to be associated with IPV.

Mental Illness and Firearm-Involved DV and IPV

Most DV situations do not involve any weapons, firearms or otherwise. In the aforementioned DOJ study, Truman and Morgan (2014) found that 77% of all DV incidents in the 10-year period they investigated did not involve any at all. Furthermore, even when weapons were involved, firearms were used less than knives and other weapons. We are confident readers will discover similar findings in their respective states as they seek to identify local norms. There also does not appear to be any compelling research linking firearms in the home to DV; however, as clinicians, we must be aware of and concerned with factors associated with fatal outcomes in these situations. Another case-specific or moderating factor to pay attention to when assessing firearm-related risk in DV situations is when the aggressor is a member of law enforcement. It is notable, however, that there is likely a high degree of underreporting in this group. Nevertheless, when 43 police-perpetrated homicide-suicides were examined between 2007 and 2014, most victims were either current or former female partners, nearly all perpetrators were males who used their service weapon to commit the offenses, and the incidents occurred within the context of DV (Klinoff et al., 2015).

With respect to intimate partner homicide (IPH), the most salient risk factors aside from direct access to guns have been found to be history of threats with a weapon (not necessarily a gun), nonfatal strangulation, controlling behaviors, and forced sex/ rape (Spencer & Stith, 2020). Homicide-suicides have not been studied in much depth but appear to have certain characteristics worth noting; namely, the majority of them

Ψ Most DV situations do not involve any weapons, firearms or otherwise. However, with respect to intimate partner homicide, the most salient risk factors aside from direct access to guns have been found to be history of threats with a weapon (not necessarily a gun), nonfatal strangulation, controlling behaviors, and forced sex/rape.

occur within spouse or ex-spouse situations, involve older couples (above 40 as compared to 30s in IPH), and include a firearm (Banks et al., 2008).

It is also important to remember that, aside from fatal outcomes, guns can be used to intimidate or otherwise threaten, even in the absence of physical harm. In fact, this is the more common use of guns in IPV scenarios (Sorenson, 2006). While the presence of a firearm does not necessarily lead to abuse, it is a notable risk factor in homes where DV is already present. However, as we have previously pointed out:

It is unclear whether access to the weapon is a risk factor in and of itself or if firearm use is a characteristic of a certain type of offender who is more likely to commit severe and repeated acts of domestic abuse. (Pirelli et al., 2019, p. 236)

The presence of a firearm in and of itself is insufficient to draw an overarching conclusion about risk and, therefore, other case-specific risk factors must be considered (i.e., easy or likely gun access is a potentially moderating variable). Alcohol misuse remains a particularly salient example. In fact, risk for homicide is increased with partners who had gun access and misused alcohol (Banks et al., 2008; Campbell et al., 2003). Other case-specific factors that increase risk for homicide in the presence of firearms include child custody situations and situations wherein the victim left or threatened to leave, or the victim was recently assaulted (Farr, 2002).

MENTAL ILLNESS AND SUICIDE

In 2019, there were 47,511 suicides in the United States—one of the top 10 causes of death (https://www.cdc.gov/mmwr/volumes/70/wr/mm7008a1.htm). Firearms were the cause of half of these suicides, whereas other methods included suffocation (13,563; 29%) and poisoning (6,125; 13%). Suicide attempts and completed suicides are underreported for various reasons, not the least of which is stigma. However, interfacing with suicidal clients is not particularly uncommon for many medical and mental health providers like us. Suicide-related behaviors can range in severity from parasuicidal, self-injurious behaviors to bona fide attempts. When working with clients in various clinical contexts, it is important to recognize that not all clients with mental illness are suicidal. Simply having a mental illness in and of itself is insufficient to make a determination of risk for suicide, or to even assume that suicidality is present. However, findings from numerous meta-analyses demonstrate that certain mental illnesses, such as mood or affective disorders (e.g., major depressive disorder and bipolar disorder), are more closely associated with suicide, as well as substance use disorders, psychotic disorders, and personality disorders (e.g., Arsenault-Lapierre et al., 2004; Too et al., 2019). As clinicians, however, we need to focus less

> Ψ As clinicians, we need to focus less on labels and more on identifying our clients' risk and protective factors, to facilitate risk management and reduction efforts.

on labels and more on identifying our clients' risk and protective factors, to facilitate risk management and reduction efforts.

In Chapters 4 and 5, we will take a closer look at assessing suicide risk and how such relates to our work in both therapeutic and evaluation contexts. We advocate for the incorporation of a formal suicide risk assessment measure, such as the Columbia Suicide Severity Rating Scale (C-SSRS; Posner et al., 2009), which can guide our decision-making processes by incorporating evidence-based factors associated with suicide risk, including risk factors, warning signs, and protective factors. All three sets of considerations are important to assess, as doing so provides information not only about

> Ψ We advocate for the incorporation of a formal suicide risk assessment measure, such as the Columbia Suicide Severity Rating Scale (C-SSRS).

suicide risk, in general, but also about the imminence of such risk, specifically. The C-SSRS includes specific warning signs including suicidal thoughts, thoughts with method, intent, and intent with specific plan.

We must also consider risk management in the context of professional liability. As we indicated in Chapter 2, in the *Reporting Duties of Medical and Mental Health Professionals* section, we must be intimately familiar with our ethical and legal obligations in these contexts. Our respective duty-to-protect-and/or-warn laws set the parameters for our responsibilities when our clients pose an elevated risk. Laws and policies can outline the steps medical and mental health professionals need to take at various stages, but they are not cookbooks and discretion cannot be legislated or otherwise predetermined. Therefore, it is incumbent

> Ψ Laws and policies can outline the steps medical and mental health professionals need to take at various stages, but they are not cookbooks and discretion cannot be legislated or predetermined. Therefore, it is incumbent upon us as clinicians to conduct effective suicide (and violence) risk assessments.

upon us as clinicians to conduct effective suicide (and violence) risk assessments (see Chapters 4 and 5).

The remaining factors on the C-SSRS guide us in determining a person's more general risk for suicide, to include any past suicidal or self-injurious behaviors, recent activating events (e.g., divorce, legal trouble), and more recent clinical issues such as hopelessness, substance abuse, major depressive episode, or command hallucinations to hurt oneself. Assessing for protective factors is equally important in this context. Although an individual may present with various risk factors, they may simultaneously believe that suicide is immoral, or have a perceived responsibility to their family, which can be highly protective. Thus, we must always conduct a comprehensive assessment, going beyond the warning signs and into details, such as one's plan, intent, means, and access to the means. Let us now take a close look at the link between mental illness and gun-involved suicides.

Mental Illness and Firearm-Involved Suicide

Of the aforementioned 47,511 suicide-related deaths in the United States in 2019, half (23,941) were firearm-involved (https://www.cdc.gov/mmwr/volumes/70/wr/mm700 8a1.htm). Indeed, using a firearm to attempt suicide increases the likelihood of lethality (Fowler et al., 2015). Even though the link between firearms and suicide is appreciably greater than that which pertains to interpersonal violence, it is also nuanced. As indicated above, research findings over the years have established that rates of suicide are higher among those with mental illnesses. However, mental health symptoms do not explain why those who have access to firearms are more likely to die by suicide via firearms (Sorenson & Vittes, 2008). While there is a strong association between the presence of a gun in the home and suicide (e.g., Conwell et al., 2002; Dahlberg et al., 2004), it is important not to infer causality. As we have highlighted and will continue to highlight throughout this book, correlation does not equal causation. In fact, findings from several studies have revealed that those with firearms in their homes are no more or less likely to have suicide risk factors as compared to those without guns in their homes (e.g., Betz et al., 2011; Ilgen et al., 2008; Miller et al., 2009), and others have also found there is no difference between rates of gun access, gun carrying, and safe storage among people with and without lifetime mental illnesses (Ilgen et al., 2008). Still, firearm access among those with severe mental illness constitutes a serious potential risk factor for suicide (Baumann & Teasdale, 2018). Although this area of literature continues to develop, the effect that easy gun access to firearms has on those with mental illness is not well understood, outside of the context of mental health crises.

In consideration of these issues, what may be most important to consider is acute, transient mental health crisis situations that include emotional distress rather than mental illness per se. Such situations are commonly associated with suicide and related behaviors and attempts, especially in the context of alcohol use (Powell et al., 2001). In fact, about a quarter of suicide attempts were decided in less than 5 minutes (Simon et al., 2001). Thus, it has been suggested that impulsivity, rather than

> Ψ What may be most important to consider is acute, transient mental health crisis situations that include emotional distress rather than mental illness per se.

mental illness per se, may be a distinguishing factor between those who own and those who do not own a firearm (Sorenson & Vittes, 2008). Overall, it may be much more productive to place emphasis on time-sensitive risk in preventing firearm-related suicides rather than broadly focusing on mental illnesses or diagnoses.

All that said, military, law enforcement, and correctional personnel are part of notably at-risk groups in terms of firearm-involved suicide risk—at appreciably greater risk than their civilian counterparts. For instance, over 90% of law enforcement suicides, to include correctional officers, are gun-involved (Swedler et al., 2015; Violanti et al., 2012).

EMERGING ROLES FOR MEDICAL AND MENTAL HEALTH PROFESSIONALS

In the final chapter of our 2019 book *The Behavioral Science of Firearms*, we identified and reviewed 30 main findings, wherein implications for practice, research, and policy were set forth for each. We encourage the interested reader to reference that text and will highlight some particularly relevant findings here. For instance, guns have historically been a part of our American culture and the Second Amendment of the Constitution remains a frequently and fervently discussed topic. Remember: guns are omnipresent in our pop culture (i.e., throughout our movies, television, video games, and music) and approximately 100 million people in this country are gun owners (i.e., one-third of the population).

As mental health and medical professionals, we have a responsibility to conduct both suicide and violence risk assessments with our clients, and this necessitates a sufficient degree of knowledge regarding firearms and firearm safety. Such is consistent with our Know, Ask, Do (KAD) model for developing professional competence, which we outline in Chapter 4. Here, let us introduce the emerging roles relevant to us as medical and mental health professionals before we take a deeper dive in the remaining chapters of this book. Namely, in the next two chapters, we provide a more comprehensive and detailed guide for practitioners in therapeutic contexts and in conducting firearm-specific forensic mental health assessments (FMHAs) and, in Chapter 6, we set forth ethical considerations for clinicians.

Despite the ubiquity of firearms in U.S. culture, medical and mental health professionals, by and large, do not receive formal education on firearms or firearm subcultures. However, we are required to develop professional competence in other areas, to include cultural competence. Such is emphasized in our education, training, and continued education, but firearm-specific competence has been overlooked. As we discussed in the *Introduction* section of this book, the education, training, and practices of medical and mental health professionals vis-à-vis firearms are sorely lacking (e.g., see Carney et al., 2002; Nagle et al., 2021; Price et al., 2007, 2009, 2010; Simpson, 2021; Slovak et al., 2008; Traylor et al., 2010; Yip et al., 2012).

We have designed this book to fill these significant gaps—to help develop the professional competence of medical and mental health professionals in the firearm-related arena, to include cultural competency. When working with clients, it is important not to make assumptions about their views on guns and related issues, just as it is equally important for us not to impose our personal views on them. As we address in greater detail in Chapter 6, the onus is on us as clinicians to ensure our personal views do not interfere with our ability to provide ethical and effective services. In most cases, consultation is key when ethical dilemmas arise; however, there are often limitations when trying to consult in areas whereby professional competence is so notably underdeveloped. Nevertheless, identification and management of our biases is essential as clinicians. We all have biases, but we must seek to determine how they might impact our work with clients. It is also critically important to remember that bias can also affect teaching, research, and policymaking efforts. Too often it seems the ideals of professional and cultural competence, ethics, and related responsibilities are solely focused on clinical practice.

Of course, as practitioners, many of us are serving on the frontlines—having to assess violence and suicide risk and making critically important decisions and recommendations based on such. Even if many of our clients are not gun owners, firearm-specific risk must be assessed every time we assess our patients' violence and suicide risk levels. Furthermore, we are likely to be called upon more and more in various other contexts, as gun laws and policies are increasing in many states across the country. Increases in flags, restrictions, and confiscations for gun applicants and owners will only result in *increased* involvement by medical and mental health professionals. Some of this involvement is being directed by lawmakers, law enforcement, and the courts, although much of it will actually be sought by gun applicants and owners filing appeals or seeking the restoration of their gun rights otherwise. The ruling in *Tyler v. Hillsdale County Sheriff's Department* (2014) is illustrative and likely representative of what is to come in terms of gun rights restoration in the United States (see the *Gun Rights Restoration and Relief from Disability* section in Chapter 2).

> Ψ Even if many of our clients are not gun owners, firearm-specific risk must be assessed every time we assess our patients' violence and suicide risk levels.

> Ψ Increases in flags, restrictions, and confiscations for gun applicants and owners will only result in increased involvement by medical and mental health professionals.

As medical and mental health professionals, we are needed in these contexts. However, we are neither inherently equipped nor adequately trained to assess firearm-specific risk at present. It is well established that our cultural competence is a central component of our professional competence and is, therefore, at the forefront of our education and training. However, discussions of cultural competence tend to focus on such factors as race, ethnicity, religion, gender, and sexual orientation, as well as more specific subgroups or subcultures within each of these areas.

To this point, firearm-related subgroups have been largely overlooked in formal medical and mental health education and training contexts, despite the fact that one-third of the country's population consists of gun owners—and many more have some direct or indirect connection with firearms otherwise. In Chapter 1, we discussed seven overarching firearm-related subcultures that we believe are relevant to consider:

1. Second Amendment groups
2. Shooting sport groups
3. Rod and gun clubs, hunting clubs, and shooting ranges
4. Gun control, gun violence prevention, and anti-gun groups
5. Military, law enforcement, and corrections
6. Members of gangs, organized crime and other criminal organizations
7. Victims of firearm-related suicide, violence, or domestic violence

The good news is that most, if not all, of us have experience with patients from one or more of these groups. What is needed, though, is to be able to work with these patients within a cultural competence framework when gun-related issues arise and call for such. It is worth reminding the reader to revisit the section *Taking Steps to Develop Firearm-Related Cultural Competence*, also in Chapter 1. For the remainder of the present chapter, however, we will consider the various functions of our roles as practitioners in the areas of firearm access, violence, DV and IPV, and suicide. Finally, we provide some thoughts as to our roles in the context of firearm law and policy. The roles we have in these areas continue to develop and emerge along with more stringent gun control laws, and the persistent focus in our society on the link between gun use and ownership suitability and mental health.

Violence

As we noted earlier in this chapter, one-third of U.S. gun deaths are homicides and homicide rates have remained stable for over two decades. We also know that active shooter incidents result in less than 1% of all firearm-related deaths, annually. However, such low–base-rate, high-impact events often have relatively higher death tolls and significant emotional impact. Although national statistics are important to consider, as practitioners, local norms are of particular importance (namely, the statistics within our respective states and counties) as firearm-related statistics can vary greatly. The use of local norms is a standard of practice in our respective fields because it is important to account for variability in data related to characteristics such as gender, ethnicity, socioeconomic status, and area of residence. We emphasize throughout this book, particularly in Chapters 4 and 5, the importance of not using a one-size-fits all approach to assessing our clients' risk levels. As such, it is important for us to consider case-specific factors, such as motivating or destabilizing factors, and triggering events. We must also ask ourselves about the kind of violence we are particularly concerned about in a given case—again warranting a contextualized and individualized risk assessment approach.

Predicting future violence or much anything else is essentially impossible; therefore, prediction-based models of assessment do not offer utility in this context. Instead, as we will detail in Chapter 5, medical and mental health practitioners should use a prevention-based risk assessment approach that is focused on risk management and reduction. A risk prevention–based approach offers an opportunity to implement interventions, which may be modified as needed. Again, none of us can predict the occurrence of a future event, violent or most otherwise, with any sufficient accuracy. It is incumbent upon as clinicians to be transparent about our limitations and to convey such to relevant clients and audiences.

For these reasons and more, it can be quite beneficial to use published frameworks, models, and measures when conducting assessments. Of course, we developed our KAD model to provide overarching guidance for clinicians in developing firearm-related competence. In Chapter 5, we present our framework for those conducting forensic evaluations to assess for firearm ownership suitability (i.e., the Pirelli Firearm-10, or PF-10). For those tasked with assessing risk in school settings, we suggest the use of the Comprehensive School Threat Assessment Guidelines (CSTAG), a leading model developed by Professor Dewey Cornell and colleagues (Cornell, 2018). The CSTAG, formerly the Virginia Model for Student Threat Assessment, was updated and is grounded in contemporary theory and has empirical support—from both field tests and controlled studies (see https://education.virginia.edu/faculty-research/centers-labs-projects/research-labs/youth-violence-project/comprehensive-school). The model is generally designed for a threat assessment team approach, but it also has referential utility for those of us functioning as individual providers. We elaborate further in Chapter 5, where we provide further guidance on conducting FMHAs more generally.

> Ψ When possible, use published frameworks, models, and measures for risk assessments. We developed our Know, Ask, and Do (KAD) model to provide overarching guidance for clinicians in developing firearm-related competence, and the Pirelli Firearm-10 (PF-10) framework for those conducting forensic evaluations to assess for firearm ownership suitability. We recommend using the Comprehensive School Threat Assessment Guidelines (CSTAG) when assessing and managing risk in educational settings.

Still, while potentially useful, no model can capture everything that may be relevant in a given case. For instance, in the context of school-based threat or risk assessments, there are factors relevant to extract from the literature (e.g., damaged masculinity, marginalization, self-image, psychosocial development). Too often, academic issues per se are the focus in educational settings. This is certainly axiomatic and understandable; however, they should not be the sole focus. Other very important issues, such as a student's psychosocial development, cannot be overlooked, as such may be the student's primary concern—and potentially the source of problems, both existing and those to come. In other words, we must go beyond considerations of issues like bullying alone and seek to gain an understanding of students' perceptions of their self-image, social status, and views on masculinity and related developmental concepts.

A final point more broadly related to interpersonal violence is that most people who own firearms are law-abiding citizens who do not present with any particular risk of engaging in violence. Again, simply owning a gun does not change that and it certainly does not *cause* someone to be violent. It is a potentially moderating variable, as we will address in greater detail in Chapter 4. Nevertheless, we still must inquire about lethal means when assessing risk. In this regard, it may have relevance to inquire about types of firearm(s), ammunition available, storage practices, and who has access to the gun(s) in question. For reference, Chapter 1 serves as a primer and includes information on types of guns and ammunition, and Chapter 2 addresses storage, transportation, and access issues to be aware of when considering patients' behaviors and perspectives. Also, we cannot overstate the importance of becoming familiar with our respective state and local laws pertaining to storage, transportation, and particular aspects of prohibited gun hardware (and ammunition). Moreover, while the entire book is devoted to developing professional competence in firearm-related matters, we squarely address issues of cultural competence vis-à-vis firearm-related subcultures in Chapter 1 and ethical considerations associated with our own views and procedures in Chapter 6.

Domestic Violence and Intimate Partner Violence

As we highlighted both in this chapter and in Chapter 2, where we explored DV- and IPV-related prohibitions, the majority of these situations do not involve any weapon at all. However, the presence of firearms has been associated with fatalities and firearms are often involved in DV-related homicides and homicide-suicides. As practitioners, when encountering patients with current or historical DV-related issues, it is imperative to consider firearms as a potentially moderating variable. While most DV scenarios are quickly resolved, we must assess for the presence of factors related to poor nonlethal and lethal outcomes (e.g., history of threats with any weapon, strangulation, controlling behaviors, or forced sex). There are additional case-specific factors to be aware of in this context as well, such as child custody problems, a female victim indicating she was leaving, physical assault in the past year, and an abuser having substance use problems (e.g., Farr, 2002). Thus, as with suicide and violence risk assessment, we must extend well beyond simply asking if someone has access to a gun and engage in a more comprehensive assessment (see Chapters 4 and 5). Of note, practitioners working with those in the military, law enforcement, and corrections must familiarize themselves with specific risk factors and vulnerabilities inherent to these groups, which are particularly associated with poor DV (and suicide) outcomes. As outlined in Chapter 1, these are recognized firearm-related subcultures and, in Chapter 4, we go a step further and address considerations for treatment with them.

In Chapter 2, we reviewed the legal underpinnings of DV-related firearm prohibitions at the state and federal levels. We also noted gun violence restraining orders, wherein firearms are removed, at least temporarily. As practitioners, we need to know our states' statuses with respect to protective order laws, especially when working with clients with DV histories. Although there is some research to suggest that protective orders in certain DV situations may be effective, there are also many problems associated with the enforcement of such orders across jurisdictions. A history that includes a protective order is a risk factor, but it may not be a particularly salient one in a given case at a particular time because many are filed and quickly dismissed, and many have been filed in relation to complaints that are not necessarily of any real substantive concern. Although such warrants attention, the mere presence of a protective order in the past is not enough to draw from, as we need to investigate the details of the situation and seek to identify risk factors at that level. Of course, there are situations wherein a protective order is never filed, and this may even occur in high-risk matters. There are myriad reasons for this, and we may even find ourselves in situations whereby clients are consulting with us as they decide if they will file one. As with any law, it behooves us to be aware of our specific state and jurisdictional laws regarding protective orders, such as what they entail and our duty-to-warn-and/or-protect responsibilities should certain information be disclosed during patient contacts (see Chapter 2).

Suicide

As we mentioned earlier in this chapter, the primary link between mental illness and firearm deaths is suicide. Less than half of the suicides in the United States are with guns, but two-thirds of gun deaths are suicides. In Chapters 4 and 5, we more closely examine a comprehensive approach to assessing suicide risk in both evaluation and therapeutic contexts. As mental health and medical practitioners, we need to be well versed in suicide risk assessment and have plans for interventions readily available for clients who are at any notable degree of risk. As with violence and DV, the presence of a gun is a potentially moderating risk factor and, as such, our assessments must extend beyond simply asking about access to firearms. These situations may be uncomfortable for many of us; therefore, it is imperative we acquire the proper firearm-related education and develop preparedness in this regard to make clinically, ethically, and legally competent decisions when needed. Of course, there are variables that can mitigate or increase firearm-involved suicide risk even in crisis situations, such as support of removal of the lethal means, and gun safety and storage practices more generally (see Chapters 1 and 5).

Historically, foundational concepts related to guns, including but not limited to gun safety, have not been taught in medical or mental health programs, thereby leading to significant gaps in firearm-related professional and cultural competency. Indeed, this book is intended to fill such gaps. A critical component of suicide and violence risk is considering gun safety. Practitioners in acute care settings may encounter this more frequently and, therefore, may need to engage in means-restriction counseling more than others (see Chapter 4). That said, those who work in emergency rooms and crisis centers have a primary task of evaluating both suicide and violence risk and therefore should be regularly asking about firearms. Nevertheless, all of us need to be aware of how to address a potential range of gun-related issues that may arise in our respective practices. This reality prompted us to develop our KAD model.

Suicide prevention efforts typically need to be multifaceted, to include assessment and intervention components—and they often involve multiple people, professionals and those from clients' personal lives. However, suicide risk assessment and management principles taught to medical and mental health professionals almost never include discussion of guns and gun safety, despite the notable association between firearms and suicide. As we address in Chapter 6, it is our ethical responsibility to practice within our areas of competence. Therefore, firearm-related competence needs to be considered an essential area of competence by our professions. As such, there is an urgent need for medical and mental health professionals to obtain the training, education, and skills necessary to navigate the complexities of gun-related issues in clinical practice.

Firearm Law and Policy

Outside of our clinical roles, we may be called to consult with policymakers who are working on firearm-related initiatives. Once we develop sufficient professional and cultural competence in this arena, we can collaborate with them to ensure efforts are evidence-based and practical. That said, policymakers need to be aware that relatively few professionals have developed sufficient levels of professional (and cultural) competence to adequately address firearm-related issues even at the ground level, in practice. It is our responsibility to be transparent about our glaring limitations and to work hard to overcome them moving forward.

In Chapter 2, we explored various federal and state laws involving guns. Many existing and proposed laws focus on categorical prohibitions rather than seeking to facilitate evidence-based processes aimed at identifying those who are at elevated risk of engaging in firearm-involved violence or suicide. The policy analysis research on the effectiveness of firearm-related laws is rather miniscule, particularly given the significant attention and efforts associated with their development. There are also unintended consequences of firearm-related policies, especially when associated with mental illness. Simply put, the added stigmatization fuels problems. For instance, people may not seek mental health treatment due to the fear of jeopardizing their gun rights. It is not difficult to accept the likelihood of such a deterrence effect on civilian gun applicants and owners because we have already seen it play out quite clearly and strongly in law enforcement, correctional, and military groups. It is faulty to assume that attaching increased access to mental health treatment to firearm-related legislation would increase help-seeking when, in fact, it is likely to deter it. It is essential for everyone, practitioners and policymakers alike, to be aware of such barriers to treatment and to recognize the sources of such. We must focus on these concerns moving forward.

RECOMMENDED FURTHER READING

American Psychological Association. (2013). Gun violence: Prediction, prevention, and policy. http://www.apa.org/pubs/info/reports/gun-violence-prevention.aspx

Cornell, D. (2018). *Comprehensive School Threat Assessment Guidelines*. School Threat Assessment Consultants LLC.

Elbogen, E. B., & Johnson, S. C. (2009). The intricate link between violence and mental disorder: Results from the national epidemiologic survey on alcohol and related conditions. *Archives of General Psychiatry*, 66(2), 152–161. https://doi.org/10.1001/archgenpsychia try.2008.537

Fowler, K. A., Dahlberg, L. L., Haileyesus, T., & Annest, J. L. (2015). Firearm injuries in the United States. *Preventive Medicine*, 79, 5–14. doi:10.1016/j.ypmed.2015.06.002

Johnson, K. L., Desmarais, S. L., Van Dorn, R. A., & Grimm, K. J. (2015). A typology of community violence perpetration and victimization among adults with mental illnesses. *Journal of Interpersonal Violence*, 30(3), 522–540. https://doi.org/10.1177/0886260514535102

McGinty, E. E., Kennedy-Hendricks, A., Choksy, S., & Barry, C. L. (2016). Trends in news media coverage of mental illness in the United States: 1995–2014. *Health Affairs*, 35(6), 1121–1129.

McGinty, E. E., & Webster, D. W. (2016). Gun violence and serious mental illness. In L. H. Gold & R. I. Simon (Eds.), *Gun violence and mental illness* (pp. 3–30). American Psychiatric Association.

Wintemute, G. J. (2015). Alcohol misuse, firearm violence perpetration, and public policy in the United States. *Preventive Medicine*, 79, 15–21. https://doi.org/10.1016/j.ypmed.2015.04.015

4

Firearm-Related Issues in Therapeutic Contexts

IN THIS CHAPTER, we present considerations related to the emerging roles of treating and evaluating medical and mental health clinicians in relation to firearm-related issues. It is first important to acknowledge that those of us engaging in clinical practice have been addressing many of these issues, directly and indirectly, for quite some time in various work settings and contexts. In the first section of this chapter, we discuss the ways in which we might address guns during *treatment* contacts with our patients. In this regard, we outline considerations when conducting mental health intakes, screenings, and routine assessments in both outpatient and inpatient settings. We then present the Know, Ask, Do (KAD) framework, which we developed in recent years to provide guidance for clinicians addressing gun-related issues in practice (see, e.g., Pirelli & Gold, 2019). We then discuss issues that may arise when patients request "clearance" to own firearms as well as considerations associated with restoration of their gun rights. We subsequently present firearm-related considerations in the context of treating and evaluating those in law enforcement, corrections, military, and related professions. In the second section of this chapter, we discuss mental health *evaluations* in outpatient and inpatient mental health settings that are clinical in nature—as opposed to forensic evaluations, which we address in the next chapter (Chapter 5).

ADDRESSING GUNS DURING TREATMENT CONTACTS

For some of us, speaking about guns with our patients is second nature, akin to discussing what they did over the weekend; in fact, such may very well have included a firearm-related activity. On the other hand, there are some of us who reside in states or regions where discussing guns is simply not part of the culture and is even considered taboo. As we noted in Chapter 1, there is wide variability in rates of gun ownership across the United States, and there are numerous types of firearm-related subcultures. Therefore, our respective levels of comfort with and our patients' receptiveness to addressing gun issues can vary greatly. While our particular role and scope of service in a given matter dictates if and how we should address gun-related issues, there are certain principles and considerations with which we should all be familiar. The concepts we present in the sections that follow are generally applicable across a range of jurisdictions, and clinical settings and disciplines. In this section, we will discuss con-

> Ψ A major tenet of our Know, Ask, and Do (KAD) model is identifying when a patient has *likely* access to a gun—not simply potential access, which many, if not most, of our patients would have.

siderations for mental health screenings in inpatient and outpatient settings, followed by a more specific discussion on what can be helpful to KAD when a patient has *likely* access to a gun—not simply potential access, which many or even most of our patients would have. We also address considerations related to situations in which patients request a

gun-specific "clearance" as well as considerations for treating law enforcement, corrections, military and related professionals. However, as with all policies and procedures, it is important for us to be aware of our specific jurisdictional requirements and prohibitions with respect to asking patients about guns.[1]

As medical and mental health practitioners, many of us assess, or at least screen for, the presence of potential mental health problems during initial sessions or at some predetermined intervals. Typically, we ask our patients questions related to their experience of anxiety-related or depressive symptoms, including but not limited to suicidality. We may do this directly or by having them complete intake, screening, or health update forms. For example, some of the more formal mental health assessments that arise in practice are those conducted prior to patients undergoing elective, semi-elective, or emergency procedures (e.g., bariatric, organ donation, transplants, neurosurgery), as well as when mental health–related concerns are raised otherwise (e.g., postpartum depression). Let us illustrate the ways in which gun-related issues may arise during more routine intake and screening sessions with our patients in the following section.

---

[1] On February 16, 2017, a federal appeals court ruled on what has been referred to as Florida's "Docs v. Glocks" lawsuit (American Civil Liberties Union [ACLU], 2017). The court issued two majority opinions and held that portions of the law threatened loss of license to doctors based on their conversations with patients, which violates the doctors' First Amendment rights. Since then, at least 10 other states have tried and failed to pass similar bills ("Allow doctors," 2017), although some have passed laws related to the doctor–patient relationship (e.g., in Missouri: MO Rev Stat § 571.012, 2015). Namely, the Missouri law indicates doctors cannot be legally compelled to ask patients about guns, record data pertaining to them in medical records, or notify government agencies about who owns them. For more information on laws pertaining to guns and the doctor–patient relationship, the interested reader is directed to Appelbaum (2017b).

Conducting Mental Health Intakes, Screenings, and Routine Assessments

Inpatient and Outpatient Settings

While there is a general push for community-based care in the United States, inpatient settings continue to be important for a number of people who experience mental health–related issues (e.g., hospitals, medical centers, psychiatric facilities). Of course, inpatient substance abuse treatment detox and rehabilitation centers are also widespread throughout the country, and so-called 28-day programs have become a mainstay in many respects. In fact, until the deinstitutionalization movement began in the mid-1950s, inpatient settings were the primary treatment environments for those with significant mental health problems in the United States. As a result of the civil rights movement and the advent of more effective psychotropic medications, however, the number of people in America's public psychiatric hospitals in 1955 (558,239) decreased 92% to 71,619 by 1994 (Torrey, 1997). One of the unintended consequences, though, has been the surge of incarceration for those with psychiatric conditions, so much so that correctional institutions have been referred to as "the last mental hospital[s]" (Gilligan, 2001) and "the *de facto* state hospitals" (Daniel, 2007). The Los Angeles County Jail and Rikers Island in New York actually became two of the largest psychiatric inpatient facilities in the United States, housing approximately 3,000 mentally ill inmates each (Torrey, 1999; Torrey et al., 1992, 2010). Moreover, psychiatric facilities have closed in many states while their correctional facilities expand to house mentally ill offenders (see, e.g., Sharp, 2016; Yates, 2016).

Some of our patients who have been or would have otherwise been civilly committed to an inpatient facility may be subject to *outpatient* civil commitment provisions; this essentially consists of involuntary, court-ordered treatment requirements to which they must adhere in the community. All states except Connecticut, Maryland, Massachusetts, and Tennessee, as well as the District of Columbia, have assisted outpatient commitment laws, which is commonly referred to as *assisted outpatient treatment* (see, e.g., Treatment Advocacy Center, 2014). These plans are designed to reduce recurring hospitalizations, arrests, and incarceration. Specialized mental health courts and jail diversion programs have also been developed in many jurisdictions to accomplish similar goals for nonviolent offenders. Indeed, probation and parole departments have been mandating mental health, substance abuse, anger management, and domestic violence programming for many years. In addition, consumer- or peer-run programs have been around even longer. For example, Alcoholics Anonymous (AA) has been internationally available to people for approximately 100 years. Others include those geared toward substance abuse and gambling (e.g., Narcotics Anonymous [NA] and Gamblers Anonymous [GA]) as well as those for people with dual diagnoses (i.e., clinical syndromes and substance use disorders)—often referred to as "co-occurring" or "mentally ill chemical abuser" (MICA) programs.

An outpatient mental health service that readily comes to mind is that of independent, or "private," practices, which may include the provision of individual, group, couples, and family treatment services. The importance of outpatient mental health services has become widely recognized and there are now many other types of community services, programs, and facilities that fall under an *outpatient mental health* classification as well. For instance, many employers have employee assistance programs (EAPs) and some even maintain their own in-house mental health services. Students in the United States often have even greater access to mental health care than the average citizen given that college counseling centers are available on campuses, and school psychologists and child study teams provide services to students, staff, and parents at the elementary, middle, and high school levels. There are also outpatient mental health clinics, which may be privately run but are often associated with hospitals and agencies like the U.S. Department of Veterans Affairs (VA). In addition, there are residential programs (e.g., group homes) and independent housing-related services for those with mental health needs, which represent a critical part of discharge planning for those being released from inpatient settings.

Some of us may also engage in on-site services, such as at patients' homes or in institutions or facilities in which they are residing (e.g., correctional, medical, and mental health facilities; schools; nursing homes). Other options include intensive outpatient programs (IOPs) and partial hospitalization arrangements, which encourage patient autonomy and independence in the community. A more contemporary outpatient treatment type is that of telehealth, which involves the delivery of treatment services remotely, online. Indeed, the COVID-19 pandemic has resulted in a significant expansion of telehealth services across the country and across medical and mental health subdisciplines.

Regardless of where or precisely how we practice, the provision of an appropriate and effective treatment is contingent upon an effective assessment. General mental health screenings are typically conducted in inpatient and outpatient medical, mental health, and correctional settings, and are typically accomplished by having patients complete intake forms and checklists that inquire about various symptoms and conditions. However, more recently, it has become commonplace to integrate mental health considerations into primary care practices due to the relationship between mental and medical health problems. Historically, some clinicians subscribed to the theory of mind–body dualism à la Descartes, whereby the mind and body were considered to be distinct entities. However, most of us now embrace their interconnected nature because the mind–body connection has been scientifically well established. Perhaps the most basic examples are that we shed tears when we feel sad and blush when we feel embarrassed. More complex examples include medically unexplained illnesses, such as chronic fatigue syndrome, fibromyalgia, multiple chemical sensitivity, and irritable bowel syndrome. Indeed, these are some of the particularly challenging conditions those of us in primary care settings may encounter with some regularity (see, e.g., Edwards et al., 2010; Johnson, 2008). There are certainly many more symptoms that we are commonly called upon to address as well, such as general muscle, back, chest, stomach, and joint pain as well as headaches and fatigue. In fact, psychological stress is related to 75% to 90% of all doctor visits, it is a factor in five of the six leading causes of death, and it has caused a $1 trillion health epidemic—above the cost of cancer, smoking, diabetes, and heart disease combined (Robinson, 2013). It is also important to note that more than 10% of Americans in the community take psychotropic medications, which is nearly double the amount of people who were prescribed such in the late 1980s into the early 1990s (Munsey, 2008). Moreover, this number does not include those who are institutionalized or incarcerated or who are prescribed general medications for psychiatric purposes. Of course, we must also consider the high number of people who abuse prescription medications and substances, more generally.

> Ψ Regardless of where we practice, the provision of an appropriate and effective treatment is contingent upon an effective assessment.

Our professions have come to realize that many mental health problems occur on a continuum. This is especially true for traits associated with personality disorders, but certainly those related to clinical syndromes as well. For instance, most of us have experienced some level of distress, anxiousness, moodiness, and sadness at times. These are normal experiences and often situationally based. However, medical professionals seek to screen for abnormal levels of these experiences, particularly when their patients' daily functioning is affected, or they experience discomfort above and beyond what is expected in certain contexts. For example, it is normal to become sad and cry following the death of a pet, but only to a point. In most cases, we would expect such feelings to be generally manageable and remit within months. On the other hand, it would be classified a clinical problem if the person could not leave the house for 6 months and experienced suicidal thoughts because of the loss. That said, there is no blanket set of behaviors or feelings that we can ascribe to all situations to determine what is reasonable, as there can be unique circumstances in each case. Thus, we need to embrace a *context-specific* and *culturally competent* approach to our assessments to account for the variability among patients and situations. Still, there is a generally accepted range of so-called normal experiences we expect to see in certain circumstances, which are largely based on societal, cultural, and subcultural norms. As such, those of us working in outpatient settings have an important role in our society because we often have the first and the most contact with people in the community relative to other helping professionals.[2] This presents us with a critical responsibility and

> Ψ We need to embrace a *context-specific* and *culturally competent* approach to our assessments to account for variability among patients and situations. Still, there is a generally accepted range of so-called normal experiences we expect to see in certain circumstances, which are largely based on societal, cultural, and subcultural norms.

---

[2] It is important to remember, though, that mental health–related issues are often first addressed at spiritual and religious centers in the community, including at churches, temples, and mosques. Many groups have meetings and retreats that can pull for discussion of emotional experiences, and some even

opportunity: to provide care to those in need—either by providing treatment directly or by making referrals to other professionals who can.

There is a fairly extensive range of inpatient and outpatient mental health services in the United States. Many of us work in inpatient or outpatient facilities or service programs geared specifically toward psychiatric evaluation, stabilization, and treatment (e.g., emergency and crisis units and centers). In these contexts, in particular, we must be well versed in suicide and violence risk assessment. While private facilities theoretically have more control as to who they accept and treat, it is safe to say that many of those working in these settings will encounter a relatively diverse clientele with respect to their histories and interests. As such, it is also a safe assumption that many of us will interface with patients who have some connection with firearms, directly or indirectly, as our patients may be in community-based, outpatient, or inpatient systems at any given time. They may also be involved with more than one type of system over time, either via transfer during a particular time period or at different time points in their lives. Although firearms may not be a primary concern in a given case, it is important for us to possess professional and cultural awareness of firearm-related subcultures and issues, especially in high-stakes scenarios (e.g., assessment of violence, domestic violence, and suicide risk). Thus, the importance of our education and training on firearm-related issues in these contexts cannot be understated. That said, we are also in a time of professional specialties and subspecialties, and increased options for those seeking mental health support in the community. Therefore, we must be prepared to work with a diverse set of patients. We are very likely to encounter firearm-related issues or, at least, patients from one or more firearm-related subcultures—yet another reason driving the need for education and training on these issues and with these groups (see Chapter 1, *Developing Cultural Competence by Recognizing Firearm-Related Subcultures*). We outline considerations for conceptualizing firearm access in clinical

provide more formal individual, couples, and family counseling. Indeed, pastoral counseling is a mainstay in most religions, whereby ministers, rabbis, priests, imams, and other psychologically trained religious leaders provide therapeutic services to their members. According to the Counseling Center (n.d.):

> Pastoral counseling is a unique form of counseling which uses spiritual resources as well as psychological understanding for healing and growth. Certified pastoral counselors are licensed mental health professionals who also had in-depth religious and/or theological education or training. Clinical Services are non-sectarian and respect the spiritual commitments, theological perspectives and religious traditions of those who seek assistance without imposing counselor beliefs onto the client.
>
> Some people feel more comfortable working with pastoral counselors and other spiritual and religious persons, particularly when dealing with loss, illness, and marital and family conflict.
>
> It is also the case, however, that they often have the opportunity to provide counseling for positive, preparatory reasons in the absence of problems—unlike most of us (e.g., Pre-Cana courses for couples seeking to marry in the Catholic faith). While religion, spirituality, or faith is not important to all of our patients, we must recognize when it is and provide our services in a culturally competent manner for those who do find it important. This may even include coordinating with spiritual and religious leaders, particularly when working with particular subcultures and in certain community enclaves.

assessments in a section that follows: *Viewing Gun Access as a Potentially Moderating Risk Factor*. However, we first turn to a brief outline of some of the key foundations of mental health screenings, more generally.

Mental Health Screenings: Purpose, Methods, and Thresholds

When we conduct intakes, we are screening for active mental health problems that may warrant more immediate clinical attention, and we also seek to identify relevant historical factors that can inform our understanding of current issues as well as those that may arise in the future. In addition, we inquire about family mental health histories due to the strong genetic connection, or loading, of certain mental health conditions. Understanding patients' presenting problems and histories helps to inform our case conceptualizations and, therefore, our preliminary hypotheses as to what may be causing, or at least contributing to, medical and mental health–related issues they may be experiencing. A strong case conceptualization accompanied by viable working hypotheses is essential to provide effective treatment and avoid implementing clinically contraindicated interventions. As such, sound assessment is the cornerstone of sound treatment, be it during the course of an initial screening or a more in-depth evaluation. Indeed, an effective mental health screening is one that clearly identifies those with obvious psychiatric issues as well as so-called gray area cases, but it is one that also does not lead to unnecessary flagging of those without such problems. Put differently, we must try to maintain an appropriate balance between false positives and false negatives in our screening procedures, whereby we accept a greater number of false positives at this initial stage. In other words, it is better to recommend a more comprehensive or specialized evaluation if we believe a patient has a mental health condition that may warrant therapeutic interventions rather than overlooking it. Therefore, screenings can be considered effective when they prompt us to refer patients for additional assessment, particularly when their presenting problems are unclear or otherwise outside of our areas of professional competence.

There are three particularly relevant clinical considerations here given that we, as clinicians, often have (1) different methods of screening for mental health problems, (2) different thresholds as to what constitutes a problem, and (3) different ways of handling situations that reach problematic levels. To illustrate, some of us may have patients complete a self-report questionnaire along with their other intake paperwork (e.g., background, Health Insurance Portability and Accountability Act [HIPAA] and privacy forms) and follow up when applicable, whereas others may directly ask patients mental health–related screening questions during session. Either way, if we are not using published psychological measures with empirical support, our assessments may be susceptible to a fair amount of subjectivity. First, there is likely significant variability with respect to the domains we are addressing. For instance, some of us may primarily screen for depression and suicidality without attending to the numerous other conditions that may be affecting our patients. Remember that the DSM-5-TR spans over 1,000 pages and includes approximately 300 disorders.[3] Of course, our patients may be dealing with issues or exhibiting behaviors that do not fit neatly into a DSM diagnosis per se. Second, if we are not using published measures with relevant norms and research bases, (quantitatively) scoring items will have little relevance and can often be misleading. Therefore, we are likely solely relying on *unstructured* clinical judgment when deciding that our patient has a mental health issue warranting further evaluation (see the *Violence Risk Assessment* section of Chapter 5 for a detailed discussion of this issue). This is not necessarily a major problem at the initial mental health screening stage. Problems can ensue, however, when we jump directly from screening to treatment, particularly when psychiatric issues are not glaringly obvious or serious. This relates to the third consideration: How do we handle what we believe to be "positive" mental health screens? Again, many positive screens should lead to referrals for a more comprehensive mental health evaluation and not necessarily immediate treatment in the absence of such. Indeed, patients would not begin chemotherapy without a thorough radiological examination. Think: clinical (manual) breast exams

> Ψ Many "positive" mental health screens should lead to referrals for a more comprehensive mental health evaluation and not necessarily immediate treatment in the absence of such.

and mammograms or digital rectal exams and colonoscopies. Depending on our own thresholds and levels of professional competence in assessing and treating mental health problems, we may choose to monitor a patient, refer out for a full and more specialized assessment, treat immediately, or even refer out for treatment—such as for psychotherapy or pharmacotherapy.

Later in this chapter, we go into some depth about what is involved in more comprehensive clinical and medical evaluations centered on evaluating mental health problems (see the *Conducting Mental Health Evaluations and Comprehensive Assessments* section below). But what about assessing for risk, specifically? As medical and mental health professionals, we are required to assess and manage the risk of harm our patients may pose to themselves or others. We may also act when we become aware of certain domestic abuse–related incidents, including but not limited to child and elder abuse. Duty to warn and protect laws vary among jurisdictions. Therefore, it is essential to know our respective state laws in this regard; namely, when patient–client confidentiality may be broken (legally, with immunity) and the ways in which we can discharge our duty to warn and protect. We discuss these issues further in Chapter 6. What is critical to remember, though, is that all such laws are predicated on the assumption that an *appropriate* risk assessment was conducted. In other words, while we have the legal protection to disclose

---

[3] It is also very important to remember that diagnostic labels are overwhelmingly nonspecific because of the significant heterogeneity *within* diagnostic categories given the many possible symptom combinations for various conditions. Perhaps the title of Galatzer-Levy and Bryant's (2013) publication in the Association for Psychological Science's journal, *Perspectives on Psychological Science*, illuminates this issue best: "636,120 Ways to Have Posttraumatic Stress Disorder."

protected health information (PHI) if we believe a patient is at imminent risk to engage in self-harm or harm to an identifiable third party, the procedures that brought us to that decision are still subject to scrutiny and must be based on acceptable practice standards and the law. Although introducing guns to the equation should not appreciably change our risk assessment procedures, we may be affected by it. This issue is what we refer to as *weapon focus*,[4] or when the mere notion of potential firearm access diverts our attention and leads us to change our typical procedures. To be clear, we certainly believe there are many instances when we should address guns and gun-specific issues—indeed, this entire book is devoted to such. However, this is a content- and not process-related consideration in most cases. In the next chapter (Chapter 5), we discuss firearm-specific evaluations and present a unique set of procedural recommendations. However, here we are generally addressing the ways

> Ψ "Weapon focus" in this context refers to a scenario whereby the mere notion of potential firearm access, or even firearms more generally, diverts our attention and leads us to change our typical procedures. It is essential to maintain consistency in our clinical practices while incorporating firearm-related considerations, just as we do when providing services in other respects (e.g., trauma-informed).

in which we, as medical and mental health professionals, can incorporate firearm-related considerations and content into our existing risk assessment procedures.

Viewing Gun Access as a Potentially Moderating Risk Factor

One particularly important tenet is to think of gun access as a *potential* risk factor when assessing a patient's risk, just as we do with other factors, such as alcohol use. In other words, alcohol can be used responsibly or irresponsibly, and the mere fact that someone has access to it does not in and of itself provide us with sufficient information to make an informed professional decision about their risk level. In fact, as we will continue to point out in this book, most (if not essentially all) of our patients have potential access to a gun at any given point; therefore, it is often important to differentiate between *potential* and *likely* access—or what is sometimes referred to as *easy access*. Nevertheless, a key question to ask ourselves is: What differentiates a patient/gun owner who we determine to be at risk to harm themselves or others with it and a patient/gun owner not deemed to be at risk for such misuse? Just as there may be a correlation between alcohol use and various concerning outcomes, we cannot simply rely on that notion to justify a therapeutic or legal intervention *for this patient, at this time, given these circumstances*. In other words, risk assessments must be context-specific. While we need to be aware of the research associated with certain risk

---

[4] The concept of "weapon focus" in the mental health and law context refers to the notion that eyewitnesses to crimes involving weapons often divert their attention to the weapon and pay less attention to other aspects of the scene (see Loftus et al., 1987). Of note is this effect has also been demonstrated with unusual objects and not solely weapons (e.g., Pickel, 1998).

Ψ Easy or likely firearm access should be viewed as a potentially moderating risk factor considered in context rather than as a stand-alone high-risk factor without context. To be able to identify and differentiate risk levels among clients, especially gun owners, our assessments must be context-specific. Namely, with a focus on *this patient, at this time, given these circumstances.*

Ψ An *idiographic* assessment approach seeks to identify and account for individual differences, or case-specific factors, while also incorporating more general, empirically derived variables. A *nomothetic* approach primarily seeks to compare the individual at hand to a representative group or population (i.e., a normative sample).

factors and behaviors, we must integrate such into an *idiographic assessment* that includes patient-specific factors, so we can make an informed decision about the person in front of us. Indeed, more general factors and normative sample data are important to consider (i.e., in line with a *nomothetic assessment* approach). Reviewing the risk factors commonly associated with suicide is illustrative. The Centers for Disease Control and Prevention (CDC; 2021) indicates that a combination of the following individual, relationship, community, and societal factors contributes to suicide risk:

- Family history of suicide
- Family history of child maltreatment
- Previous suicide attempt(s)
- History of mental disorders, particularly clinical depression
- History of alcohol and substance abuse
- Feelings of hopelessness
- Impulsive or aggressive tendencies
- Cultural and religious beliefs (e.g., belief that suicide is a noble resolution of a personal dilemma)
- Local epidemics of suicide
- Isolation, a feeling of being cut off from other people
- Barriers to accessing mental health treatment
- Loss (relational, social, work, or financial)
- Physical illness
- Easy access to lethal methods
- Unwillingness to seek help because of the stigma attached to mental health and substance abuse disorders or to suicidal thoughts

Questions remain, however. For instance:

- To what extent do the factors need to be present?
- Which combinations of factors are particularly relevant?
- With what level of suicide risk are certain combinations of factors associated?

Although we may tend to gravitate toward numerical ratings and cutoff scores to (ostensibly) simplify our clinical decision-making in these types of clinical assessments, we must remember that scores can lack meaning and, therefore, be misleading at times. Perhaps the best example in this context is the leading suicide risk assessment measure, the Columbia Suicide Severity Rating Scale (C-SSRS) (http://cssrs.columbia.edu/the-columbia-scale-c-ssrs/about-the-scale/). The C-SSRS has been endorsed, recommended, or adopted as the standard of suicide assessment by leading organizations such as the CDC, the World Health Organization (WHO), the U.S. Food and Drug Administration (FDA), the National Institute of Health (NIH), the Substance Abuse and Mental Health Services Administration (SAMHSA), and the U.S. Department of Defense (DoD). It has also been translated into more than 100 country-specific languages, it has an unprecedented empirical basis,[5] and, Dr. Jeffrey Lieberman, former president of the American Psychiatric Association, equated its development to the introduction of antibiotics. All that said, the C-SSRS does not rely on scores per se. While some versions allow for numerical ratings for certain items to indicate severity level, there are no "cutoff" scores and no total score for the measure is generated.[6] In other words, it is a *discretionary* measure as opposed to those that are *non*-discretionary, such as actuarial risk assessment instruments. Its website clearly reflects such:

Determining Next Steps
To use the Columbia Protocol most effectively and efficiently, an organization can establish criteria or thresholds that determine what to do next for each person assessed. Decisions about hospitalization, counseling, referrals, and other actions are informed by the "yes" or "no" answers and other factors, such as the recency of suicidal thoughts and behaviors.

The take-home message is: While we should structure our assessments in such a way to ensure we are addressing empirically supported risk factors, we cannot avoid using clinical judgment. Even standardized assessment measures that have cutoff scores derived from normative samples rely on clinical judgment to some extent (e.g., the way in which data are gathered and items are scored). We must also remember that our clinical decisions are often affected—at least in part—by external factors, such as institutional requirements, state laws, available resources, and patient-specific factors. Let us now turn our attention to case examples that illustrate coming to two different conclusions about patient/gun owners.

---

[5] http://cssrs.columbia.edu/wp-content/uploads/CSSRS_Supporting-Evidence_Book_2017-04.pdf
[6] There are numerous version of the C-SSRS, as they have been designed to be used in different contexts. For instance, there are versions for use by families, friends, and neighbors as well as for use in healthcare and other community settings. Examples include versions for use in corrections; triage steps for law enforcement; and even separate screeners for firefighters, coaches, and teachers. There are literally dozens of versions of the C-SSRS.

CASE EXAMPLE 3: JAMES BLAKELY (PATIENT/GUN OWNER "A")

James is a 44-year-old man who has been a patient for 7 years. He is married with two young children and runs a small plumbing and heating company. He is a gun owner. In fact, one of the few social outlets he has is going target shooting at the local range with friends once or twice per month. Although he has no notable history of mental health–related problems, he reported in his most recent session that he has been feeling "depressed" since his father died suddenly last month. James states that his father was his "best friend" and he just cannot accept that he is gone. Specifically, he reports a loss of appetite and interest in activities he once enjoyed, in addition to ruminating over his father's body in the casket throughout the day and also experiencing nightmares about it. He also indicates that he is "really questioning the point of life at this point," and expresses resentment toward God. He has not returned to church since the funeral service. He is clearly upset but is open to "suggestions to make it better"—especially for the sake of his young children—even if it means he should take psychotropic medication for the first time to "get through this."

　　From a diagnostic standpoint, the death of James's father and his corresponding psychological reaction to it is still rather new and his presentation seems consistent with an expected *bereavement*. Certainly, it may be the case that such symptoms do not remit and will be ultimately better explained by an adjustment or depressive disorder diagnosis.[7] Nevertheless, it is warranted to assess for suicide risk given that he presents with risk factors in this regard (i.e., relational loss, expressing hopelessness to some extent, access to lethal means). If we incorporate the C-SSRS into our assessment, however, it becomes apparent that he does not have any other notable risk factors—neither historically nor of recent concern. Also, while he presents with the aforementioned risk factors, he does not present with *warning signs* associated with suicide; he does not have a plan, intent, or desire to harm himself, for instance. Moreover, he has numerous *protective* factors in this regard; namely, he cites his wife, children, and business as primary reasons to live, and he feels a strong responsibility to them; he has a supportive family and social network otherwise; he is well engaged in work; and he also believes that suicide is an immoral act that would only make matters worse, especially for his children.

CASE EXAMPLE 4: AIDEN MURPHY (PATIENT/GUN OWNER "B")

Aiden is a 52-year-old man who has been a patient for about a year and a half, as he moved to the area once his wife filed for divorce; she remained in their home with their toddler in the adjoining town. Aiden's initial complaints were of a physical

---

[7] Please note that the so-called bereavement exclusion to major depressive disorder (MDD) from DSM-IV-TR (Criterion E, requiring 2 months to pass among other notations) was removed in the latest version of the diagnostic manual, the DSM-5. Therefore, MDD can be diagnosed subsequent to a loss regardless of the time that has passed. The diagnosis is made based on clinical judgment now, rather than (primarily) based on a prescribed time period.

nature, such that he had reported experiencing acid reflux and headaches; however, they ultimately seemed to be best accounted for by his marital distress. He only engaged in a few office visits since becoming a patient and never indicated much more than the aforementioned issues. However, during his most recent visit, Aiden reported that the divorce-related turmoil has escalated, and the associated child custody dispute has become very bitter and nasty. He now presents as somewhat disheveled with respect to his hygiene and grooming and is much more blatantly stressed than before. Of concern is that he also now reports experiencing "thoughts to end it all" daily, which is particularly alarming because he has previously mentioned that he is a gun owner.

While Aiden does not present with a readily identifiable mental health diagnosis, there are certainly a number of significant concerns here from a risk perspective. In addition to having certain general characteristics associated with suicide risk, such as being a middle-aged White male who has easy access to a gun, there are *dynamic* risk factors that raise even more specific and imminent concerns. Specifically, he is not only in the middle of a divorce process, but he has also now become engaged in a highly contentious child custody dispute. Whereas being married and having children in the home are considered protective factors, Aiden is in the opposite scenario at this point, and child custody disputes can be very damaging to all parties involved. In addition, what was likely internal distress manifesting into physical symptoms at an early point has evolved into much more obvious effects—to a point of impacting his activities of daily living (ADLs), including his hygiene and grooming. Lastly, but what is most directly concerning with respect to his risk, is that Aiden is experiencing suicidal and/or homicidal ideation daily. As such, Aiden presents with both risk factors and warning signs associated with suicide and, perhaps, homicide as well.

It is important to point out that there are case-specific factors in Aiden's situation that notably heighten his risk—factors that are not clearly listed in risk guidelines or even formal assessment measures like the C-SSRS. For instance, while both the aforementioned CDC list and the C-SSRS note the relevance of recent losses (or other significant negative events), these are intentionally broad areas to consider because of the countless types of losses people can experience. That said, the C-SSRS includes consideration of "Other Risk Factors" and "Other Protective Factors" to allow the clinician to account for even more unique case-specific factors that may be present.

Ψ Risk factors can be characterized as either dynamic or static. Static risk factors are those that do not change and, therefore, are typically historical in nature (e.g., past acts of violence). Dynamic risk factors are potentially changeable for better or worse and, therefore, are present- or future-oriented (e.g., current violent attitudes, likelihood of adhering to treatment moving forward). As such, interventions are often primarily focused on addressing dynamic risk factors because, by definition, they can potentially change (improve). In contrast to both, warning signs are those that raise imminent risk and crisis concerns, such as someone getting rid of belongings in the context of their suicidality.

Differentiating Risk Levels When Guns are Present

As we see in the case examples of James and Aiden, we can have two patients who both have easy access to guns and come to starkly different conclusions about their respective risk levels. Again, most (if not all) of our patients have potential access to a gun at any given point and, therefore, our decisions should be largely based on that assumption. Put differently, it may be a necessary yet insufficient recommendation alone to restrict a patient's firearm access. While it may be one aspect of our treatment plan, neither means-restriction counseling nor even forfeiture of guns or gun rights is likely to appreciably reduce a patient's risk level over an extended period. Rather, these may be effective short-term interventions during acute periods of crisis to essentially "buy time" and try to block lethal options while we seek to treat or otherwise address the source of the risk. This is the reason we emphasize considering firearm access as a potentially moderating factor, such that it may be significantly concerning in conjunction with other risk factors and warning signs but not others—as we have illustrated in the cases of James and Aiden above.

Ultimately, our task is to distinguish between patients who readily have access to a firearm and pose an elevated risk to themselves or others and those who also have such access, but whom we do not consider to be currently "at risk."

To be clear, we advocate for a prevention- and management-based risk assessment approach and not black-and-white thinking that leads to attempts to predict our patients' future behaviors. However, we all must develop certain thresholds for when we believe certain risk levels necessitate particular interventions. While we cannot provide a cookbook in this regard, we delineate risk assessment principles and related considerations throughout this book, such as in the section below, *What to Know, Ask, and Do (KAD) When a Patient Has Likely Access to a Gun*, and in the chapters that follow. We also provide case examples and our professional recommendations and reminders to facilitate well-informed and methodical decision-making across cases. Still, we cannot overstate the reality that the vast majority of people in our country have potential access to firearms—including those they own; those owned by family, friends, and acquaintances; and those owned and operated by law enforcement personnel, armed guards, or related professionals—or those available to rent when simply visiting a gun range. In fact, we may not even think about some of the many subtle contexts wherein guns are present. For example, there are many collegiate shooting teams and clubs, including those at Ivy League schools. In sum, guns are omnipresent in America, and we should assume all of our patients have potential access to them. In fact, guns have even been found in various jails and prisons in recent years (some examples include New Orleans: www.cnn.com/2013/04/03/justice/new-orleans-jail-video/index.html; Florida: https://www.huffingtonpost.com/2014/06/20/inmates-smuggle-gun-sue-prison-system_n_5514955.html; and New Jersey: www.nj.com/news/index.ssf/2008/10/bomb_threat_locks_down_trenton.html). Thus, it is essential that we all develop a working knowledge of what to *know*, *ask*, and *do* when we believe our patients have likely access to guns.

What to Know, Ask, and Do (KAD) When a Patient Has Likely Access to a Gun

It can be quite useful to have a framework from which to draw when we believe it is potentially relevant to ask a patient about guns or gun-related issues, particularly when he or she has likely, or easy, access to a gun (again, not simply potential access). But what do we first need to *know*? Then, what might we *ask*? Finally, what can we *do* from that point? These are the precise questions that led us to develop what we refer to as the KAD framework for medical and mental health professionals to use in practice, which we outline below (see also Pirelli & Gold, 2019). Please note that the following outline is not necessarily exhaustive and there may be certain areas you may want or need to cover based on case-specific, institutional, or jurisdictional factors. However, we developed KAD to serve as a semi-structured framework to help guide your clinical decision-making when firearm-related issues arise—at least until more formal training models are developed and become widely available.

There are four main areas in which essentially all practicing medical and mental health professionals should have a general working knowledge in relation to firearms: (1) gun culture, safety, and laws (Box 4.1); (2) when and how to ask about guns (Box 4.2); (3) how to assess risk (Box 4.3); and (4) intervention options (Box 4.4). There are certain corresponding questions we might ask patients and actions we may need to take when clinically indicated and ethically appropriate to do so. While KAD is a somewhat detailed, aspirational framework, many of us would be well served to at least acquire basic firearm knowledge related to guns and general gun safety laws, particularly those pertaining to storage and transportation.

BOX 4.1
GUN CULTURE, SAFETY, AND LAWS

1. **Cultural Competence:** Develop an awareness of:
   A. Gun-related language, terms, and definitions
   B. Clinicians' own potential biases related to patients' views on guns and ownership status
   C. Firearm-related subgroups: identify which, if any, patients belong to—include patients' gun ownership status and/or level of access, including any changes to either
   D. Local norms (e.g., rates of gun ownership, public sentiment and practices, violence and suicide rates—with and without guns, legal regulations)
2. Gun Safety Principles:Gain an understanding of clinicians' and patients' knowledge of and adherence to gun safety principles, including patients' storage, transportation, handling, and gun use practices
3. **Gun-Related Laws:** Identify clinicians' and patients' knowledge of:
   A. State laws on confidentiality and reporting (i.e., duty to warn and/or protect)
   B. Federal and state laws generally related to prohibited persons, firearms, ammunition, and magazine capacity, background checks, Castle doctrine ("stand your ground"), right to carry (RTC), transportation and storage (incl. child access prevention [CAP]), transportation, and hunting

---

BOX 4.2
WHEN AND HOW TO ASK ABOUT GUNS

1. **Local Laws and Policies**
   A. Develop knowledge and a process for:
      i. Clinicians' state- and institutional-level requirements regarding asking or counseling patients about guns
      ii. Clinicians' options when patients do not want to discuss/report guns or gun access
   B. In non-crisis situations, give patients the option to discuss/report their gun ownership status and/or level of access; maintain an open stance and invitation.
      i. For patients who decline, seek clarification as to why.
      ii. For those who are agreeable, inquire about family support and assistance and/or other storage options for firearms should a risk management plan be needed in the future.

2. **Professional Ethics and Standards of Practice**
   A. Ensure patients understand the limits of confidentiality.
   B. Exhibit a professional and cultural competence-based approach to prioritize and facilitate rapport-building, and to ensure the highest quality of care to include consistency in procedures across patients and services versus arbitrary or casual inquiries. Avoid confirmation bias and knee-jerk reactions.
   C. Ask questions that seek to gain a clinical appreciation of both the patients' group levels of acculturation and their individual differences.
   D. Know the limits of professional competence and when to refer out, especially understanding therapeutic versus forensic roles.

BOX 4.3
HOW TO ASSESS RISK

1. **General Violence and Suicide Risk Assessment Models and Principles:** When applicable:
   A. Assess violence and/or suicide risk using questions from a stepwise, semi-structured, prevention-based framework. Avoid prediction-based approaches.
   B. Include questions related to nomothetic and idiographic (case-specific) factors.

2. **Firearm-Specific Risk:** When applicable:
   A. Inquire about the nature and extent of likely (or "easy") gun access.
   B. Assess for the presence of firearm-specific risk factors to distinguish patients who are likely to engage in firearm-involved violence and suicide from those who are not.

BOX 4.4
INTERVENTION OPTIONS

1. **Remember:** If a case extends beyond your professional competence, seek consultation and/or refer out for further evaluation and/or treatment.
2. Develop an emergency plan in advance, to include options for peer consultation as well as awareness of local firearm storage options and emergency care, or crisis, services.
3. Be prepared to provide general counseling in matters that do not reach a higher risk threshold, which may include psychoeducational materials regarding risk factors, warning signs, and preventive and emergency response measures.
4. When a concerning risk threshold is reached, attempt to collaborate on a risk management plan with the patient unless it is a crisis or a duty to warn and/or protect duty is prompted.
    A. Updated inquiries about family support and assistance in this regard and/or other storage options for firearms
    B. a long series of bipolar Is an emergency risk protection order or red flag order an option for the clinician or family?
5. a long series of bipolar Document relevant information, assessment, and procedural data.
6. a long series of bipolar Recognize when no particular action is clinically warranted.

When Patients Request Gun-Specific "Clearance"

Some of us may have already been approached by patients requesting a letter or "clearance" for firearm ownership, although these occurrences are likely to be largely dependent on where we practice given the significant regional differences in perspectives and comfort levels related to gun ownership—and the laws and policies generally corresponding to such. In states like New Jersey, for example, this is a relatively common inquiry from patients who are flagged during the initial application stage. There are approximately 10 sets of inquiries on the New Jersey Firearms Purchaser Identification Card application, which include but are not limited to applicants' histories and current issues related to domestic violence, criminality (juvenile and adult), physical defect and disease, substance abuse, and mental health. Typically, an applicant will be required to produce additional, clarifying information if he or she answers affirmatively in any of these areas. That said, the verbiage for some items is quite vague; take, for instance, item 26:

> Have you ever been attended, treated or observed by any doctor or psychiatrist or at any hospital or mental institution on an inpatient or outpatient basis for any mental or psychiatric condition? If yes, give the name and location of the doctor, psychiatrist, hospital or institution and the date(s) of such occurrence.

In our experience, some applicants answer "no" but are later flagged during the next stage of the background check when information to the contrary is identified—including juvenile hospitalization admissions and the like. It is not particularly uncommon for applicants to then be denied based on "falsifying" their applications (in addition to the issue related to such), although it is relatively rare for applicants to be formally (criminally) charged. If applicants are denied, they may appeal; however, there are also police departments that do not deny applicants right away and essentially pause the process to allow them to provide clarification in the form of an updated mental health assessment for consideration. However, we have often observed departments telling applicants with more benign histories that they "just need a letter from a doctor." Essentially, these departments are looking for a doctor's "clearance," albeit one that explicitly indicates the patient is safe to own and operate firearms, and that he or she is not a danger to the public health, safety, or welfare. Please note: This can also occur in gun forfeiture matters, in which patients are seeking to have their guns returned. So, what do we do if we receive this type of request from a patient or if we are contacted by a police department?

First and foremost, we must start with what we must and must not do (i.e., what is required and what is prohibited). Namely, we must have the necessary consents or releases in place from our patients before we speak to anyone about them or their PHI, consistent with HIPAA as well as professional ethics and regulations, more generally. Of course, records can be subpoenaed or court-ordered and we can be compelled to testify in any case, theoretically, but here we are speaking of more routine requests prompted by our patients' gun applications to police departments. As such, they have very likely already consented to mental health records checks with their respective departments. Still, it is advisable for us to secure our own consents and releases from patients.

Once this procedural step has been satisfied, we can turn our focus to content—that is, what might we actually disclose?

Ψ A critical first step in the decision-making process related to the release of information is to ensure we have the necessary consents or releases in place from our patients. Certain legally driven situations may require us to release information regardless, but our patients' consent is essential in most cases otherwise.

As we highlight throughout this book, it is our overarching opinion that a patient's firearm ownership suitability is a forensic question that calls for an associated forensic evaluation. Therefore, we recommend *against* directly opining about a patient's firearm ownership suitability unless one is in a forensic role and has conducted a firearm evaluation. Instead, these inquiries should be treated just like others often brought to us by patients in personal injury, workers' compensation, disability, and even family court–related matters (e.g., parental capacity, child custody). Specifically, as treating clinicians, we can provide a treatment summary that certainly speaks to such issues as patients' presenting problems, symptoms and diagnoses, nature and course of treatment, and prognoses. Indeed, it is appropriate to note if a patient ever raised bona fide concerns about risk to self or others; however, we should not seek to connect such to the ultimate legal questions at hand. In the firearm context, this would equate to providing an opinion about a patient's firearm ownership suitability specifically, which we should not make because that is a forensic evaluation question and not a treatment-based question. There are very tangible distinctions between forensic and therapeutic roles (see Table 1 in Greenberg & Shuman, 1997) and, just as treatment providers should not opine on questions of child custody and parenting time or the proximate cause of a psychological injury in a civil tort lawsuit, they should refrain from connecting treatment data to ultimate opinions about gun ownership suitability. It is outside of a treating clinician's role and scope. Indeed, this may frustrate inquiring

Ψ The question of whether a patient is suitable for firearm ownership is a forensic question, and therefore calls for an associated forensic evaluation. Therefore, we recommend *against* directly opining about a patient's firearm ownership suitability unless one is in a forensic role and has conducted a firearm evaluation. Instead, treatment providers can provide treatment summaries, which may include such information as patients' presenting problems, symptoms and diagnoses, nature and course of treatment, and prognoses. See what we refer to as *The "Therefore" Problem* in Chapter 6.

police departments and, therefore, our patients and even their attorneys. However, it is our opinion that this is the most professionally responsible and appropriate approach to handling these types of requests. In the case example presented here, we provide an example of the type of *treatment summary* treating professionals may wish to provide in these contexts—as opposed to "signing off" on a patient's suitability for gun ownership or providing a "clearance" letter. Please note that we address firearm-specific evaluations and corresponding reports in the following chapter (Chapter 5), which are intended to directly address gun ownership suitability questions.

CASE EXAMPLE 5: TONYA SORENSON (PATIENT/GUN APPLICANT REQUESTING "CLEARANCE")

Tonya has been a psychotherapy patient for about a year and a half. She was initially referred from her primary care physician (PCP) once she began experiencing panic attacks during her pregnancy. She is 28 years old and she has no prior mental health history; she also no longer experienced panic attacks once her child was born, approximately 1 year ago. However, she has remained in psychotherapy because she finds it helpful to discuss the challenges of being a new mother, including the prospects of returning to the workforce in the near future. In the meantime, though, questions about her suitability to own a firearm have arisen because she applied for a handgun permit and reported her engagement in psychotherapy on the application. The police sergeant screening her application called her for clarification and, despite explaining the purpose and nature of her mental health contacts, the officer told her that her application will remain in "pending" status until she provides a letter from her treating therapist or a doctor indicating she does not pose a risk to public safety and is appropriate to own a gun.

Tonya has subsequently requested a "clearance" letter based on the department's request. She stated that she is seeking to purchase a small revolver to keep in the house for home defense purposes because her husband began traveling frequently for work and, therefore, she is often home alone with her infant daughter. She grew up with guns in the family and even has some experience with them, as she has gone shooting numerous times. That said, she never thought she would seek to own one, but her situation has changed, and she reached this decision with her husband with the best interests of the family in mind.

As her treating psychotherapist, what is an advisable next step? As we will detail in Chapter 6, there are many ethical considerations to take into account in this type of scenario—and, as such, there are a number of possible next steps one may take. The following is an example of a treatment summary–based letter that would be an appropriate option in this situation, albeit one that may not actually satisfy the police department's request because of the lack of firearm-specific language.

To Whom it May Concern:

Ms. Sorenson has been a patient of mine for the past 18 months, at which point she had been referred to me by Dr. Richardson, her primary care doctor, because she was experiencing anxiety attacks for the first time. Ms. Sorenson attended weekly psychotherapy sessions with me for approximately 6 months, which were then decreased to biweekly sessions for another 6 months, and now monthly sessions over the past 6 months. I initially diagnosed her with Panic Disorder without Agoraphobia, as she experienced panic attacks consisting of her heart racing, sweating, feeling as though she could not breathe, some mild chest pain, and fear that she was going to have a heart attack—and all of which was followed by worry about the next panic attack. She initially experienced these anxiety attacks approximately two times per week, but she responded well to the Cognitive Behavioral Therapy (CBT) treatment approach I implemented, and her attacks decreased notably within the first 6 weeks—to about twice per month. Ms. Sorenson was able to continue to apply CBT techniques on her own and acquired a very good handle on how to manage her anxiety. She essentially stopped experiencing panic attacks once her child was born, approximately 10 months ago. However, she continued in treatment with me (less frequently) to address some of the normal stressors associated with being a new mother. Ms. Sorenson engaged in and responded very well to treatment, and we will be terminating our work together over the next 3 weeks as a result. I am aware that she has applied for a firearms purchaser permit, and she has requested this letter to outline her mental health treatment contacts with me. Although I cannot directly speak to her appropriateness to own or use a gun,

I can certainly say that she never raised any concerns with respect to harm to herself, others, or property. She has always presented as a polite, respectful, even-tempered, and calm person. Even during her greatest struggles with anxiety early on in treatment, 18 months ago, she never raised these concerns. She continues to do very well; she has been asymptomatic for many months and her prognosis is very good.

Sincerely,

Angela M. Bautista, Psy.D.
Licensed Psychologist
NJ #74512

Restoration of Gun Rights

We address issues related to the restoration of gun rights in greater detail in the next chapter, Chapter 5, including further explaining "relief from disabilities" (RFD) evaluations. It is relevant to provide a general overview here, though, as treating clinicians are likely to encounter an increasing number of patients seeking such relief. Namely, numerous states have legal mechanisms in place for people who are prohibited from owning firearms due to their mental health histories to have their gun rights restored, provided they demonstrate present suitability. A relatively recent landmark federal court ruling is illustrative of the issue.

Specifically, in a 2014 landmark ruling, the U.S. Court of Appeals' Sixth Circuit held that Michigan's prohibition of Clifford Tyler's gun ownership based on his mental health history violated his Second Amendment rights (*Tyler v. Hillsdale County Sheriff's Department*, 2014). Mr. Tyler was a 73-year-old Michigander who had been involuntarily institutionalized 28 years earlier, in 1986, due to suicidality he experienced as a result of a very difficult divorce in his mid-40s. A current psychological evaluation report indicated that his aforementioned depressive episode was the only one he ever experienced, he currently evidenced no mental illness at all, and he had no substance abuse or criminal histories. In contrast, he had remarried and maintained employment as well as a close relationship with his two daughters from his first marriage. The evaluating psychologist opined that the 1985 episode was an isolated, brief reaction to his wife divorcing him. In 2011, Mr. Tyler attempted to purchase a handgun but was informed by the Hillsdale County Sheriff's Department that the FBI's National Instant Criminal Background Check System (NICS) indicated his prior commitment, and his application was denied in 2012. Given that Michigan did not have an RFD mechanism in place, Mr. Tyler had no recourse other than to file a lawsuit in federal court. Ultimately, the Sixth Circuit held that he should be able to exercise the right to bear arms in any state he chooses to live, regardless of whether the state has chosen to accept federal grant money to fund a relief program. The court further held that Congress designed the law to enforce prohibitions only during periods in which the person is deemed dangerous, which does not necessarily equal a lifelong prohibition. While the court did not order that Mr. Tyler's rights be restored immediately, it provided him with the opportunity to demonstrate that he had regained mental stability and that his mental illness did not pose a risk to himself or others.

As we explain further in Chapter 5, our position—and that of numerous other experts in this area and mental health organizations—is consistent with the *Tyler* ruling: Gun rights prohibitions should be based on people's risk levels and not their mental health diagnoses or histories per se. This is based, in part, on the reality that only 3% to 5% of interpersonal violence is attributable to even severe mental illness (Swanson et al., 1990, 2015) and even lower numbers are associated with firearm-involved violence (see, e.g., Gold & Simon, 2016; the American Psychiatric Association's resource documents: Pinals et al., 2015a, 2015b; and the American Psychological Association's Panel of Experts Report; American Psychological Association, 2013). In fact, people with major mental illnesses are more likely to be *victims* of violence. That said, it is the case that firearm-involved suicide is more closely associated with mental illness, and it is important to recall that two-thirds of gun deaths in the United States are suicides. However, it is also the case that the vast majority of people diagnosed with mental health conditions do not experience suicidality or engage in suicide attempts. Moreover, gun-involved violence and suicide is associated with mental health *crises*, not simply diagnoses per se. The Consortium for Risk-Based Firearm Policy was formed to bring together national gun violence prevention and mental health experts in an effort to advance an evidence-based policy agenda on the issue of mental illness and firearms, and they agreed on a guiding principle for future policy recommendations:

> Ψ Gun-involved violence and suicide is associated with mental health *crises*, not simply diagnoses per se.

Restricting firearm access on the basis of certain dangerous behaviors is supported by the evidence; restricting access on the basis of mental illness diagnoses is not. (McGinty et al., 2014, p. e22)

Still, issues related to patients' violence and suicide risk and their suitability for gun ownership and use are likely to increase for treating clinicians moving forward for multiple reasons. Namely, gun control remains at the forefront of the national discussion and has become a staple talking point for lawmakers and media outlets, which is typically amplified after a mass shooting or similarly tragic event that involves guns. As a result, some politicians have sought to increase prohibitions and restrictions on gun applicants and owners, thereby increasing the number of people flagged due to concerns pertaining to their substance use, violence or suicide risk, and mental health, more generally. As we discussed in Chapter 2, a number of states now have "red flag," or extreme risk protection order (ERPO), laws on the books that allow other citizens, including family or household members, to seek a court order to revoke the gun rights of people they believe are dangerous (https://lawcenter.giffords.org/gun-laws/pol icy-areas/who-can-have-a-gun/extreme-risk-protection-orders/). Numerous states have passed other laws that will likely lead to an increase in both gun forfeitures in other contexts (e.g., domestic violence-related incidents) and the flagging of new or returning gun applicants. For us as clinicians, increased attention to guns and gun control measures will lead to a contemporaneous increase in our involvement in gun-related matters. Of course, this is already a salient issue for those of us who provide treatment services to law enforcement, corrections, military, and related professionals—an area to which we will now turn.

> Ψ For us as clinicians, increased attention to guns and gun control measures will lead to our increased involvement in gun-related matters.

Considerations for Treating Law Enforcement, Corrections, Military, and Related Professionals

Although active and retired military, law enforcement, and correctional personnel have received formal gun training, there is often notable variability between and within these groups. This is also the case for their mental health–related training and associated awareness, including but certainly not limited to self-care principles and practices. One particularly relevant point of which many of us may not be aware is that members of these groups may have access to and routinely handle their *service* guns, but this does not necessarily translate to their (legal) suitability to do so as a civilian. For example, a military, correctional, or law enforcement officer may not have had any fitness-for-duty–related questions arise and, therefore, he or she may actively and legally possess (and even carry off duty) a service gun, but simultaneous be required to undergo a psychological firearm evaluation as a civilian to be granted permission to own a personal firearm. Let us turn to a case example to illustrate.

CASE EXAMPLE 6: OFFICER HELENA RODRIGUEZ
(LAW ENFORCEMENT–CIVILIAN CONFLICT)

Officer Helena Rodriguez, age 34, is a military veteran and has been on the Wrightstown Police Department for 7 years. She was first trained to operate fire-arms during boot camp with the U.S. Army and was regularly around firearms throughout her 4 years of active duty. She was then formally trained once again at the police academy and has carried and qualified with her service weapon every year since without incident. Officer Rodriguez does not have a particular interest in guns per se, but she is quite comfortable handling and operating them. She never really carried off duty although she has carried on duty for the last 7 years; she is now interested in at least carrying to and from work, though, because she moved and now has to pass through higher-crime areas. However, she would like a smaller handgun for off-duty carry.

Thus, Officer Rodriguez applied for a handgun permit in her township, but she was flagged during a mental health background check. Namely, a 10-day psychiatric hospital admission from when she was 16 was noted and, as a result, her residential police chief informed her that she needed a "clearance from a doctor" indicating that she was appropriate to own a firearm as a civilian. Therefore, Officer Rodriguez has entered a limbo stage of sorts, whereby she is required to carry a handgun as a law enforcement officer while her suitability to do so as a civilian is being questioned contemporaneously.

Ψ Law enforcement, corrections, military, and related professionals may have access to and routinely handle their *service* guns, but this does not necessarily translate to their (legal) suitability to do so as a civilian. It is also possible for people within these groups to have issues in their respective on-duty contexts that impact gun-related clearances and duties, which may not be conveyed to relevant parties in their civilian lives.

Officer Rodriguez's situation may be rare but certainly not unheard of—especially in jurisdictions employing strict gun laws and policies. The only mental health contacts most law enforcement personnel have had were routine psychological assessments during pre-employment stages. We provide a general overview of these and other evaluations for law enforcement, corrections, and military personnel in the next chapter (Chapter 5). Officer Rodriguez's evaluation process should essentially proceed in the same manner as for any other civilian gun applicant, although significant problems could certainly arise if a medical or mental health professional found her to be unsuitable—as such could put her career in jeopardy.

As medical and mental health professionals, we are more likely to encounter military, law enforcement, and correctional personnel when they are required to come for treatment by their employer for various reasons, including but certainly not limited to following critical incidents (e.g., officer-involved shootings) or other fitness-for-duty–related concerns. Of course, we are most likely to see members of these groups during the course of routine care and treatment; indeed, many of us may have patients who happen to be police or correctional officers, but their service contacts with us are not directly connected to their jobs. Just like anyone else, they may be presenting with general medical issues or even mental health, substance use, or other concerns that prompt a referral, such as marital problems or a work conflict.

Nevertheless, we should not assume that there is no link between their employment and medical and mental health problems simply because patients do not specifically identify work-related issues as stressors. Law enforcement, correctional, and military positions can be very stressful in and of themselves, aside from the potential exposure to traumatic experiences—both directly and vicariously. It comes as no surprise, then, that these positions are associated with the development of medical, mental health, and substance abuse problems as well as domestic violence issues and suicide. In fact, the professional literatures in these areas are quite voluminous and extend over 30 years.

The police stress literature, in particular, is vast and reflects the notable stressors to which officers are exposed, such as crimes, accidents, complaints, verbal and physical altercations, deaths, periods of notable boredom followed by intense excitement, public and political pressures, and rotating shifts. These do not include the significant intradepartmental as well as family problems that can often arise. As a result, substance use, domestic violence, and related problems may follow, including medical and mental health problems. Also, as with correctional officers and military personnel, suicide rates are often higher than those of the general public among law enforcement. Some illustrative statistics are as follows:

- A Buffalo Cardio-Metabolic Police Stress (BCOPS) study found that police officers were at elevated heart attack risk levels compared to national standards and had higher cholesterol levels, pulse rates, and diastolic blood pressure levels than recommended (Violanti et al., 2006).
- According to the National Institute on Alcohol Abuse and Alcoholism (Ballenger et al., 2011), between 11% and 16% of urban police officers drink alcohol at "at risk" levels, and more than one-third of officers have been found to engage in at least one problematic drinking behavior (Swatt et al., 2007). Some have suggested that the actual rates of alcohol abuse may even be double that of the general population, given that officers are less likely than others to report and seek help for their problems (Kirschman, 2006; Violanti, 1999).
- Police officer families have been found to have higher rates of domestic violence (DV) than non–police officer families (Cheema, 2016). In fact, the National Center for Women and Policing (n.d.) has cited research indicating that 24% to 40% of police officer families experience DV compared to 10% in the general population.
- Police officers have also been found to experience greater suicidality than the general public (Violanti, 1999). Correctional officers have been found to have even higher rates; moreover, they present with higher levels of stress and DV-related problems than police officers (Summerlin et al., 2010). In turn, substance abuse, divorce, and suicide rates are very high in correctional officer populations relative to not only the general public but also their police counterparts.
- There are also many serious concerns that face our active and retired military personnel. In the largest study of mental health risk ever conducted among the U.S. military, Kessler et al. (2014) found that 25% of approximately 5,500 active-duty, non-deployed Army soldiers had a mental health disorder, 11% had more than one illness, and 13% reported severe role impairments. The rate of

depression was five times greater than that for civilians, intermittent explosive disorder was six times greater, and posttraumatic stress disorder (PTSD) was 15 times greater.

- According to the VA (n.d.), substance use disorders (SUDs) co-occur with PTSD among veterans at very problematic rates:
  - At least 20% of veterans with PTSD also have an SUD.
  - War veterans with PTSD and alcohol problems often binge drink, which may be in response to bad memories of combat-related trauma.
  - Of Iraq and Afghanistan war veterans, 1 in 10 seen in the VA have a substance use problem.
- The U.S. Army suicide rate reached an all-time high in 2012, consistent with 2015 VA statistics indicating a rate of 20 veteran suicide deaths per day that year—a 21% greater rate than civilians—and accounting for 14% of all adult suicide deaths in the United States. Of particular note is that 67% of all veteran deaths were via firearm (VA Suicide Prevention Program, 2018).

Of course, considerations related to law enforcement, correctional, and military personnel can fill entire books specifically devoted to these issues. While a comprehensive review of these issues is outside of the scope of this book, the need to assess firearm-related factors when treating and evaluating members of these groups is clear when we consider even the brief overview presented here. Much of what we cover in this book can be applied to our practices in this regard.

CONDUCTING MENTAL HEALTH EVALUATIONS AND COMPREHENSIVE ASSESSMENTS

As previously noted, both medical and mental health professionals are often required to go beyond simply screening for mental health problems and are tasked with completing at least brief if not comprehensive assessments of patients. The purpose of such assessments may be for diagnostic purposes, treatment recommendations, or to decide whether the client may need a referral to an outside source, such as a specialist. Thus, the referral questions and depth of the assessments will vary across situations and contexts. In the following two subsections, we address procedures related to comprehensive mental health assessments occurring in outpatient settings, such as at agencies, clinics, and schools, and then the typically briefer assessments that take place in inpatient settings (e.g., hospitals).

Outpatient Mental Health

As previously mentioned, mental health services are most often sought and obtained in the community, on an outpatient basis. This may occur in settings such as mental health clinics or agencies, schools, or independent ("private") practices. Some government-run, private, nonprofit agencies also employ in-house evaluators. However, it is common for many agencies to seek outside evaluators to conduct comprehensive mental health evaluations. For instance, a mental health evaluation may be requested for diagnostic clarification, treatment recommendations, special accommodations (e.g., learning disorders, developmental disability services), or determination of appropriate residential needs. We previously discussed intake and screening assessments, but here we look closer at the role of risk assessment in the context of more comprehensive clinical assessments.

Clinicians conducting more comprehensive evaluations often have the benefit of time as well as access to collateral data. Procedurally, evaluators review available records, conduct clinical interviews with examinees, administer psychological or cognitive tests, and conduct collateral interviews with those such as family members and treatment providers. These data sources may provide information related to past and present mental health problems, including but not limited to that which pertains to violence and suicide risk. A review of available records when conducting a comprehensive mental health evaluation is procedurally necessary, as doing so can provide a wealth of information to help guide our clinical decision-making. Such may include mental health, medical, educational, and even legal records. The information therein may provide us with examinees' diagnostic histories as well as those associated with medical and mental health treatment (e.g., psychotherapy, psychopharmacological interventions, hospitalizations). In the context of guns, we want to be particularly attuned to firearm-specific risk factors (e.g., alcohol abuse problems, history of violence or suicidality, misuse of guns). Collateral interviews with family members, friends, and treatment providers can offer similar types of information and at a more granular level. In addition, collateral interviews can provide the opportunity to zero in on a specific period of time and pull back to look at factors across an examinee's lifetime.

All that said, the cornerstone of a sound mental health evaluation is a comprehensive clinical interview. Of course, time may be limited in certain settings and scenarios; therefore, it is incumbent on us, as clinicians, to be strategic and efficient data gatherers and analysts. An evaluation is an investigation into a person's history and current functioning as well as future-oriented factors. A main component is inquiring as to the onset, frequency, intensity, and management of mental health–related problems and symptoms. It is important to keep in mind that mental states can fluctuate and qualitatively change over time. An effective clinical interview will help delineate not only what are referred to as *precipitating* factors, or those that lead to the onset or exacerbation of symptoms, but also the presence of *protective* factors, or those that are associated with psychiatric and behavioral stability. This remains true even for personality traits and disorders, which tend to be more stable and pervasive than many clinical syndromes. As clinical evaluators, we may also consider administering psychological tests, provided that we have the requisite professional competence to do so. Additional information can be gleaned from psychological assessment instruments, such as the Personality Assessment Inventory (PAI) or the Minnesota Multiphasic Personality

Inventory (MMPI-2). Typically, these are administered and scored by licensed psychologists, as they usually have been trained in this regard; therefore, an outside referral may be needed in certain cases. However, there are other psychological and cognitive tests that do not require such advanced training in administration, scoring, and interpretation. For example, the Beck Inventory scales, such as the Beck Depression or Anxiety Inventories (BDI/BAI) or the Beck Scale for Suicidal Ideation (BSSI), do not require specialized training, nor do they have complicated scoring and interpretation systems. Recall the C-SSRS, described in the *Viewing Gun Access as a Potentially Moderating Risk Factor* subsection earlier in this chapter, as another example. Perhaps the most recognizable example, though, is the Mini-Mental State Examination (MMSE), which is widely used by an array of medical and mental health professionals as an initial cognitive screen in a whole host of cases.

> Ψ Time may be limited in certain settings and scenarios; therefore, it is incumbent on us as clinicians to be strategic and efficient data gatherers and analysts.

The reality that mental status and symptoms can fluctuate over time is an important consideration when conducting assessments of risk. Moreover, assessments of violence and suicide risk are often included in the context of comprehensive mental health evaluations. As previously outlined, the CDC has indicated that a combination of factors contributes to suicide risk (please refer to the *Viewing Gun Access as a Potentially Moderating Risk Factor* subsection earlier in this chapter), such as family histories of suicidality, childhood maltreatment, substance abuse, mental health concerns, and various cultural and religious factors. While many of these areas are typically covered during clinical and collateral interviews, evaluating clinicians may decide to conduct more nuanced or otherwise comprehensive risk assessments. This may be especially true when there are documented or reported histories of suicide attempts, self-injurious behaviors, threats of suicide, or violence toward others. Clinicians may choose to incorporate formal measures into their assessments but must ensure they have sufficient professional competence (i.e., qualifications) in this regard; if not, a referral for such may be indicated. Moreover, as evaluating clinicians, we need to ensure the measures are appropriate for use with the examinees and referral question at hand.

> Ψ We subscribe to and recommend using a prevention- rather than a prediction-based framework when conducting risk assessments, with the goal of developing plans to *prevent* certain types of concerning behaviors instead of trying to *predict* them.

The benefit of utilizing formal measures, such as the C-SSRS to assess suicide risk and the Historical, Clinical, Risk Management-20, Version 3 (HCR-20 V3) for violence risk, is that they provide structure and are in line with a prevention- rather than a prediction-based framework. We address this concept in greater detail throughout Chapter 5, but it is our recommendation to conduct risk assessments in this manner, consistent with the overarching goal of developing plans to *prevent* certain types of concerning behaviors instead of trying to *predict* them. Doing so also allows us, as clinical evaluators, to incorporate our clinical judgment vis-à-vis case-specific risk factors that are not accounted for on formal measures (i.e., an idiographic assessment approach). As such, the treatment recommendations and overarching risk management plan can account for the most salient risk factors—both general and case-specific.

By considering firearm access as a potentially moderating factor, we emphasize viewing it in relation to the presence of other risk and protective factors and also stress the importance of identifying the presence of *warning signs* or lack thereof. To reiterate, it is important to differentiate between *potential* and *likely* (or easy) access, and our KAD model provides guidance to clinical evaluators on what to do when a patient has such *likely* access.

When there are concerns about suicide or violence risk at hand with patients who have *likely* access to guns, additional considerations and follow-up questions are necessary to pursue. For instance, we will want to inquire about patients' gun ownership statuses and levels of access, as well as plans, intent, or desire to misuse their firearms. Information about patients' gun ownership, interests, and background (e.g., hunting, military) may arise simply during the course of gathering historical data. Such information can facilitate conversations associated with general risk-related and specific gun access–related concerns. Given that risk assessments should be context-specific, it is important to inquire as to whether patients of concern have experienced problems with firearms in the past or if any past risk for harm has been associated with firearms otherwise (e.g., threats to self or others involving guns). Again, information can be obtained through both clinical interview and collateral data sources, when possible.

Given that risk levels and mental states can fluctuate over time, short-term interventions may be called for in the context of efforts to limit access to lethal means during acute crisis, assessment, and treatment phases (i.e., so called means-restriction efforts). Thus, consistent with the KAD framework's Intervention Options, it is generally advisable to consider these options in advance, to avoid last-minute scrambling should an unexpected concern arise in a given case. As Bryan and colleagues (2011) articulated it:

> It is important to clarify what is meant by *means-restriction* and to distinguish it from the linguistically similar but conceptually different *means-restriction counseling*. Means-restriction entails the actual process of limiting or removing access to potentially lethal methods for suicide or self-harm (e.g., locking up medications, removing a firearm from the home). Means-restriction counseling, in contrast, is a process in which a clinician educates patients and supportive others about the risks associated with easy availability of means; the clinician then collaboratively assists them in developing plans to limit the suicidal individual's access to these means. The distinction between these two concepts is critical, as means-restriction counseling is well within the scope of clinical practice but

the act of physically securing a patient's lethal means (i.e., means-restriction) in most cases is not.

To highlight the difference between these two concepts, consider the common problem of suicidal patients who own or possess firearms. Clinicians should, as a general practice, not seek to physically secure or remove a patient's firearm themselves for a number of safety (e.g., having armed patients in the workplace) and legal reasons (e.g., firearm registration and possession laws). However, clinicians should routinely ask patients about firearms possession, engage them in a discussion about the risks of firearm possession when suicidal, and collaboratively develop a plan for maximizing the patient's safety . . .

In the context of the present discussion, means-restriction counseling entails two distinct but interrelated clinical actions, as outlined by the Harvard School of Public Health (2008): (1) assessing whether individuals at risk for suicide have access to a firearm or other lethal means and (2) working with them and their families and support systems to limit their access until they are no longer feeling suicidal. The first of these two actions—assessing for access to means— has received a reasonable amount of attention in the literature. It is the second of these actions—working to limit access to these means—that has been largely neglected in the clinical literature and is therefore of greatest concern to clinicians. In our experience, it is confusion about this second action that reduces the likelihood of clinicians accomplishing the first: "If I don't know what to do to limit access to means, then I'd better not ask about it." (p. 340)

Indeed, in order to work with our patients on issues of advance planning and crisis interventions, we have to have sufficient competence and confidence related to guns and gun safety. However, we know this is not the case in the medical and mental health professions. Diurba and colleagues (2020) found that although emergency department and behavioral health providers were somewhat comfortable screening for lethal means among suicidal patients, fewer were comfortable with (lethal means) counseling. Again, this is not particularly surprising given the inordinate amount of attention paid to educating and training medical and mental health professionals in relation to the absolute dearth of education and training we receive on firearms and gun safety (i.e., the primary motivation for this book).

For patients who may not be currently "at risk" per se but who have known histories of concern or who have otherwise elevated violence- or suicide-related risk levels, we may want to develop (preventive) emergency plans. This concept is akin to that of a psychiatric advance directive, such that we identify a plan of action that might involve emergency contacts in relation to gun storage options during crisis or otherwise precarious situations (e.g., DV-related concerns, risk-related concerns associated with other members of the household). Of course, a duty to warn and/or protect may be prompted when our patients are currently "at risk," which we will address in greater detail in Chapters 5 and 6. This may necessitate immediate action and cooperation of a family member or friend in securing firearms until stability is regained and, in some cases, when gun rights are restored. Regardless of the particular situation at hand, we should proactively familiarize ourselves with local, external storage options as well.

Inpatient Mental Health

There are a number of reasons for mental health assessments to be conducted in hospital settings. Some are conducted in circumstances not directly related to a mental health issue per se, such as in the context of routine evaluations for patients who will be undergoing elective, semi-elective, or even emergency procedures. Nevertheless, as with all mental health evaluations, risk of harm to self and others must be considered. Many medical facilities have a psychiatric consultation-liaison (C-L) service, whereby professionals and trainees in the areas of psychiatry, psychology, and social work conduct assessments, provide brief therapeutic interventions (treatment), set forth recommendations, and set up follow-up services for patients in need. This type of service may be called upon by medical staff concerned about their patients' mental health, but for whom such is outside of the scope of their practice. C-L services may be called to address various types of referral questions, such as to assess for the presence of specific mental health symptoms or general psychological functioning, as well as to determine which types of therapeutic and pharmacological interventions are recommended. C-L personnel may also be asked to help provide diagnostic clarity when differential diagnoses are being considered, especially because such can be unclear in medical scenarios when medical conditions may be having masking, driving, or otherwise combined effects with mental health–related issues. Certain types of symptoms cut across diagnostic labels; for instance, psychosis may be attributable to various conditions, ranging from a bona fide psychotic disorder to a urinary tract infection—among other potential sources (e.g., illicit or prescribed substances). A C-L service may also be called to assess risk when concerns for patients' suicidality arise and, ultimately, to determine if the risk levels are sufficiently elevated to warrant inpatient psychiatric unit admissions.

Generally, these types of inpatient evaluations are relatively briefer than those conducted in more specialized contexts; yet the assessment of risk should still *procedurally* parallel that of more comprehensive evaluations. Put differently, while evaluators in these contexts may not go into the same depth in particular areas of inquiry, overarching risk assessment principles must be met. To reiterate, risk assessments should include consideration of risk and protective factors and, certainly, warning signs. Moreover, it is generally advisable to gather data from different types of data sources to the extent possible (e.g., clinical interview, collateral interviews and records, medical and psychological testing). There are limitations in most assessment contexts and there are often constraints when working in acute care settings, particularly when time is of the essence and resources are not readily available. In these situations, there may be no possibility of conducting psychological testing or even collateral interviews. Collateral data from sources such as family members, treatment providers, and medical or mental health records may simply be unavailable, making clinical interviews and assessments with patients very important. Still, it is generally recommended to seek collateral information when possible. This is especially true when there may not be imminent risk, without warning signs, but clinicians may have some concern and intervention is necessary. Assessment measures like the C-SSRS can still be useful in these contexts, as they provide guidance and structure in our efforts to identify risk factors. Then, follow-up questions can be asked to contextualize any present risk and determine if the presence of a firearm acts as a notable moderating risk factor "for this particular client at this time."

More comprehensive assessments may be conducted on inpatient psychiatric units and a prevention-based risk assessment is essential for discharge planning. Such can include the involvement of relatives or connected others who can help ensure that someone with *likely* access to firearms is restricted from them when they return home—at least until a period of stability is achieved. This procedure would be similar to that which may completed during a more comprehensive evaluation on an outpatient basis. Of course, legal interventions may also be put in place to restrict gun access (e.g., gun forfeiture or confiscation, revocation of gun rights).

RECOMMENDED FURTHER READING

Appelbaum, P. S. (2017a). Does the Second Amendment protect the gun rights of persons with mental illness? *Psychiatric Services, 68*(1), 3–5.

Appelbaum, P. S. (2017b). "Docs vs. Glocks" and the regulation of physicians' speech. *Psychiatric Services, 68*(7), 647–649.

Columbia Lighthouse Project. (n.d.). *A unique suicide risk assessment tool.* https://cssrs.colum bia.edu/the-columbia-scale-c-ssrs/about-the-scale/

Galatzer-Levy, I. R., & Bryant, R. A. (2013). 636,120 ways to have posttraumatic stress disorder. *Perspectives on Psychological Science, 8*(6), 651–662.

Gold, L. H., & Simon, R. I. (Eds.). (2016). *Gun violence and mental illness.* American Psychiatric Association.

Pirelli, G., & Gold, L. (2019). Leaving Lake Wobegon: Firearm-related education and training for medical and mental health professionals is an essential competence. *Journal of Aggression, Conflict and Peace Research, 11*(2), 78–87. https://doi.org/10.1108/JACPR-11-2018-0391

5

Forensic Mental Health Assessment and Firearm-Specific Evaluations

FIREARM-SPECIFIC EVALUATIONS ARE part of a particular class of forensic mental health assessments (FMHAs). In addition to needing to be grounded in FMHA principles, we have also contended these evaluations "represent a unique class of assessments with a particular set of considerations" (Pirelli et al., 2015, p. 250; see also Pirelli & Witt, 2015, 2017; Wechsler et al., 2014, 2015). Our ongoing research and practice in this area has made us even more confident in characterizing this as a subspecialty area that requires a specific type of professional competence, to include cultural competence. In this chapter, we first provide an overview of FMHA as an overarching specialty area of clinical practice, and then turn to a detailed outline of firearm-specific evaluations and their respective considerations. Namely, we discuss conducting evaluations in the context of initial and return gun applicants; mental health expungements; and gun forfeiture and reinstatement matters, such as in "red flag" and related scenarios. In addition, we provide an overview of risk assessment models and approaches, which can be applied to gun-related evaluation contexts. Specifically, we address violence, suicide, and firearm-specific assessments, to include the use of the evaluation framework we have developed over the last decade: the Pirelli Firearm-10 (PF-10). Lastly, we set forth considerations for conducting evaluations for law enforcement, corrections, and military personnel.

Ψ Firearm-specific evaluations are part of a particular class of forensic mental health assessments (FMHAs) with a unique set of considerations.

FORENSIC MENTAL HEALTH ASSESSMENT

Modern forensic subspecialties within the medical and mental health professions had their start over 100 years ago. They have significantly developed over the last 50 years, in particular, with the advent of numerous formal educational and training programs throughout the country as well as specialized journals, associations, and related professional outlets. In order to understand more advanced principles in this context, it is important to first be able to distinguish between forensic and therapeutic specialties. Therefore, let us start with examples of how they are defined in psychiatry and psychology.

Per the American Academy of Psychiatry and the Law's "Ethics Guidelines for the Practice of Forensic Psychiatry" (2005):

> Forensic Psychiatry is a subspecialty of psychiatry in which scientific and clinical expertise is applied in legal contexts involving civil, criminal, correctional, regulatory or legislative matters, and in specialized clinical consultations in areas such as risk assessment or employment. These guidelines apply to psychiatrists practicing in a forensic role. (I. Preamble Commentary section)

According to the American Psychological Association's "Specialty Guidelines for Forensic Psychology" (2013), forensic psychology

> refers to professional practice by any psychologist working within any subdiscipline of psychology (e.g., clinical, developmental, social, cognitive) when applying the scientific, technical, or specialized knowledge of psychology to the law to assist in addressing legal, contractual, and administrative matters. (p. 7)

There are forensic subfields across medical and mental health disciplines. For example, recognized practice areas include those in forensic science, nursing, social work, counseling, and, of course, in relation to pathologists and medical examiners. The main question here, though, is: What differentiates forensic specialists from those engaging in the more traditional, therapeutic roles associated with the aforementioned medical and mental health professions?

Two seminal articles written by Greenberg and Shuman (1997, 2007) are illuminating, as they compared and contrasted the role of the therapeutic clinician with that of the forensic mental health evaluator and outlined 10 distinct differences between therapeutic and forensic roles:

1. Identifying the client
2. Relational privilege
3. Cognitive set and evaluative attitude
4. Areas of competency
5. Nature of the hypotheses tested
6. Scrutiny applied to the information utilized

7. Amount and control of the structure
8. Nature and degree of "adversarialness"
9. Goal of the professional
10. Impact of critical judgment by the psychologist

We encourage readers to review all 10 of these areas, regardless of whether they practice in primarily forensic or therapeutic roles. In fact, it may be even more useful for clinicians who do not engage in forensic work per se and who do not identify as forensic practitioners—because it is important to identify the bounds of one's practice. Put differently, it is important for treating medical and mental health professionals to be aware of the lines between forensic and therapeutic roles and tasks. Patients and the myriad parties who may be involved in their lives in some way (e.g., employers, schools, attorneys) come to clinicians with many wide-ranging requests; therefore, we must know what we can and cannot do as well as what we should and should not do— and why (see e.g., Chapter 4—*Case Example 5: Tonya Sorenson*). While a full review of the areas delineated by Greenberg and Shuman is outside of the scope of this chapter, it is useful to highlight the points that are particularly relevant to most, if not all, of us as clinicians.

First, we must identify who our direct client is in a given scenario. For those of us who provide treatment, this is usually obvious: the patient receiving the treatment. In psychotherapy contexts, our "client" may also be couples or families, as a unit. However, identifying our clients in forensic scenarios is often less straightforward, and it is also common to have multiple clients. For instance, our clients may simultaneously include an examinee (e.g., a defendant), a retaining attorney, a court, and even the community at some level, even though the retaining attorney may be our direct, or primary, client. As such, it is essential to identify the client(s) in each professional service context because doing so provides the foundation and associated considerations for our work moving forward. We need to know, for example, with whom we have a relational *privilege*.

> Ψ An essential preliminary step for a practitioner is to identify the direct client.

Legal privilege refers to the privacy protections for communications between certain parties. We must protect our patients' confidentiality unless our obligations related to duty to warn and/or protect are prompted (à la *Tarasoff v. Regents of the University of California*, 1976); however, we cannot guarantee absolute privacy in essentially any context given that we can be subpoenaed or court-ordered to produce our records and testify at any point. When we engage in forensic roles, privilege may exist in limited ways and circumstances, such as within the context of an attorney–client relationship (e.g., some of our data and communications may be protected under attorney work product provisions). On the other hand, there is no such privilege in most administrative matters or court-ordered evaluations. Needless to say, confidentiality afforded to examinees in forensic contexts is usually quite limited. These nuances related to privilege in both therapeutic and forensic situations are important for us to know for many reasons, not the least of which is because we have to explain them during informed consent processes.

Greenberg and Shuman's third distinction—cognitive set and evaluative attitude— clearly distinguishes therapeutic from forensic practice. In treating roles, we usually try to be supportive, accepting, and empathic, whereas in forensic roles we seek to be as neutral, objective, and (personally) detached as possible. Some may even argue that empathy "gets in the way" in forensic practice, in line with the concept of *moral disengagement* relevant to forensic, correctional, and other clinical contexts. While others have contended that empathy and even humor is appropriate in forensic contexts (Brodsky & Lichtenstein, 1999; Brodsky & Wilson, 2013), or at least not as detrimental as once thought (Vera et al., 2019), it remains the case that clinicians' attitudes and approaches toward forensic clients are often distinct from their attitudes and approaches toward patients in treating contexts.

Greenberg and Shuman's fifth noted difference between therapeutic and forensic work relates to the nature of the respective hypotheses tested. Namely, as treatment providers, we test hypotheses associated with our patients' complaints and related treatment goals, including considering differential diagnoses, family history and dynamics, and other relevant themes that may arise during treatment. In contrast, as forensic practitioners, we test hypotheses related to specific psycholegal questions (e.g., an examinee's mental capacity to make medical, legal, and financial decisions; the proximate cause of an examinee's psychological injury). Therefore, forensic practitioners must have a relatively sophisticated level of legal knowledge and, of course, they must be able to operationally define and clinically assess the relevant aspects of psycholegal constructs. For example, those of us who evaluate allegedly incapacitated adults in legal guardianship cases must know how to appropriately assess examinees' competence-related abilities (i.e., expressing a choice, understanding, appreciation, and reasoning) within the context of particular legal standards.

The overarching difference between therapeutic and forensic roles in relation to hypothesis testing is connected with Greenberg and Shuman's ninth distinction: the goal of the professional in each relationship. Specifically, as treating professionals, our primary goal is essentially to help our patients get well, feel better, or otherwise improve or reach particular goals, which is starkly different from our scope when functioning in a forensic evaluation role. As forensic evaluators, our main goal is to address psycholegal questions to ultimately assist legal triers of fact (i.e., judges or juries) or to otherwise provide information to those tasked with making decisions in a given matter (e.g., attorneys, agencies, administrators).

Having the foundational knowledge of what constitutes *forensic mental health* and the distinction between therapeutic and forensic roles in clinical practice is essential to understanding FMHA concepts. FMHA is the evaluation of the emotional, behavioral, and cognitive functioning of a person whose mental state is an issue in a legal proceeding (Heilbrun, 2001). While medical and mental health practitioners have conducted these types of assessments for over 100 years, there have been particularly significant advancements in the FMHA arena in the second half of the 20th century, including the publication of contemporary and seminal resources such as Goldstein (2001, 2007); Greenberg and Shuman (1997, 2007); Heilbrun (2001); Heilbrun et al. (2009, 2014); Lieberman and Krauss (2009); Melton et al. (2018); Otto et al. (2014); and Weiner and Otto (2013). In addition, the reader is directed to reference the professional ethics codes and guidelines set forth across our disciplines (medical and mental health), which we review in a fair amount of detail in Chapter 6.

Although it is critical for practitioners to have sound clinical education and training, our society has valued and relied upon specialists for quite some time. Indeed, the forensic subspecialty is just one of many other clinical specialty areas in medical and mental health

Ψ There are numerous distinctions between therapeutic and forensic roles. For instance, in therapeutic roles, we provide treatment to someone (i.e., the client) and focus on treatment goals and gains. We produce progress notes and treatment summaries and, if requested, can be called to testify as fact witnesses. In forensic roles, we can provide treatment in some instances, but we are typically asked to conduct evaluations with examinees and our primary clients are usually retaining parties (e.g., attorney, court). Our goals are not associated with helping examinees improve, but rather, to address psycholegal or related referral questions. We produce forensic reports and serve as expert witnesses.

practice (e.g., developmental, educational, geriatric, neuro, sports). As a result of the proliferation of research and formal education and training in these fields, we have entered a time of subspecialties, such that having knowledge of clinical and forensic principles is essentially a *prerequisite* for many areas of more nuanced practice. Put differently, although we may be well versed in general clinical and forensic concepts, that alone does not ensure our competence to engage in all areas of practice or with all types of clients. For example, a forensic evaluator may be very skilled at conducting criminal responsibility, or so-called insanity evaluations, but not sufficiently competent to conduct child custody evaluations. Moreover, some practitioners only provide psychotherapy services in forensic contexts (e.g., court-mandated sex offender treatment), whereas others do not engage in treatment at all. The potential nuances are seemingly endless because practitioners have a wide range of professional competencies and interests, and there are also jurisdictional factors that come into play, such as state laws and court procedures that necessitate certain types of services and prohibit or otherwise restrict others. To be sure, we have entered into a period of subspecialties for a variety of reasons. Therefore, we have consistently

Ψ As a result of the proliferation of research and formal education and training in these fields, we have come to enter a time of subspecialties, such that having knowledge of clinical and forensic principles is essentially a *prerequisite* for many areas of more nuanced practice.

contended that firearm-specific evaluations should be grounded in clinical and FMHA principles, but they have unique features that require those who conduct them to develop and maintain a particular type of professional and cultural competence.

FIREARM-SPECIFIC EVALUATIONS

Dating back to our earliest publications in this area, we have contended that firearm evaluations should be considered a specific type of FMHA (e.g., see Pirelli et al., 2015). However, the medical and mental health professions and their corresponding educational and training programs remain in the very early stages of endorsing and adopting this conceptualization. In fact, it is likely most have yet to even consider the issues at hand. Nevertheless, the American Psychiatric Association's workgroup has previously set forth both a position statement and a resource document on guns and mental health. Namely, Pinals et al. (2015a) outlined five areas and 18 subareas reflecting the Association's 2014 "Position Statement on Firearm Access, Acts of Violence and the Relationship to Mental Illness and Mental Health Services." There are two areas particularly related to the types of firearm-specific evaluations that we discuss in this section. The first area is:

> Reasonable restrictions on gun access are appropriate, but such restrictions should not be based solely on a diagnosis of mental disorder. Diagnostic categories vary widely in the kinds of symptoms, impairments, and disabilities found in affected individuals. Even within a given diagnosis, there is considerable heterogeneity of symptoms and impairments. Only a small proportion of individuals with a mental disorder pose a risk of harm to themselves or others. The APA supports banning access to guns for persons whose conduct indicates that they present a heightened risk of violence to themselves or others, whether or not they have been diagnosed with a mental disorder. (p. 196)

The second area is:

> Given that the right to purchase or possess firearms is restricted for specific categories of individuals who are disqualified under federal or state law, the criteria for disqualification should be carefully defined, and should provide for equal protection of the rights of those disqualified. There should be a fair and reasonable process for restoration of firearm rights for those disqualified on such grounds. When restrictions are based on federal law, disqualifying events related to mental illness, such as civil commitment or a finding of legal incompetence, are reported to the federal background check database (National Instant Criminal Background Check System; NICS). Some states have expanded the scope of disqualifying events to be reported to NICS to include non-adjudicated events, such as temporary hospital detentions.

a. Non-adjudicated events should not serve as sufficient grounds for a disqualification from gun ownership and should not be reported to the NICS system. The adjudicatory process provides important protections that ensure the accuracy of determinations (such as dangerousness-based civil commitment), including the right to representation and the right to call and cross-examine witnesses.

b. Rational policy with regard to implementation of such restrictions calls for the duration of the restriction to be based on individualized assessment rather than a categorical classification of mental illness or a history of a mental health related adjudication.

c. Although the restrictions on access to firearms recommended in items 1 and 2 above would decrease the risk of suicide and violence in the population, extending restrictions to individuals who voluntarily seek mental health care and incorporating their names and mental health histories into a national registry is inadvisable because it could dissuade persons from seeking care and further stigmatize persons with mental disorder.

d. A person whose right to purchase or possess firearms has been suspended on grounds related to mental disorder should have a fair opportunity to have his or her rights restored in a process that properly balances the person's rights with the need to protect public safety and the person's own well-being. Accordingly, the process for restoring an individual's right to purchase or possess a firearm following a disqualification relating to mental disorder should be based on adequate clinical assessment, with decision-making responsibility ultimately resting with an administrative authority or court. (p. 197)

As noted, Pinals and colleagues (2015b) also authored the "Resource Document on Access to Firearms by People with Mental Disorders," wherein they reviewed the connection among psychiatric disorders, firearms, suicide, and violence; issues related to registries of prohibited purchasers as a strategy to prevent firearm-involved suicide and violence; restricting access to guns during periods of mental health crisis; and privacy protections in the context of firearm-related mental health registries. As they indicated, "Diagnosable mental disorders are present in an overwhelming proportion of people who commit suicide. However, the vast majority of violence in our society is not perpetrated by persons with serious mental disorders" (p. 1). As they further articulated it, "Concerns about discrimination are further heightened when the statutory exclusion is categorical rather than being based on an individualized risk determination" (p. 3). Thus, they warned of the potential of deterring people from seeking help out of fear of losing their gun rights. They also reiterated the need for a fair gun rights restoration process, whereby psychiatric evaluations and testimony should be required because

> Ψ Firearm-related violence and suicide is associated with mental health crises, not simply psychiatric diagnoses per se.

they can "describe and interpret the individual's mental health history and current mental health status, and the effects of treatment and other factors on improvement or exacerbation of the person's condition" (p. 3). In addition, Pinals and colleagues advocated for removing guns from those deemed to be at significant, imminent risk to themselves or others (i.e., those who are in crisis), and applaud states with such legal mechanisms. As they put it:

> [B]y focusing on immediate risk, rather than on a person's mental health history, they are more carefully tailored to prevent firearm violence and suicide . . . they address dangerousness per se, and discard the mistaken premise that acute violence risk is associated exclusively or primarily with mental disorder; these laws thereby avoid the discrimination inherent in statutes that exclusively target people with mental disorders . . . they clearly establish the legal framework for psychiatrists and other clinicians to inform police of an apparent danger and the accompanying need to remove firearms. (pp. 3–4)

Both the APA's position statement and resource document were seminal, as they succinctly and cogently presented some of the main, contemporary issues relevant to guns and mental health. They provide a strong foundation for medical and mental health practitioners in this way and set the stage for all of us as clinicians, researchers, and educators to form corresponding practice, research, and teaching principles in this area. In the remaining aspects of this section, we go steps further by applying many of these foundational concepts—as well as those from the FMHA arena and mental health, more generally—to inform our practice entailing firearm-specific evaluations. Specifically, we will now turn to discussions pertaining to evaluations of gun applicants; assessments in mental health expungement contexts; and evaluations of those in reinstatement/gun forfeiture matters. These areas are followed by a presentation of formal assessment models and approaches as well as considerations for conducting evaluations for law enforcement, corrections, and military personnel.

> Ψ Firearm-specific evaluations include assessments of those at the gun permit application stage, those in mental health expungement contexts, and those in reinstatement/ gun forfeiture matters.

Gun Applicants

Initial and return gun applicants may be flagged by officers in charge of screening applications due to their self-reports on applications or during criminal and mental health background checks, or as a result of statements made by character references. Applicants may be flagged for one or more reasons, including but not necessarily limited to concerns associated with their legal, mental health, or substance use histories. It is important to highlight the fact that this applies to all gun applicants and not solely those who are applying for their first permit. For example, in New Jersey, a person may apply for a firearms purchaser identification card at age 18 but can only purchase a long gun and not a handgun at that time. At age 21, the person may apply for up to three handguns at a given time. However, he or she cannot purchase more than one every 30 days and must purchase them all within 90 days, with the opportunity for an additional 90-day extension (see Firearms and Weapons, 2002). That said, departments will conduct a completely new set of background checks—criminal and mental health—and treat an application as if it were an initial one if at least 1 year has passed since the last handgun application and approval. It is also the case that a completely new set of background checks and a new application will be required when someone simply requires a change of address on their New Jersey firearms purchaser identification card because identification cards in New Jersey are issued by police chiefs in each respective municipality (or by the state police when there is no local police department). Moreover, even though no permits are needed for long guns and there is no limit on the amount one may purchase in New Jersey with a firearms identification card, the seller will run a check during the transfer process.

Therefore, to summarize: New Jersey residents are subject to numerous criminal and mental health background checks over time even if they have undergone them recently, as they can be prompted by even the most benign events (e.g., changing their address). As a result, initial applicants can certainly be flagged because of their legal, mental health, and substance use histories, but so can return applicants. As we will address in the following section, some of this may be circumvented by securing a mental health expungement. However, such would generally only apply to criminal and inpatient mental health and substance misuse histories. In other words, a person who engaged in routine outpatient treatment for mental health or substance use–related problems can be flagged over and over again without any option for reprieve, thereby putting them in a potentially worse position to secure their gun rights compared to those with histories of criminal charges or even involuntary civil commitments. While procedures vary across jurisdictions, the language used in applications and relevant forms is often quite broad. As we noted in Chapter 4, item 26 on the New Jersey Application for Firearms Purchaser Identification Card and/or Handgun Purchase Permit reads:

> Have you ever been attended, treated or observed by any doctor or psychiatrist or at any hospital or mental institution on an inpatient or outpatient basis for any mental or psychiatric condition? If yes, give the name and location of the doctor, psychiatrist, hospital or institution and the date(s) of such occurrence. (New Jersey State Police [NJSP], 2009)

There is ostensibly room for interpretation here, particularly when patients have seen a mental health professional for family or couples therapy, or even individually for a relatively benign issue. There may be further confusion for applicants who were required to engage in a work-related evaluation, ranging from routine pre-employment assessments to fitness-for-duty evaluations. For instance, what about law enforcement

Ψ Certain jurisdictions with stringent gun laws readily flag existing gun owners who need to complete additional applications at various points (e.g., in New Jersey, for change of address or handgun permits).

officers who are required to see someone after a critical incident, such as a shooting? In fact, there are many potential situations that can arise whereby a person needs to see a mental health professional for reasons other than treatment for a psychiatric condition (e.g., divorce and child custody matters, employment matters—such as workers' compensation, employment harassment, discrimination, and wrongful termination cases). Rather than lay out all of the potential scenarios our patients may encounter, let us refocus on the primary issue at hand for us as clinicians: Our patient/gun applicants who get flagged for any one of a whole host of reasons will likely need to produce documentation showing their appropriateness for firearm ownership. As we highlighted in the section *When Patients Request Gun-Specific "Clearance"* in Chapter 4, police departments may simply ask one of our patients to "get a letter from a doctor" in this regard. However, recall that such is unlikely to be based on a firearm-specific assessment and, therefore, may have limited to no use for this specific purpose. Moreover, we should not opine on ultimate psycholegal issues, such as appropriateness for gun ownership, if we have not specifically assessed for such (see *Case Example 5: Tonya Sorenson* in Chapter 4). Therefore, we provide a framework for these types of firearm-specific evaluations for gun applicants in the *Risk Assessment Models and Approaches* section below. First, however, let us turn to an overview of mental health expungements in the firearm ownership context.

Mental Health Expungements

People may seek expungements for various reasons, such as to secure employment; namely, by having criminal records effectively removed to ensure they will not be flagged during background checks made by potential employers. This is consistent with the ideals of so-called second-chance reintegration policies and efforts that have been set forth by U.S. legislators and presidents in recent years, intended to allay the notable employment barriers that accompany even the more benign criminal histories. In this same vein, many states have laws that allow for the expungement of certain records. Federal offenses are typically more difficult to expunge, and any relief would likely be in the form of pardons, which are rarely granted. As is the case for most laws and policies, there are significant nuances in expungement laws across the country; therefore, we must specifically look to those in each of our own states to be properly informed.

Some states may permit the expungement of mental health records, which typically pertains to involuntary civil commitment records from mental health institutions or facilities. Those seeking expungement of these types of records need to satisfy statutory requirements for the respective states in question. For instance, in New Jersey, a person must demonstrate that their mental health problems have either "substantially improved" or are "in substantial remission" (Application for Relief, 2009). To do so, the person must file a "verified complaint" for expungement of the civil commitment record in a New Jersey Superior Court along with the applicable civil commitment, mental health, and criminal history records as well as with a report and/or certification of a licensed psychologist or psychiatrist indicating the person is not a danger to self, others, or property—and their condition has either substantially improved or is in substantial remission. The person must also provide character letters from employers, family members, and/or friends speaking to the person's standing in the community. Copies of this filing are also provided to the county adjuster, prosecutor, and the medical director from the relevant institution. A court hearing will follow, whereby a judge must determine if the person is unlikely to act in a manner dangerous to the public safety and that the expungement is not contrary to the public interest. Of particular note: If an expungement is granted, it effectively means the commitment did not occur and the person may answer questions to that effect accordingly (i.e., the person can indicate that they have not been civilly committed).

So, how do mental health expungements play out in firearm ownership contexts? In a nutshell, their effects are potentially limited because, while they allow people to indicate they were not committed on official forms, applications, and the like, they still may need to report they were treated at some point—such as to screening officers who specifically ask about their mental health histories. We must also keep in mind that, if a person has already applied for a gun permit, a screening police department will already know about the mental health history, thereby making an expungement relatively ineffectual in most cases—at least at that stage. Some people proceed anyhow, with their futures in mind, particularly if they plan on moving to another municipality or state.

There is another major issue to highlight here, though: Evaluating mental health professionals will come to find out about examinees' mental health histories, whether they have been expunged or not, provided they conduct thorough evaluations and examinees are forthcoming. While people may rightly believe that law enforcement agencies and other relevant parties who run background

Ψ Mental health expungements may have limited utility as a practical matter. While expungements allow people to indicate they were not psychiatrically committed on official forms, applications, and the like, they still may need to report they were treated at some point—such as to screening officers who specifically ask about their mental health histories. In addition, the municipality in question may already be aware of the incident(s) in question, essentially making the expungement irrelevant—at least for the time being. Interested readers are directed to the following site, which has information on expungement laws and restoration rights for states across the United States: http://ccres ourcecenter.org/state-restoration- profiles/50-state-comparisonjudicial- expungement-sealing-and-set-aside/.

checks will not be privy to expunged records, such can still come up during the course of a comprehensive clinical assessment and, therefore, police departments may very well come to find out about said histories anyhow. Moreover, some jurisdictions allow state attorneys (and therefore judges) to not only have access to expunged records but also to use them as bases for denials. Of course, each situation and jurisdiction may be different in terms of the information that can and will be available to certain parties; therefore, it is incumbent upon us, as evaluating clinicians, to learn the nuances and expectations in a given case prior to accepting and moving forward with it. This can present very precarious scenarios vis-à-vis addressing, managing, and conveying information related to expunged records. In sum, while we certainly are not (and cannot) providing legal advice, we humbly reiterate that mental health expungements may only have limited value in the gun ownership context, overall.

Gun Rights Restoration Matters: Forfeiture, Reinstatement,
"Red Flag," and Related Scenarios

Another specific type of firearm evaluation is that which pertains to those seeking to have their gun rights restored, or reinstated, to include confiscated firearm permits, licenses, and/or guns. While this can occur when law enforcement becomes aware of a range of issues related to any one of a state's prohibitor areas, two of the more common situations are those involving domestic violence (DV) and psychiatric crisis. Historically, such a process would typically unfold in one of two ways: (1) when police inquire about guns during the course of their response to a house call or (2) when a professional entity notifies police that a person of concern is a gun owner (e.g., medical and mental health professionals as well as community agencies such as child protective or battered women's services). As we discussed in Chapter 2 and noted in Chapter 4, though, some states have also begun to implement orders that allow other citizens, including family or household members, to seek court orders to revoke persons' guns—often referred to as "red flag" laws, extreme risk protection orders (ERPOs), and gun violence restraining orders (GVROs). These policies are likely to increase the number of gun forfeitures in those states and, therefore, lead to a simultaneous demand for increased involvement by medical and mental health professionals in these matters.

Ψ Some states have begun to implement orders that allow other citizens, including family or household members, to seek court orders to revoke persons' guns and gun rights—often referred to as "red flag" laws, extreme risk protection orders (ERPOs), and gun violence restraining orders (GVROs).

As noted, it has traditionally been the case that forfeiture-related issues arise when law enforcement is called to a residence and officers find out that guns are present. In particular, DV-related calls can prompt officers to ask about the presence of guns in the home even if particular situations did not involve firearms or even threats associated with guns. That said, officers typically cannot take a person's guns without their permission or without either a court order or justification consistent with emergency procedures. Anecdotally, we have found that officers will often preliminarily seek the permission of gun owners (or that of their significant others) to voluntarily hand over their firearms for "safekeeping"—although doing so does not guarantee the departments in question will return the items in the same (informal) fashion. To the contrary, it is not uncommon for departments to require the same types of proofs they would request from a flagged applicant (e.g., medical and mental health records, including a certification indicating the person is safe to own and handle firearms). It is also not uncommon for prosecutors' offices to become involved and even seek the indefinite denial of gun rights.

We have also noted that, in other cases, the question of gun ownership may come about during outpatient or inpatient mental health screenings. Of course, police may be present for some of these cases (e.g., on-site assessments by mobile response teams or during evaluations at crisis centers or emergency rooms), but it is more likely they would be contacted by concerned medical or mental health professionals after the fact—as a result of information that arises during mental health intakes or treatment sessions. In other words, in situations wherein our duty-to-warn or duty-to-protect obligations are prompted (à la *Tarasoff*). We address these issues in greater detail in Chapter 6, but it is certainly worth emphasizing how important it is for us to know our jurisdictions' laws and requirements in this context because breaking client confidentiality is a very serious matter and the parameters of such can vary greatly from state to state. It is fair to say, though, that, as treating and examining medical and mental health professionals, we are typically required to break confidentiality and engage in some level of action when we believe patients pose imminent risk to identifiable third parties or themselves.

The variability across jurisdictions usually comes into play insofar as *how* we are to discharge our duty to protect and/or warn. In New Jersey, for example, we can do so by engaging in one or more of the following four actions: (1) arranging for our patient's voluntary admission into a qualified psychiatric facility; (2) initiating involuntary commitment procedures to a qualified psychiatric facility; (3) advising local law enforcement of the patient's threat and the identity of the intended victim; and/or (4) warning the intended victim (Health care professionals, immunity from civil liability; duty to warn and protect, 2019). Of note is that parents or guardians must be notified if the person of concern or a potential victim is less than 18 years old. Incidentally, New Jersey also now requires that, in addition to engaging in one or more of the above, medical and mental health professionals must notify chief law enforcement officers of the municipalities in which the patients reside or the superintendent of the state police if they live in municipalities without full-time police departments.

The question for us in this section, however, is: How does a gun forfeiture and reinstatement matter differ from firearm evaluations with initial or return applicants, or those conducted in the context of mental health expungement petitions? A primary distinction is that, in reinstatement evaluations, there tends to be increased attention to the person's risk of engaging in future acts of violence or self-injurious behavior—particularly given the events or issues that led to the revocations in the first place (e.g., DV incidents; psychiatric crises leading to suicide attempts; destruction of property). Therefore, in a reinstatement evaluation, we are particularly focused on a person's suitability to own and operate guns in light of the specific concern or event that led to the revocation of the gun rights, which is certainly different than our typical scope during a more routine evaluation of an applicant.

Of course, suicide and violence risk are relevant areas to assess in essentially all firearm-related evaluations, but other factors related to gun ownership may be just as important to consider—especially when an examinee does not have a history of engaging in violence or self-injury. Namely, it is also important to ascertain the reason why a person is seeking the permit or license, the person's experience with guns, plans for use and storage, and plans for developing increased competence and seeking continuing education regarding firearm use and safety. While these areas may not be directly connected to a state's legal standard, they can be relevant to a person's suitability, more generally. This is particularly important in jurisdictions that have rather broad statutory language (e.g., the issuance of a firearm permit would not be contrary to public safety, health, and welfare). We explain their potential significance in the *Risk Assessment Models and Approaches* section that follows. The take-home message here, though, is that these other factors are more likely to be overshadowed by the referral incidents in reinstatement evaluations. Let us turn to a case example to illustrate.

> Ψ Gun forfeiture and reinstatement matters (i.e., gun rights restoration) differ from firearm evaluations with initial or return applicants, and from those conducted in the context of mental health expungement petitions. A primary distinction is that, in reinstatement evaluations, there tends to be increased attention to the person's risk of engaging in future acts of violence or self-injurious behavior—particularly given the events or issues that led to the revocations in the first place (e.g., DV incidents, psychiatric crises leading to suicide attempts, destruction of property).

CASE EXAMPLE 7: JONATHAN ASTOR (GUN RIGHTS RESTORATION)

Jonathan is 31 years old and has been around guns throughout his life. He was introduced to them in the Boy Scouts as an adolescent and has continued to engage in trap and skeet shooting as well as general target practice. He secured his firearms purchaser permit at age 18 and has been a member of a rod and gun club since. He owns three shotguns, which he uses for trap and skeet shooting, and two handguns he usually brings to the 25-yard indoor range near his home. Jonathan maintains his firearms unloaded in a safe in his basement and ammunition in a separate locked case. Over the last 6 months, Jonathan and his fiancé, Amy, have experienced difficulty in their relationship. They had been dating for nearly 8 years without any notable problems but began to argue with some regularity once they got engaged—primarily about issues related to their wedding plans and the like. The tension ultimately escalated to a troubled point and their fights became physical for the first time. Namely, 2 weeks ago, Amy pushed Jonathan when he made a comment about her mother's involvement in the wedding plans during a heated argument and he responded by screaming at her, pushing her back, and throwing a small potted plant against the wall. Amy immediately ran to her room and called her father, who then contacted the police. The dispatcher reportedly asked if there were guns in the home and Amy's father answered affirmatively. Approximately 10 minutes later, two police officers responded to the home and separated Amy and Jonathan. Although they found no basis for an arrest, the officers asked Jonathan if he would leave the home to "cool off," at least for the next couple days, to which he agreed. They also asked if he would allow them to take his firearms for "safekeeping." He balked initially, but ultimately agreed when they told him he could have them back "once everything settled down" in his relationship. The officers asked both parties if they wanted to file formal complaints or seek temporary restraining orders (TROs), but both declined. Within a few days, Jonathan returned home, and he and Amy decided to start couples therapy. They did so and, after a few weeks, Jonathan went to the police department to reclaim his guns. However, they stated he would need to provide a certification from a doctor indicating that he is safe to own and operate them. The couple's therapist was unwilling to issue such a certification, but the department indicated he needed such from a doctor anyhow. They also informed Jonathan that they referred his situation to the county prosecutor's office, who was considering issuing a formal denial. Given the situation, Jonathan hired an attorney who advised him to find a forensic mental health evaluator who could assess his suitability, issue a report, and testify, if needed.

This case is not particularly uncommon in the firearm ownership context, especially because relationship dynamics and sentiments can change dramatically and suddenly, but can return to baseline rather quickly as well. Thus, it is not uncommon for protective orders (e.g., TROs) to be dismissed or otherwise dropped soon after they are sought and granted. Moreover, the person who initiated such may even be the strongest advocate for the reinstatement of their partner's gun rights and property (e.g., firearms, ammunition). It is important to highlight the fact that *misdemeanor* DV and IPV scenarios have a fairly weak correlation with firearm-related violence. That said, every situation requires an independent assessment that takes the context into account, as there are particular risk factors associated with firearm-involved violence and suicide in these situations. For example, a number of factors have been found to be associated with lethal DV, including but not limited to prior history of DV; marital estrangement;

Ψ *Misdemeanor* DV and IPV scenarios have a fairly weak correlation with firearm-related violence.

obsessive-possessiveness, including extreme jealousy, stalking, and suicide attempts or threats; threats to kill; and child custody disputes (Johnson et al., 1999). Although this is not an exhaustive list, it is useful to recognize that it includes a set of factors that are distinct from many (non-fatal) DV and IPV situations, which illustrates the importance of attention to nuance and context when assessing risk.

The situation involving Jonathan and Amy presented in this section did not involve a firearm, the threat of using one, or even causing severe bodily harm otherwise. Recognizing such is not to minimize what happened or even suggest that extreme violence or suicide could not occur at a later point. Of course, we are not mind readers and none of us has a crystal ball. In fact, *we advise against employing a prediction-based risk assessment approach* anyhow. Therefore, while we do not try to predict any future event, we seek to identify risk and protective factors—and, ultimately, *likely scenarios*, as we highlight in the *Risk Assessment Models and Approaches* section that follows. The key is to focus on probabilities rather than possibilities because, essentially, anything is possible.

As for Jonathan and Amy, they never had a problematic relationship, but they began to experience difficulties in the context of planning their wedding. Arguments ensued and they engaged in some pushing for the first time. In conducting a gun rights restoration evaluation of Jonathan, the particular focus would need to be on their relationship dynamics and any additional DV-related risk and protective factors we can identify. However, we still recommend conducting a comprehensive mental health firearm evaluation in which a full range of firearm-specific and prohibitor factors are also addressed—just as in the case of an initial or return applicant. It

> Ψ Focus on probabilities rather than possibilities because, essentially, anything is possible.

is also important to note that the use of formal risk assessment measures will be possible in many restoration, or reinstatement, matters because the behaviors and statements in question will likely meet their definitions of violence, DV, or those related self-injury concerns.

RISK ASSESSMENT MODELS AND APPROACHES

In this section, we provide an overview of violence, suicide, and firearm-specific risk assessment frameworks, which are sometimes also referred to as "models" or "approaches." Although evaluators can employ unstructured, semi-structured, or structured approaches, it is not advisable to conduct an unstructured risk assessment for various reasons, which we will highlight in the subsections that follow. Of additional note is that our conceptualization of evaluating firearm ownership suitability includes accounting for firearm-specific factors *in addition* to those related to examinees' response styles, interpersonal violence risk, suicide risk, mental health, and substance use. Simply put: Firearm evaluations must be grounded in contemporary risk assessment principles. This is important because the legal standards we are ultimately addressing in these contexts are primarily based on prohibitors related to violence and suicide risk. Of course, potential concerns related to acciden- tal injury and death due to improper storage or handling are quite relevant (e.g., child access prevention issues) and should be considered in these assess- ments as well, but the overarching focus in gun evaluations tends be risk to self or others via purposeful, or intentional, acts. Nevertheless, we reiterate our posi-

> Ψ Firearm evaluations must be grounded in contemporary risk assessment principles. They should be at least semistructured (never unstructured), and violence and sui- cide risk assessments are *necessary but not sufficient* components.

tion that assessing violence and suicide risk per se in firearm evaluations is *necessary but not sufficient* given that many, if not most, examinees who will come to us would have not engaged in behaviors associated with violence or self-injury—and, as such, additional factors should be addressed to conduct comprehensive firearm evaluations. Before we turn to firearm-specific assessment models, we provide a general overview of violence and suicide risk assessment models and approaches to illustrate how the mental health field has developed in these regards and, ultimately, how such has laid the foundation for conducting firearm evaluations.

Violence Risk Assessment

Formal violence risk assessment models were developed throughout the 20th century and specific approaches to assess risk have been characterized as first, second, third, and fourth generation (Bonta & Andrews, 2007). The first-generation method con- sisted of what has been referred to as *unstructured professional judgment*, which was used during most of the first half of the 1900s (Grove et al., 2000; Rice, 1997). In fact, this is not much of a method at all, as mental health professionals simply use their clinical intuition to make judgments about examinees' risk levels based on interview and other available data. However, by the 1970s, actuarial, evidence-based assessment instruments had been developed for use in place of the unstructured approach (Bonta & Andrews, 2007). This is considered the second generation of risk assessment. The empirical research related to violence risk proliferated and particularly focused on iden- tifying correlates of violence and violent recidivism, which were then included as items on various actuarial measures. As such, actuarial measures tend to rely on the scoring of static (i.e., historical, stable) factors that have been found to be correlated with vio- lence and violent recidivism. However, the inclusion of static factors is not what makes something an actuarial measure, although the concept may be frequently confused. Rather, a measure is characterized as actuarial if the procedure involves adding item scores to produce a cumulative or total score that is then linked to a probability, or quantitative estimate, of risk (Heilbrun, 2009). An example of an actuarial measure is the Violence Risk Appraisal Guide (VRAG; Harris et al., 1993; Quinsey et al., 1998).

Given that research demonstrated actuarial risk assessment instruments were supe- rior to unstructured clinical judgment when predicting violence (Bonta & Andrews, 2007; Heilbrun, 2009), a professional debate ensued over the utility of clinical decision-making at all. Indeed, Paul Meehl (1954) compared clinical versus statistical prediction in his seminal book, which has been frequently cited to support the notion that actuarial methods are best and clinical decision-making is faulty; it is not uncommon to still hear some say that "clinical decision-making is no better than chance." However, these sentiments are often based on a misinterpretation of the professional research and commentary in this context. Namely, it is *unstructured* clinical judgment rather than *structured* clinical judgment that is being (negatively) referenced in the context of clinical prediction and decision-making (Westen & Weinberger, 2004).

Nevertheless, there are at least three notable shortcomings of second-generation, or actuarial, measures:

1. They are atheoretical.
2. They often heavily or exclusively rely upon static, or historical, risk factors and, therefore, they do not account for recent or current changes in patients that may affect risk levels (i.e., *dynamic* risk factors, such as treatment progress and current mental state).
3. Psychometric properties are characteristics of data and not tests; therefore, it is necessary to have research on specific normative samples to be able to generalize a person's score properly.

Realizing these limitations, test developers and researchers began to account for dynamic risk factors (i.e., current, changeable), which led to the development of third-generation risk assessment measures and guides that include both static and dynamic factors as well as those associated with risk management and reduction (Andrews et al., 2006; Bonta, 2002; Bonta & Andrews, 2007). Structured professional judgment (SPJ) measures are a part of this classification, as they include empirically derived static and dynamic risk factors; however, they are coded rather than scored. In other words, even when numbers are used for coding purposes (e.g., 2 = present, 1 = partially present, 0 = absent), they are not intended to be aggregated and, therefore, no total scores are generated for clinical use.[1] In fact, a significant concern can arise from

> Ψ It is not uncommon to still hear some say that "clinical decision-making is no better than chance." However, these sentiments are often based on a misinterpretation of the professional research and commentary in this context. Namely, it is *unstructured* clinical judgment rather than *structured* clinical judgment that is being (negatively) referenced in the context of clinical prediction and decision-making.

---

[1] Confusion can arise when researchers combine item scores to generate total scores for so-called research purposes—while simultaneously advising against such for clinical uses. Typically, researchers do so in an effort to analyze certain psychometric properties associated with the internal structure of the measure (e.g., construct validity) rather than properties related to its use in the real world (e.g., predictive validity). However, clinicians can misinterpret the research in this way by simply pointing to the fact

even a single risk factor on an SPJ measure, leading to a high-risk determination (e.g., an examinee making a substantive threat at present).

One example of an SPJ measure is the Historical, Clinical, Risk Management-20, Version 3 (HCR-20ᵛ³; Douglas et al., 2013). The inclusion of dynamic risk factors is important because it provides us with the ability to consider how examinees' current functioning and risk factors affect their risk levels, and it also allows us to consider how a change in such factors may impact these levels. Nevertheless, it is essential to consider both static and dynamic risk factors as well as protective factors when assessing violence risk– and to focus on *prevention* rather than *prediction*. As Skeem and Monahan (2011) articulated it:

> Ψ The inclusion of dynamic risk factors is important because it provides us with the ability to consider how examinees' current functioning and risk factors affect their risk levels, and it also allows us to consider how a change in such factors may impact these levels. In fact, it is essential to consider both static and dynamic risk factors as well as protective factors when assessing risk—and to focus on *prevention* rather than *prediction*.

The violence risk assessment field may be reaching a point of diminishing returns in instrument development. We might speculate that incremental advances could be made by exploring novel assessment methods, including implicit measures (Nock et al., 2010) or simple heuristics (Goldstein & Gigerenzer, 2009). But specific structured techniques seem to account for very little of the variance in predictive accuracy. If we are approaching a ceiling in this domain, there clearly are miles to go on the risk reduction front. We hope that forensic psychology shifts more of its attention from predicting violence to understanding its causes and preventing its (re)occurrence. (p. 41)

Moreover, as we will reiterate in the suicide risk assessment subsection that follows, we are not able to predict certain important outcomes with particular accuracy. Perhaps the title of the American Psychological Association's November 2016 press release speaks for itself in this respect: "After Decades of Research, Science Is No Better Able to Predict Suicidal Behaviors." Such was based on a meta-analysis of 50 years of research conducted by Franklin and colleagues (2017), who analyzed 365 studies and concluded that suicide risk prediction was "only slightly better than chance

---

that researchers, even measures' developers themselves, calculate total scores and correlate them with particular variables. This may provide evaluators with a false sense of protection vis-à-vis procedural credibility, despite not using measures in the way they were intended. For instance, SPJ measures are not intended to be used as actuarial measures; in fact, doing so is in direct contrast to the SPJ conceptual framework. Indeed, SPJ measures were developed *to avoid* such a method. The fact that some researchers, even measures' developers themselves, have done so for a particular research purpose does not give clinicians a pass to use said measures in a conceptually and clinically inappropriate manner. Researchers and practitioners share responsibility in being transparent and articulate when outlining their methods, as not to confuse others across professional disciplines and roles.

for all outcomes" and "predictive ability has not improved across 50 years of research" (p. 187). This finding provides substantial support for employing a prevention- rather than prediction-based approach when assessing risk, such as taking an SPJ approach, for instance. SPJ guidelines typically include developing both risk formulations and likely scenarios (see Hart et al., 2016). In practice, various techniques may be used to generate a risk formulation, and one such method is to identify factors that drive, (dis)inhibit, or otherwise impact the likelihood that someone will engage in violence (i.e., risk and protective factors). Once we have created a useful formulation of the case at hand, we can begin to focus on risk moving forward. Once again, we are not trying to predict any future events, but rather we seek to develop potential, realistic events that may unfold based on the risk and protective factors we have outlined. As Hart and colleagues (2016) articulated it:

> Ψ Various techniques may be used to generate a risk formulation; one is to identify factors that drive, (dis)inhibit, or otherwise impact the likelihood that someone will engage in violence (i.e., risk and protective factors). Once we have created a useful formulation, we can begin to focus on risk moving forward. We are not trying to predict future events, but rather, we are seeking to develop potential, realistic events that may unfold based on the risk and protective factors we have outlined.

We must ask ourselves, what kind of violence am I worried that the person might commit? What will he do, to whom, and why? What might be the psychological or physical harm suffered by others? Where and when is he likely to perpetrate such violence? Is the risk acute in nature, limited to certain times or situations, or is it chronic? How certain or confident am I that this kind of violence might actually occur? The process of answering these questions allows us to use narrative cognition to evaluate the plausibility of the scenario in the light of what we know about violence and people in general, and more specifically about the person we are evaluating and his or her history of violence. We must remember that all scenarios, as stories of a future that has not yet and may never occur, are fictional. The goal is not to predict what will happen, but rather to consider systematically what might happen. For evaluators, scenario planning may be considered a form of thought experiment or *Gedankenspiel* about what kinds of violence a person might perpetrate in the future, a way to do one's mental "due diligence" with respect to violence risk . . .

There is an art to developing scenarios. For example, they should not be too specific or detailed. We should ask, could this type of violence occur in a different way, or with a different outcome, or under different circumstances? If so, we can broaden one scenario to encompass several variations on a single theme. Also, we should avoid generating too many scenarios, else case management planning is cumbersome. We start by considering our greatest fear or concern, then consider the next largest, and so forth. At some point, the remaining fears or concerns are relatively minor and, in this respect, more or less indistinguishable. There is no need to proceed further. Good plans are focused on primary hazards; it is impossible to develop plans that take into account every possible outcome. Although artful, scenarios developed in this way should not be perceived by others as fantasy or wild speculation, but rather as descriptions of negative outcomes that are plausible or reasonable in the light of general knowledge, professional experience, and the facts of the case at hand. (p. 656)

As is clear, this risk assessment approach lends itself to identifying and implementing interventions focused on violence risk management and reduction—and not prediction. As we indicated in Chapter 3, we also encourage our fellow clinicians and other professionals working both in private practice and group settings, such as schools, clinics, hospitals, and businesses, to consider the Comprehensive School Threat Assessment Guidelines (CSTAG; Cornell, 2018). The CSTAG, formerly the Virginia Model for Student Threat Assessment, is grounded in contemporary theory and has empirical support—from both field tests and controlled studies (see https://education.virginia.edu/faculty-research/centers-labs-projects/research-labs/youth-violence-project/comprehensive-school). Although it was developed for responding to student threats of violence, we believe the CSTAG has utility in a wide range of contexts that call for risk assessments, including but certainly not limited to truncated assessments during treatment sessions. While we are not advocating for the misapplication of these guidelines or for their use in any unintended manner, they provide a useful framework from which to draw. Namely, the steps outlined in the model reflect a stepwise, decision-making approach to assessing risk that is both efficient and grounded in strong risk assessment principles. Specifically, the CSTAG consists of five steps once a threat arises:

1. Evaluate the threat.
2. Attempt to resolve the threat as transient.
3. Respond to a substantive threat.
4. Conduct a safety evaluation for a very serious substantive threat.
5. Implement and monitor the safety plan.

A key component of the CSTAG is distinguishing between *transient* and *substantive threats*. Transient threats can be quickly addressed and triaged because they are those that reflect an expression of emotions rather than the substantive intent to do harm to others. Within the context of their model, Cornell and colleagues have provided guidance in this regard by illustrating a continuum of threats—in escalating fashion from figures of speech, jokes, fleeting expressions of anger, attention-seeking/boasting, thrill of causing a disruption, to attempt to intimidate, or warn of impending

> Ψ It is important to distinguish between *transient* and *substantive threats*. Transient threats can be quickly addressed and triaged because they are those that reflect an expression of emotions rather than the substantive intent to do harm to others.

violence. We strongly recommend readers to review the available publications on the CSTAG, including under its former name—the Virginia Model—to gain a more thorough and detailed understanding of what goes into each of the aforementioned steps.

Suicide Risk Assessment

As we highlight throughout this handbook, two-thirds of gun deaths are suicides; therefore, it is essential to outline suicide risk assessment principles in this context. As with interpersonal violence, the suicide and self-injury–related literature is longstanding and extensive. Thus, we refer the interested reader to the more comprehensive review we previously published (i.e., Pirelli et al., 2019, Chapter 6). One particularly important point to highlight is that some contemporary theories diverge from earlier ones in many respects. For instance, in their interpersonal theory of suicide, Van Orden and colleagues (2010) conceptualized suicide as being caused by the simultaneous presence of two interpersonal constructs: *thwarted belongingness* (social isolation) and *perceived burdensomeness* (e.g., in the context of family conflict, unemployment, and physical illness). As they noted, older theories, such as that of Shneidman (1985, 1987, 1998), focused on individual factors, with "psychache" (i.e., psychological and emotional pain that reaches intolerable intensity) as the primary causal factor of suicide. However, according to Van Orden et al. (2010):

> In contrast to Shneidman's model, we propose that the need to belong is the need central to the development of suicidal desire, consistent with the wealth of findings linking social connectedness to suicidal behavior.

Thus, the interpersonal theory is consistent with past theoretical accounts of suicidal behavior through its proposal for a key role for social connectedness. However, the interpersonal theory diverges from previous theories in its proposal that an unmet "need to belong" (Baumeister & Leary, 1995, p. 1) is the specific interpersonal need involved in desire for suicide. (p. 582)

Ψ Van Orden and colleagues (2010) conceptualized suicide as being caused by the simultaneous presence of two interpersonal constructs: *thwarted belongingness* (social isolation) and *perceived burdensomeness* (e.g., in the context of family conflict, unemployment, and physical illness). In contrast, older theories focused on individual factors, with "psychache" (i.e., psychological and emotional pain that reaches intolerable intensity) as the primary causal factor of suicide.

This is important to us as clinicians to recognize because individual factors in the context of "psychache" should not be necessarily assumed to be causal in the context of suicide attempts or completed suicides. Various other longstanding assumptions are viewed differently than they once were as well. For example, we should also not automatically assume the presence of fear leading up to the act of self-harm. In fact, decreased fear of death has been regarded as a risk factor in some contemporary suicide risk assessment models in relation to what is referred to as the *acquired capability* for suicide. The relevant interaction here is that of *increased* pain tolerance and *reduced* fear of death. In fact, fear of death or dying because of pain and suffering is an empirically based primary protective factor associated with decreased risk of suicide attempt or death by suicide (e.g., see the Columbia Suicide Severity Rating Scale [C-SSRS]; Posner et al., 2011).

As we discussed in Chapter 4, the C-SSRS is perhaps the leading suicide assessment measure available: It has been endorsed by many national organizations, it has extensive empirical support (see the Columbia Lighthouse Project, 2020), and its development has been equated to the advent of antibiotics. Given that it is advisable to move away from a prediction-based approach and toward a prevention-based, or risk management and reduction approach, the C-SSRS is a great option. It lends itself to such and is similar to SPJ measures in that it incorporates empirically based risk and protective factors but does not try to quantify and aggregate them in an actuarial manner. There are numerous versions of the measure available because it has been designed and modified to be used by a very wide range of people across many settings and contexts, including by families, friends, and neighbors; first responders; government personnel; healthcare professionals; military personnel; school personnel; correctional professionals; and researchers. Even within these groups, there are nuanced versions that apply to different timepoints of interest and the like. For our purposes, we provide a brief overview of the "Risk Assessment" version for healthcare professionals.

On the Risk Assessment version of the C-SSRS, the first five areas pertain to suicidal and self-injurious behavior; namely, whether there have been preparatory acts or actual suicide attempts in the past 3 months or in one's lifetime, or other self-injurious behaviors without suicidal intent. The second section covers five areas related to suicidal ideation over the past month, to include thoughts and intent to die by suicide. The third section accounts for recent activating events, such as recent losses and other negative events, including legal, financial, or relationship problems as well as pending incarceration, homelessness, or current or pending isolation. The fourth section contains four areas associated with one's treatment history; namely, previous mental health diagnoses and treatment, hopelessness or dissatisfaction with treatment, noncompliance with treatment, and a history of not receiving treatment. The fifth and lengthiest section pertains to the person's recent clinical status. There are 15 areas to account for in this section, such as hopelessness; various serious mental health symptoms and episodes; highly impulsive behavior; substance misuse; perceived burden on family or others; chronic pain; homicidal ideation; aggressive behavior; method for suicide available; refusal or inability to agree to safety plan; a history of sexual abuse; and family history of suicide. The sixth section addresses recent protective factors, such as identified reasons for living; feeling a responsibility to family or others as well as living with family; having a supportive social network or family; being fearful of death or dying due to pain and suffering; believing suicide is immoral; and engaging in work or school.

There are also two additional open-ended sections on this version of the C-SSRS in which other risk and protective factors can be included, and a final section to describe any suicidal, self-injurious, or aggressive behaviors with their corresponding dates. It is readily apparent why the C-SSRS has utility in suicide risk assessments: It is comprehensive, empirically based and supported, and very user-friendly and efficient for a wide range of clinical applications. Still, formally addressing these factors is necessary but insufficient in firearm-specific evaluations. Just as examinees may not have engaged in violence in the past, they may not have a history or presentation associated with suicide-related concerns. Therefore, incorporating something like the C-SSRS would be one component of a what is a much more comprehensive firearm-specific evaluation.

FIREARM-SPECIFIC ASSESSMENT

Firearm-specific evaluations are a type of FMHA and, therefore, need to be grounded in the principles we have outlined throughout this chapter. However, there are unique aspects to gun evaluations above and beyond risk assessments and other types of FMHAs that evaluators need to consider and incorporate in order to be comprehensive. First and foremost, when a person's firearm ownership suitability comes into question as a result of a mental health-related concern, it has essentially become a forensic issue. Therefore, an evaluator must assess the association between the purported mental health problem and an examinee's appropriateness to own and operate a firearm. As with many types of FMHAs, the presence of a bona fide mental health–related issue must first be established. This is a *threshold* issue. In other words, if there is no mental health–related problem, there can certainly be no connection between such and suitability for firearm ownership. It is important to emphasize here, though, that we are speaking rather broadly in terms of constitutes a "mental health–related concern." For our purposes in this context, we are referring to factors associated with violence risk, DV and IPV risk, suicide risk, mental health, and substance use. Indeed, our firearm ownership suitability model includes these domains in addition to accounting for response style and various firearm-specific factors. There is another model to consider when conducting certain types of firearm-specific evaluations as well, published by Gold and Vanderpool (2016), which we will now review before turning to our model.

> Ψ When a person's firearm ownership suitability comes into question as a result of a mental health–related concern, it has essentially become a forensic issue. Therefore, an evaluator must assess the association between the purported mental health problem and an examinee's appropriateness to own and operate a firearm. Like most other FMHAs, the presence of a bona fide mental health–related issue must first be established (i.e., a *threshold* issue).

Relief from Disability

Gold and Vanderpool (2016) set forth over a dozen sets of inquiries to incorporate into relief from disability (RFD) evaluations. Their assessment framework is consistent with the Consortium for Risk-Based Firearm Policy's (2013a, 2013b) recommendations in addition to the principles Heilbrun (2009) set forth in his book on best practices in risk assessment. Within the context of their framework, Gold and Vanderpool present 16 sets of questions for the evaluator to incorporate, corresponding to the following areas of inquiry: the reason the person is seeking restoration of their gun rights; identifying the factors associated with the prohibition in the first place, including if such pertains to concerns about firearm misuse, mental health, violence, suicide, or substance misuse; assessing adherence to and the impact of mental health treatment, if applicable; identifying various static and dynamic risk and protective factors; and determining if access to guns would increase risk.

Ψ Gold and Vanderpool (2016) set forth over a dozen sets of inquiries to incorporate into relief from disability (RFD) evaluations. Their framework as consistent with the Consortium for Risk-Based Firearm Policy's (2013a, 2013b) recommendations in addition to the principles Heilbrun (2009) set forth in his book on best practices in risk assessment.

Pirelli Firearm-10

Firearm evaluation models need to be sufficiently flexible to meet the demands of a range of gun ownership–related cases and associated legal standards. Therefore, we have developed our model, the Pirelli Firearm-10 (PF-10), consistent with an SPJ approach. Unstructured clinical assessment approaches should not be used because they are simply subpar and empirically inferior to more structured evaluation formats. Actuarial approaches are certainly better to use than unstructured approaches and may have utility in certain contexts but would fall short in most gun ownership evaluation contexts for a number of reasons. For instance:

1. They are based on the concept of prediction rather than risk management and prevention, which would be contraindicated in the context of trying to accurately assess risk in such considerably low-base-rate behaviors as firearm-involved violence and suicide.
2. They often rely on static, or historical, risk factors rather than present- and future-oriented dynamic factors.
3. They require the aggregation of item scores to be compared to a normative group, and we simply do not have sufficient data in this regard in this arena.
4. Their use is often dependent on the examinees having engaged in certain behaviors (e.g., interpersonal violence) that would not be applicable to many, if not most, firearm applicants.

Ψ The Pirelli Firearm-10 (PF-10) is a framework we developed consistent with an SPJ assessment approach.

It is a 10-domain framework to be used in conjunction with a semistructured interview to facilitate clinical decision-making in firearm-specific evaluations. The PF-10 includes gun-specific and response-style domains, in addition to those more generally associated with gun ownership–related prohibitors and concerns (e.g., violence, DV, suicide, mental health, substance use).

Again, actuarial measures may have some utility in certain firearm evaluation matters, such as for those seeking reinstatement after a problematic incident, but they are likely to lack utility, regardless, by not accounting for the full range of factors relevant in firearm-related matters. Indeed, a more flexible yet evidence-based approach is needed in these matters, but it must also be one that is comprehensive (i.e., inclusive of all relevant factors). Namely, it is beneficial to utilize an evaluation framework that is semi-structured in nature and includes a set of domains in line with research findings, forensic assessment principles, and legal standards. We developed the PF-10 in this manner and also in such a way that is sufficiently flexible for evaluators to incorporate additional, supplemental measures as needed (e.g., measures of violence, DV, and suicide risk; response style; psychopathology; substance use problems). Moreover, a firearm evaluation framework must formally address firearm-specific factors. These fundamental perspectives led to the development of the PF-10.

In addition to covering the types of areas included in the aforementioned RFD framework, the PF-10 contains gun-specific domains associated with an examinee's history of exposure to firearms; knowledge of and perspectives on gun safety and related regulations; personal experience with guns; and intent for use, storage, and continued education. The PF-10 also calls for the consideration of an examinee's *response style*, consistent with forensic assessment principles. The PF-10 was developed as an SPJ guide designed to assist practitioners conducting firearm evaluations with civilian gun applicants or with those seeking to have their gun rights reinstated. However, it may also have utility in other types of firearm-related matters, such as in evaluations with law enforcement, correctional, governmental, and armed security personnel.

The PF-10 is a 10-domain framework to be used in conjunction with a semistructured interview to facilitate clinical decision-making in firearm-specific evaluations. This framework also calls for the consideration of data from other sources typically included in FMHAs (e.g., record review, collateral interviews, psychological testing). The 10 domains are as follows and will be described in greater detail below:

1. Reason for seeking licensure/reinstatement
2. Exposure to firearms
3. Knowledge of and perspectives on firearm safety precautions and relevant firearm regulations

4. Firearm use: experience, intent for use, storage, and continued education
5. Response style
6. Violence risk
7. Domestic violence and intimate partner violence risk
8. Suicide risk
9. Mental health
10. Substance use

Domain 1: Reason for Seeking Licensure/Reinstatement

When vetting a potential referral and prior to accepting it, we must first determine if the examinee is an initial or return applicant or someone seeking reinstatement in the context of a gun forfeiture matter (i.e., gun rights restoration). Clarifying the referral question is an important first step in essentially all evaluation contexts because it sets the stage for the rest of our involvement and associated actions (and inactions). Indeed, we must determine if we have sufficient professional competence and are willing to take the referral in the first place. If so, having a clear understanding of the reason for the referral will guide our next steps along the hypothesis-testing process that is forensic assessment.

Referral incidents associated with gun forfeiture matters are often those that have occurred more recently than situations for which initial applicants are flagged. Therefore, they often come with more acute concerns related to violence, DV, psychiatric stability, and substance use. Of course, by definition, they also include the assessment of someone who was already a gun owner, perhaps for many years. On the other hand, there are flagged applicants who have never owned or even used a firearm. There are certainly cases whereby an existing gun owner is flagged when trying to secure an additional permit or firearm, as particular databases become available over time and lead to a hit on a background check (i.e., what we refer to as "return applicants").

For example, take Mr. Jones, who has owned guns for 10 years without incident but was flagged when he sought to purchase another firearm because a brief childhood psychiatric hospital visit arose during a routine background check. This can happen in certain jurisdictions even if the record has never come up before. It may very well be the case as well that no actual records from the hospital admission are available, particularly when many years have passed because of recordkeeping policies and even the possibility of a facility's closure.

The overarching issue is that an examinee wants to be able to own and operate a firearm, and it is useful for us to know why—in addition to why the person is being blocked from doing so at this time. It is also necessary to ask about the jurisdiction at hand—namely, if the referral incident occurred in a different place from where the matter is now being addressed. Moreover, it is important to identify the immediate or foreseeable decision-makers as to the gun rights in question, and to determine if there are specific issues or particular (legal) language that needs to be addressed in the evaluation and corresponding report. It is also recommended to ask if an examinee has ever applied for a firearm before or if there have been any prior gun-related concerns or forfeitures, which may be further addressed in the domains that follow.

Remember: The nature of our questions and associated case conceptualizations can differ for those seeking a firearm for hunting purposes versus home defense or self-defense, and even from those who wish to engage in shooting sports. However, we should not impose our moral judgments in any case. Rather, our primary role within the context of this domain is to assess the *rationality* of an examinee's expressed intentions from a clinical perspective. Therefore, we are to focus more on an examinee's thought *process* as opposed to the particular *content* of the person's answer. Of course, a certain reason offered for wanting to be a gun owner can be problematic on its face, such as one reflecting overtly paranoid or otherwise psychotic thinking. However, a fair amount of latitude should be given to examinees when trying to understand why they want to own guns. Put differently, it should not matter to us as evaluators if gun rights are being sought for hunting, shooting sports, home defense or self-defense, or for any other legal purposes—again, unless clinical, case-specific concerns arise. Still, given that an examinee's rationale is our primary focus, we also must recognize that a concerning thought process may be reflected in the context of essentially any reason for seeking ownership.

In addition, asking about the specific type of firearm being sought can also inform our questions as well as our professional opinions. For instance, we know that handguns are more likely to be involved in homicides than long guns, which is an example of an important piece of information that might factor into our ultimate case conceptualization. Indeed, a homicide can be committed with any type of gun, but the base rates differ, and our opinions should incorporate consideration of such rates. It is also for this reason that evaluators who choose to conduct firearm-related evaluations receive continuing education as needed to develop and maintain their professional and cultural competence. For example, consistent with our KAD model, it is important for us as evaluators to become familiar with firearm-related language and considerations. For example, it can be important to know particular terms, such as *AR-15* and *semiautomatic*, and even the general ammunition counts in boxes for certain caliber guns. If we do not have such perspective and our evaluations are not appropriately contextualized, we can evidence bias and perpetuate misinformation via ill-informed opinions.

Domain 2: Exposure to Firearms

As we address in some detail in Chapters 1 and 6, cultural competence is a core component of professional competence. Ascertaining the type and level of exposure a person has had to firearms can help provide context to such cultural considerations. Furthermore, exposure to guns often impacts perspectives on firearm-related issues. For example, hunting is an integral aspect of some people's family histories and heritage. It may also be the case that law enforcement and military family histories are notable for certain people. Indeed, there are others who have been *negatively* exposed to guns in their lives, such as in the context of being around criminal activity or being affected by gun-involved violence or suicide at some level. Of course, there are many people who have had no direct or indirect exposure to guns in their lives at all.

As we indicated in the previous item, within the context of the overarching purpose of the PF-10, there are really no right or wrong answers here per se. While certain types of negative exposures (e.g., gun-involved interpersonal violence, gang activity) may be correlated with concerning outcomes and positive or prosocial exposures may be associated with favorable outcomes (e.g., gun safety), neither set of considerations is likely to be dispositive of gun ownership in and of themselves. Therefore, exposure is a factor we consider as one part of this more comprehensive PF-10 framework. Someone does not have to have any exposure to be considered suitable for firearm ownership, just as negative exposures do not necessarily make someone unsuitable. Again, the purpose here is to gain a better understanding of an examinee's history and perspectives, which may help inform our ultimate opinion about the person's appropriateness to own and operate guns. As such, within this domain, evaluators should inquire about the *type* and *nature* of direct and indirect exposure examinees have had to firearms throughout their lives. In this way, it is important to review the firearm-related subcultures we outlined in Chapter 1 (see also Pirelli & Witt, 2017). Please note, this domain is distinguishable from domain 4 (below), which pertains to a person's direct *experience* owning or operating guns.

Domain 3: Knowledge of and Perspectives on Firearm Safety Precautions and Relevant Firearm Regulations

There are certainly gun-related proficiency tests in certain jurisdictions for various reasons (e.g., hunter safety and concealed carry handgun courses), but this domain is not intended to be a test in any way. Instead, here, we are once again focused on gathering information to ultimately opine as to a person's firearm ownership suitability from a clinical perspective. Assessing an examinee's attitudes is an important step in the consideration of the person's *dynamic* violence and suicide risk factors.

Still, this domain should also include a review of any gun safety, education, or instructional courses in which the examinee has engaged. However, similar to the aforementioned domains, we are not looking for a person to meet a particular threshold or cutoff. Rather, we are seeking to gain a sense of an examinee's knowledge of and perspectives on relevant gun safety principles and regulations, primarily to ensure that they do not present with any notable concerns in this regard.

Put differently, a novice with little to no factual knowledge of gun safety principles or laws should not necessarily raise clinical concerns in the context of this domain; however, the person's *views* about such might. For instance, we are not speaking of a person's overarching thoughts on the Second Amendment or the like, but rather an expressed blatant disregard for gun safety principles or laws. In other words, someone may certainly disagree with a particular policy, but still indicate they intend to adhere to it. That said, we are also not law enforcement agents and, therefore, we are not seeking to investigate if someone has engaged or intends to engage in some level of lawbreaking. Think of how we handle situations whereby our clients tell us they smoked marijuana or ran a red light while driving; indeed, we typically would not necessarily become alarmed and would certainly not report these types of reported infractions. Similarly, examinees may report certain types of gun-related indiscretions or (minor) infractions. Instead of allowing our own views on guns to color our opinions, we should consider information within the context of the overarching evaluation and stay within its scope. In this case, we would likely be looking for *patterns of concerns* related to the person's gun ownership suitability and not run with a single piece of data, particularly one that may be relatively minor.

Nevertheless, gun owners should still, at least, have a general awareness and understanding of basic gun safety and laws. For example, those who have children in the home at any point should have a working knowledge of child access prevention (CAP) and storage laws. In addition, examinees should have a general understanding of gun carrying and transit laws. Again, we are not seeking to "test" an examinee's knowledge, but these types of inquiries are relevant when assessing a person's overall judgment and decision-making abilities. For instance, an examinee may be unaware of particular restrictions or requirements but be able to explain how to go about gathering the necessary information related to such. This domain highlights the importance of evaluators becoming familiar with relevant gun safety principles and laws—to be able to, in turn, adequately understand examinees' levels of knowledge.

Domain 4: Firearm Use: Experience, Intent for Use, Storage, and Continued Education

Within the context of this fourth and final firearm-specific domain, we seek to gather information about an examinee's direct experience operating or otherwise handling guns, in addition to the person's intended use, storage, and continued education moving forward. Consistent with the first three domains, whether someone has ever used or even come in contact with a gun is not a clinical concern. Regardless, it is important to inquire about examinees' intentions related to firearm use, storage, and education. It can still be helpful to include this information to provide context for examinees who have interacted with guns as well.

Namely, it can be informative to know that someone has interacted with guns for many years without incident, particularly during a referral incident period. Of course, someone can still engage inappropriately with a firearm in the future, but such may be more suggestive of out-of-character behavior driven by situational factors rather than a pattern of irresponsible behavior in the past. Although acts of negligence and poor responses to high-stress situations can both result in negative outcomes, data must be put into context to focus our assessment. It is generally unlikely for an examinee to be at high risk of engaging in every type of problematic behavior, particularly with a gun. Therefore, we can narrow down our concerns vis-à-vis the most *likely scenarios* that lie ahead by contextualizing our assessment.

Two additional components of this domain relate to an examinee's intent for use and storage, which are directly relevant and applicable to everyone we assess because they shed light on gun safety, consistent with the National Rifle Association's gun safety rules. There may be additional relevant considerations in a particular case as well, such as how children in the home will be introduced to and educated about the presence of a firearm or if anyone with likely access has any notable risk factors of concern in this context (e.g., history of violence, serious mental illness, and/or substance misuse). On one end of the continuum, someone may respond in a manner that raises concerns about their firearm ownership suitability. It is one thing for a person to have broken a law, perhaps naively, and it is quite another for someone to express complete disregard for gun safety principles and regulations, especially those related to proper use and storage. Novices may not have the precise language or laws down, but they should certainly be able to demonstrate an intent to properly use and store firearms.

As for the final component related to continuing education, examinees are not be legally required to engage in such in many cases. There are a number of exceptions, though, such as hunters and those who have carry permits in certain jurisdictions. Therefore, we should review collateral records that may be available and applicable, such as firearm-related certifications or test results—along with course certificates and related materials (as in domain 3 in relation to gun safety, more specifically). That said, this is another aspect of the evaluation that should not be counted against a person from a clinical perspective. Nevertheless, continuing education remains a relevant area of inquiry, as it can provide additional context to this comprehensive firearm ownership suitability evaluation. That said, it is worth highlighting that the response to this component is expected to comport with an examinee's intended use. While minimal competence is essential for all gun owners, we would expect appreciably greater levels from those who operate guns regularly compared to those who are unlikely to ever use their guns at all. As clinicians, we are not looking to assess examinees' firearm-related proficiency, but rather gauge their suitability for firearm ownership and use based on their behaviors and thought processes related to such.

Domain 5: Response Style

Consistent with FMHA best-practice standards, assessing an examinee's response style is an essential component given the potential for secondary gain in these types of evaluation contexts. However, it would be insufficient to consider only one type of response style (e.g., malingering) when evaluating examinees because there is a fairly wide range of ways people may approach evaluations and respond to questions. It would also be incorrect to assume people are honest across the board. There is a voluminous and longstanding research literature essentially indicating that we all lie at some level and with some regularity. Dr. Richard Rogers is a preeminent scholar in this area of study and has published the seminal text, *Clinical Assessment of Malingering and Deception*, which is now in its fourth edition. In its opening line, he noted: "Complete and accurate self-disclosure is a rarity even in the uniquely supportive context of a psychotherapeutic relationship" and, also, "Most individuals engage in a variety of response styles that reflect their personal goals in a particular setting" (p. 3; Rogers & Bender, 2018). Furthermore: "In summary, all individuals fall short of full and accurate self-disclosure, irrespective of the social context" (p. 4). As he and his collaborators indicate, there is much to consider vis-à-vis response styles across settings and examinee populations.

Given the importance of assessing response style in FMHAs and mental health assessments, more generally, we have made this a standalone domain within the PF-10 framework. As such, evaluators should formally assess examinees' response styles when possible. There are various ways to accomplish this, such as incorporating a psychological assessment measure that contains validity scales. Doing so can have utility in various ways because such measures can provide additional information related to the violence, suicide, mental health, and substance use domains that follow.

While most of us are likely familiar with the concept of malingering, it would actually be quite unlikely for an examinee in a firearm ownership–related matter to malinger; if anything, we would expect a person to want to present as healthy and stable. To the contrary, it would be much more likely for an examinee to engage in what is referred to as *positive impression management*, or portraying oneself in a socially desirable manner—free of shortcomings and mental health–related problems. This is not a particularly uncommon finding in certain types of forensic assessments, such as in parenting and fitness-for-duty evaluations, whereby people want to come across as healthy and well adjusted.

As evaluators, we must also remember that we should typically not base our opinions on single data points, with the exception of particularly compelling information (e.g., an examinee threatens to engage in violence or self-harm). Moreover, we must not paint an examinee with broad strokes, as an elevated score on a validity scale does not mean the person responded in such a manner to every inquiry during an evaluation. In actuality, an examinee can engage in numerous types of response styles within a single set of inquiries; they may be forthcoming to one question, lie on the next, and minimize in response to a third. Human interactions can be very complex and nuanced, which we must recognize. Nevertheless, it remains appropriate for us to assess response style and account for it in our assessment because it can facilitate our decision-making related to the weight we ascribe to available data when forming our opinions. Of course, data from psychological testing represent only one source; we must seek to gather data from multiple sources, including from the clinical interview and collateral sources, to determine the levels and nature of convergence or divergence.

Ψ In the context of assessing response style in gun evaluations, it is more likely for examinees to engage in *positive impression management* or portraying themselves in socially desirable ways—free of shortcomings and mental health–related problems—as opposed to negative impression management, malingering, or the like.

Domain 6: Violence Risk

Most acts of violence are not attributable to even severe mental illness. It is also the case that many examinees we will see, particularly initial and return applicants (as opposed to those in gun forfeiture matters), have not engaged in any known acts of violence per se. In fact, eight out of 10 felonies in state courts are classified as non-violent (Bone, 2010). Still, interpersonal violence risk is a central concern in firearm-related matters; indeed, it is those who have engaged in such violence who are typically cited in the context of gun control discussions—and not those who die by firearm-involved suicide (despite the numbers being double that of homicides and other gun-involved deaths combined).

As we addressed in the *Violence Risk Assessment* section earlier in this chapter, this area of study and practice has developed significantly in recent decades. Perhaps most notably, we have moved from engaging in unstructured to more structured evaluation approaches and, also, from seeking to predict dangerousness to assessing risk. Although we are not particularly accurate at predicting future acts of violence (or many other behaviors for that matter), there is certainly support for employing formal risk assessment and management frameworks into our evaluations (e.g., see Federal Bureau of Investigation, 2016; U.S. Secret Service, 2021). That said, assessing violence (and suicide) risk is an essential yet insufficient component of a comprehensive firearm evaluation. Presumably, that is a tenet with which most would agree, but the question remains: How can we best assess risk?

It is important to reiterate that many examinees will not have engaged in an act of violence per se, thereby rendering a number of formal violence risk assessment measures unusable in the typical fashion. This would be particularly true for *actuarial* measures, which are theoretically more mechanical in terms of their administration, scoring, and interpretation. This is yet another reason we subscribe to an SPJ approach. In addition to being empirically driven and semi-structured, an SPJ approach provides more flexibility to evaluators, particularly in matters such as these. Namely, the HCR-20[v3] (Douglas et al., 2013) has utility (even as an *aide-mémoire*) in many firearm-specific evaluations by including both static and dynamic empirically based items related to violence risk. Still, our gun evaluations need to be sufficiently context- and case-specific, consistent with an idiographic assessment approach. Exclusive reliance on nomothetic data (data derived from larger, representative groups) and broad-based concepts will lead us to overlook potential case-specific factors and nuances that can be rather distinguishing and, therefore, essential to consider in gun-related matters.

A guide like the HCR-20[v3] accounts for potential violence-related risk factors associated with an examinee's past, present, and future. Specifically, its historical section (H) comprises areas related to past violence, antisocial behavior, relationships, employment, substance use, mental health diagnoses, traumatic experiences, violent attitudes, and treatment or supervision response. Its clinical section (C) addresses current levels of insight, violent ideation or intent, mental health symptoms, instability, and treatment or supervision response. The third section accounts for risk management (R) areas, or future-oriented factors to consider, such as professional services and plans, living situation, personal support, treatment or supervision response, and stress or coping. In total, there are 20 empirically driven factors associated with violence risk. That said, the HCR-20 [v3] is not firearm-specific and, therefore, violence risk does not necessarily equal firearm-involved violence risk in this context. Therefore, we must go further and account for case-specific factors, the professional literature, and local norms to adequately cover this domain on the PF-10.

Evaluators must also be specific in relation to risk; namely, risk to *whom? when? where? why?* This type of clinical decision-making process is what Douglas and colleagues (2013) refer to as creating "likely scenarios"—that is, providing a context and accounting for *motivators, disinhibitors,* and *destabilizers.* For instance, a primary motivator in a particular matter may be a person's intense desire to seek revenge. Disinhibitors may relate to the person's negative self-concept, isolated lifestyle, lack of insight and awareness, and lack of empathy. Destabilizers may be disturbed perceptions about the target of the anger, impaired judgment, and unremitting, obsessive thoughts. This violence risk assessment model and type of case conceptualization may be applicable and quite useful in the context of assessing various types of violence risk, including, but not limited to, DV and IPV (i.e., domain 7).

Domain 7: Domestic and Intimate Partner Violence Risk

Although the vast majority of DV and IPV matters do not involve guns at all, the removal of firearms is often a priority when such issues arise (e.g., taking them out of the home). Indeed, so-called red flag laws have been modeled after restraining, or protective orders, in DV-related matters for a reason. Nevertheless, current or past DV or IPV is an explicit firearm ownership prohibitor in many legal statutes throughout the country and, as noted, restraining orders typically prompt the immediate revocation of guns and gun rights. However, it is important to highlight the fact that, empirically, it is the more serious and particularly violent scenarios that are tied to fatal, or lethal, DV incidents rather than those that are nonviolent or minimally so (e.g., misdemeanors and dismissed or dropped restraining orders).

As with all types of risk, we must conceptually parse the idea of whether an examinee made a threat from the actual question for us as clinical evaluators: Does the person *pose* a threat?

By the time someone has come to our attention in these matters and when DV is in question, it is axiomatic to say that the person has at least allegedly engaged in certain concerning behaviors. We are not the trier of fact, though, and it is not within our purview to determine what did or did not happen in the past. While we consider all relevant data related to such, our primary focus is to assess risk, which is a future-oriented opinion—albeit one that takes into account past, current, and future-related considerations. While "red flag" laws are being implemented more and more throughout the United States, fewer than half of the states have them on the books at this point. Still, every jurisdiction has some mechanism to issue protective orders, and there are many laws that provide discretion to law enforcement officers and judges to manage and otherwise intervene in DV-related matters.

From a risk assessment standpoint, we can incorporate formal measures, guides, and frameworks into our evaluations when an examinee is charged with or even accused of engaging in violence. For instance, we may use certain general violence risk assessment measures in these cases or a DV-specific measure, such as the Spousal Assault Risk Assessment, Version 3 (SARA; Kropp & Hart, 2015) or the Domestic Violence Risk Appraisal Guide (DVRAG; Hilton et al., 2008). The SARA is a structured professional judgment measure developed by the same group who created the HCR-20[v3], whereas the DVRAG is an actuarial measure. As such, we would recommend the former, consistent with our SPJ framework and consistent with the way in which we assess violence (domain 6) and suicide risk (domain 8) via the PF-10. The Centers for Disease Control and Prevention (CDC) also provides a potentially useful resource of measures that may be useful for evaluators who are assessing DV-related concerns (Basile et al., 2007).

Regardless of how we decide to assess risk in this regard, it is necessary to emphasize that DV-related risk does not necessarily equate to firearm-involved DV risk per se. Speaking to this more specific type of risk requires an additional analysis and incorporation of case-specific factors, local norms, and the literature associated with firearm-involved DV. When considering DV-related risk, in general, it is important to consider perpetrator and victim factors (e.g., risk factors and vulnerabilities, respectively); behavioral factors (e.g., history of physical violence); and environmental and situational factors (e.g., ongoing child custody dispute).

It is particularly important to remember that fatal DV incidents typically include notable power and control dynamics as well as acts of particularly serious violence (e.g., choking, beating). Of course, we may be concerned by other behaviors and even verbal threats and the like, but if we are guided by base rates at some level, our initial operating position should be that a firearm is one of the least likely issues of concern in DV situations across the board. Our primary goal as evaluators is to try and identify the relatively few who may engage in firearm-involved DV, which is no easy feat. Once again, attempts to predict are ill advised; therefore, we need to assess risk in the contextualized fashion we have continued to discuss throughout this handbook. As such, we are seeking to account for general DV-related risk factors as well as those associated with fatal DV. One potentially useful conceptualization was set forth by Frye and colleagues (2006), who distinguished between *situational couple violence* and *intimate terrorism*, whereby a person uses violence to impose coercive control over another. Johnson et al. (1999) identified specific factors present in lethal DV situations, which are very important to attend to, especially in firearm-related matters: prior history of domestic violence; marital estrangement; obsessive-possessiveness, including extreme jealousy, stalking, and suicide attempts or threats; prior police involvement; prior criminal history of the perpetrator; threats to kill; substance use problems; protection orders; acute perceptions of betrayal; and child custody disputes (see Johnson et al., 1999).

Domain 8: Suicide Risk

As we have highlighted multiple times in this handbook, the majority of gun deaths in the United States each year are suicides. Firearm-involved suicides occur at a much higher rate than gun deaths resulting from interpersonal violence, in general, and at an exponentially greater rate than deaths from "mass" shootings. As clinicians, the importance of assessing suicide has been deeply ingrained in our education and training from the start, and it is regularly reinforced. Perhaps the only other area given as much attention in our clinical training is that of privacy and confidentiality, à la the Health Insurance Portability and Accountability Act (HIPAA) of 1996 and related considerations. Most of us have likely learned that firearm access is a primary risk factor to consider when assessing suicide risk. However, we urge a seemingly slight yet substantive adjustment to this concept; namely, it is *likely access* that is important to try and ascertain because the vast majority of people have potential access to a gun. In addition to the fact that at least one in three homes have firearms in the United States, it is relatively easy to gain access to a gun otherwise—legally (e.g., going to a gun range) or illegally (e.g., stealing one or buying one as a prohibited person, or what is called a *straw sale*). Therefore, the first concept we should adjust in our minds is that of likely access rather than access, simply.

Another important concept is that of likely access as a potentially *moderating* variable, or factor. This is a particularly salient consideration for those conducting firearm-specific evaluations because clinicians in therapeutic and general assessment contexts may not need to engage in such nuanced evaluations. In other words, their duty to protect or warn may be incurred at an earlier point in the assessment process and they may simply not need to set forth such detailed inquiries. Of course, it will still be essential to try to ascertain if someone at elevated risk has likely gun access, but it may not be a factor that tips the scale with respect to the person's level of risk per se. Rather, it may serve as an additional consideration related to the associated interventions needed to promote safety (e.g., it may be a piece of information conveyed to law enforcement). This is contrasted with a firearm-specific evaluation, such as a gun ownership evaluation incorporating this PF-10 framework, whereby even likely access to a gun is a given.

Put differently, it would not be useful to consider firearm access as a risk factor in gun evaluations because they, by definition, assume the person will have access—indeed, it is the point of the assessment. Therefore, we should consider likely access to be a potentially moderating variable, whereby we seek to determine if such access *combined* with other factors in a given case would elevate an examinee's suicide risk. This is true when assessing violence risk as well, including DV risk.

As such, a comprehensive suicide risk assessment includes the identification and analysis of risk factors, warning signs, and protective factors. It is important to remember, though, that the presence of suicide risk factors does not necessarily mean an examinee is at elevated risk of firearm-involved suicide. It is for this reason that we promote an empirically based, context-specific evaluation that accounts for general and case-specific factors as well as local norms. A good starting point would be to incorporate a formal suicide assessment measure into the PF-10 evaluation framework, such as the C-SSRS (Posner et al., 2011) or the Suicidal Behaviors Questionnaire-Revised (Osman et al., 2001). There is a fairly wide range of published suicide risk assessment measures available to clinicians and they can be used in essentially all cases because they do not necessarily require that the examinee has engaged in self-injurious behavior or a suicide attempt, or even that they experience suicidal ideation (i.e., in contrast to violence risk assessment measures). Even if suicide risk is not a particular concern in a given case, it is still advisable to at least cross-check known risk factors because of the strong connection between suicide and firearms within the context of gun deaths.

Domain 9: Mental Health

Despite public perception that mental illness is associated with firearm-involved (interpersonal) violence, the connection is actually quite weak. The real association, statistically speaking, is between mental illness and firearm-involved suicide. This is an important nuance because it demonstrates the problem with speaking of the connection between "gun violence and mental health." These terms are overly broad and rarely defined in public discourse, which can be misleading or otherwise cause confusion. Nevertheless, mental health is necessary to address within the context of this PF-10 model when assessing firearm ownership suitability. It is warranted given the overarching relationship between mental health–related problems and firearm-involved suicide, and also because we subscribe to an idiographic assessment approach that accounts for case-specific factors. In other words, even though there is a weak (statistical) relationship between mental illness and firearm-involved violence, such is not to say that it is not a particular concern for a particular examinee before us. Accounting for potentially significant variables is very much in line with best practices in risk assessment; jumping to conclusions based on faulty assumptions is not. As is the case in research endeavors, it is generally best to account for variables and analyze their potential significance in a given context as opposed to dismissing them or, worse, simply accepting them as fact.

As evaluators in firearm matters, we must differentiate between incorrect assumptions and empirically based information, and we also need to go well above and beyond broad concepts and labels. There are more than 300 disorders listed across more than 1,00 pages in the *Diagnostic and Statistical Manual of Mental Disorders*, Fifth Edition Text Revision (DSM-5-TR; American Psychiatric Association, 2022), and a large segment of the population will meet criteria for a diagnosable mental health condition at some point in their lives. It is also the case that diagnoses can be unbelievably heterogenous, as the DSM-5 classification system is based on symptom combinations or clusters. Perhaps Galatzer-Levy and Bryant's (2013) analysis is most illustrative in this regard; namely, they found there are 636,120 possible symptom combinations that can lead to a diagnosis of posttraumatic stress disorder (PTSD) via the previous DSM edition, the DSM-5. Most other diagnoses allow for a wide range of symptom combinations as well. For these reasons and more, a diagnosis alone usually lacks utility in firearm evaluations (and many other FMHA contexts). In fact, a diagnosis can be misleading, particularly when not adequately explained at the symptom and functional level, and when left to interpretation—especially by laypersons, but also by medical and mental health professionals. This reality, combined with the fact that statistically few people diagnosed with a mental health condition engage in any type of interpersonal violence, particularly that which involves a gun, requires us to closely consider the concept of mental illness in firearm-related matters.

Most mental health conditions have no particularly noteworthy connection to interpersonal violence or suicide. Remember that the DSM-5-TR includes a wide range of conditions, such as learning disorders, eating disorders, sleep disorders, phobias, and various other diagnoses that have no general, statistical connection to violence or suicide. Moreover, even those that have been found to be more associated with these issues (e.g., disruptive, impulse control, and conduct disorders; antisocial personality disorder; substance use disorders (SUDs); bipolar and related disorders; depressive disorders) are not necessarily predictive of any violent or self-injurious event, with or without guns. This is why we must assess the examinee from a functional perspective, whereby we first seek to ascertain if a mental health condition is present; if there is, we then determine its impact or lack thereof on the person's firearm ownership suitability. Of course, there are certain symptoms and diagnostic presentations that are likely to be troublesome on their face, such as certain schizophrenia spectrum and other psychotic disorders as well as paranoid, aggressive, or similarly concerning features. Acute substance misuse and suicidality are additional examples of obviously problematic presentations.

Nevertheless, in most cases, the presence of a mental health diagnosis alone is an inadequate criterion to set forth an opinion that someone is clinically inappropriate to own or operate guns. We need to focus on psychiatric crises more so than diagnoses. Significant efforts have been made to destigmatize mental illness over many decades, including the advent and evolution of the Americans with Disabilities Act of 1990 (ADA) and its 2008 revision (ADA Amendments Act of 2008). Long gone are the days when the mere presence of a mental illness blocks someone from being afforded certain legal rights or due process (e.g., a diagnosis does not per se equate to incompetence to make certain legal, medical, vocational, financial, or educational decisions). Therefore, as evaluators, we need to consider each examinee's symptom presentation in conjunction with other risk factors and across diagnostic categories. Once again, consider mental health as a potentially moderating variable rather than one that is dispositive of firearm-involved violence or suicide risk. As a practical matter, this is another reason why traditional psychological assessment instruments may have utility in firearm evaluations—such as personality assessment inventories or cognitive tests—if we believe these types of mental health–related issues may impact an examinee's suitability for firearm ownership (e.g., poor decision-making associated with cognitive deficits or psychosis). These are potentially important areas to cover in what is a comprehensive assessment approach incorporating the PF-10 framework.

Domain 10: Substance Use

As noted within the context of the aforementioned mental health domain (domain 9), certain substance use–related conditions are particularly concerning; in particular, active problems with substance misuse have been found to be associated with various types of interpersonal violence and self-injurious behavior. With respect to firearm misuse, specifically, acute and chronic alcohol misuse situations should raise considerable concerns. Less clear and ostensibly compelling are histories related to such, more broadly.

First and foremost, please note that we are using the term *misuse* and not simply *use* when discussing historical considerations, as a wide range of people have used a substance at least once in their life—even as benign as trying alcohol. In most cases, trying a substance in the past is unlikely to be a notable concern, in and of itself. As evaluators, we are primarily looking for histories that involve bona fide substance misuse, including those that rose to a level of substance dependence. The DSM-5-TR no longer differentiates between what was once referred to as substance abuse and that of dependence; now, someone essentially has an SUD, or they do not.

Per the DSM-5-TR, dependence was removed because it was easily conflated with addiction, even though tolerance and withdrawal are normal responses to various substances and are not necessarily indicative of an addiction per se. Thus, specifiers are used to indicate the level of severity of the condition (i.e., mild, moderate, severe) as well as particular features (e.g., perceptual disturbances). There are also additional specifiers that can be especially important in FMHAs such as firearm evaluations; namely, indicating if the condition is *in early remission* or *in sustained remission*, and if the person is *on maintenance therapy* or *in a controlled environment*. Sobriety is often considered a lifelong process for those with notable SUDs, but these specifiers can help form our case conceptualization and, therefore, facilitate our functional analysis in a given matter.

Of course, most substances are mind-altering at some level and can lead to impairments in various areas of daily functioning. This is why it is important to consider the misuse of all substances and not just alcohol. Still, as with other mental health–related issues, a functional assessment is warranted. It is also important to highlight the ongoing prescription medication problem in our society. There are many people taking medications "as prescribed" but, in actuality, they may have been overprescribed in the first place. If so, such can certainly lead to impairments—even though the person is not technically abusing or misusing anything. There are also considerations related to the more recent legalization of marijuana and even medicinal marijuana, which has become an issue that varies state by state. Therefore, evaluators must remember not to focus solely on the legality of a substance but, again, on the way in which it impacts the examinee's *functioning*—especially in the context of firearm use and ownership.

As with other domains within the context of our firearm evaluation framework, assessment of substance use–related issues is a necessary yet insufficient first step. Identifying a potential concern in this regard is unlikely to be enough of an issue to halt our analysis. Of course, we can imagine exceptions, such as someone who is actively abusing alcohol at concerning levels. Then again, this person is unlikely to be seeking our services in a firearm ownership suitability context in the first place.

A relatively more likely scenario would involve a gun *forfeiture* matter, whereby someone recently lost gun rights because of a particularly concerning incident in which substances played a role (e.g., a DV-related issue that involved heavy drinking by the gun owner just months ago). This type of situation can be quite challenging, especially if the person in question is challenging the notion that he has or ever had a problem with substance misuse. If so, we would first want to decide if we believed that such a problem, or condition, was (or is) present—but, most importantly, we need to determine if the substance use is a significant enough risk factor in the context of firearm suitability, regardless of whether a formal diagnosis is indicated. Questions relevant from a functional firearm evaluation perspective are those such as: *Did the examinee interact with guns during the same time period they misused substances? If so, was there firearm misuse?* It can be compelling to identify that a person was not inappropriate or irresponsible with guns even when they were actively abusing substances. Indeed, the main concern in this context is if the examinee will simultaneously misuse substances and firearms at a future point. However, we should generally put more stock into what we already know has happened in this regard as opposed to what we predict might happen, consistent with an SPJ approach like the PF-10 framework.

Evaluations for Law Enforcement, Corrections, and Military Personnel

Although the PF-10 framework was originally developed for use with civilians, it is sufficiently adaptable and flexible to be incorporated in assessments with law enforcement, corrections, and military personnel. To be clear, a member of any one of these groups may be presenting to us as a civilian in a given matter anyhow and, therefore, we should proceed in the same manner as we would with most other examinees in those instances. Certainly, police and correctional officers as well as members of the military seek personal gun rights (and firearms) at times, and they often must apply in the same way as their civilian counterparts. As such, our clinical-forensic procedures should be comparable if not the same in most cases. However, there are additional and sometimes very different considerations when law enforcement, corrections, and military personnel are engaging in assessments with us for reasons associated with their employment, such as in the context of pre-employment evaluations and fitness-for-duty evaluations (FFDEs).

> Ψ Although our PF-10 framework was originally developed for use with civilians, it is sufficiently adaptable and flexible to be incorporated into assessments with law enforcement, corrections, and military personnel. Indeed, members of these groups are required to qualify periodically (i.e., meet shooting proficiency requirements), and some may be carrying essentially at all times—or, at least, regularly interacting with guns.

According to the International Association of Chiefs of Police (IACP) Preemployment Psychological Evaluation Guidelines (2014):

[A] preemployment psychological evaluation is a specialized examination to determine whether a public safety applicant meets the minimum requirements for psychological suitability mandated by jurisdictional statutes and regulations, as well as any other criteria established by the hiring agency . . . In most jurisdictions, the minimum requirements for psychological suitability are that the applicant be free from any emotional or mental condition that might adversely affect the performance of safety-based duties and responsibilities and be capable of withstanding the psychological demands inherent in the prospective position. (p. 1)

The IACP also indicates the assessment should include a job analysis, testing, an interview, and a review of relevant background information:

Information about the required duties, responsibilities, working conditions, and other psychologically relevant job characteristics should be obtained from the hiring authority prior to beginning the psychological evaluation. This information should be directed toward identifying skills, behaviors, attributes and other personal characteristics associated with effective and counterproductive job performance. (p. 3)

Again, incorporating a framework such as the PF-10 may have utility as well given that police officers are required to carry guns in the United States and correctional officers need to own and operate them. Paradoxically, evaluators do not necessarily formally address firearm-related issues in their pre-employment assessments. Our hypothesis is that firearm-related questions are not a main aspect of these evaluations, if they are incorporated at all. That said, it is an obviously important area to address given that guns and these careers literally go hand in hand. There are various other positions that require the ownership, handling, and even carrying of guns as well (e.g., federal and state government agents; private employees, such as armed guards). It seems axiomatic to consider firearm-related factors in pre-employment evaluations with law enforcement, corrections, and military personnel as well as with those seeking employment with private agencies requiring gun handling and use—just as we would with those in civilian firearm ownership contexts. There is simply no compelling clinical distinction.

Nevertheless, it is likely much more common that firearm-specific factors are addressed in FFDEs, which are typically sought when an employee raises concerns in some way (e.g., engaging in irresponsible or threatening behavior) or after a particularly concerning incident or situation in the workplace (e.g., an assault). The IACP (2013) has also developed guidelines for these matters, defining a psychological FFDE as:

a formal, specialized examination of an incumbent employee that results from (1) objective evidence that the employee may be unable to safely or effectively perform a defined job and (2) a reasonable basis for believing that the cause may be attributable to a psychological condition or impairment. The central purpose of an FFDE is to determine whether the employee is able to safely and effectively perform his or her essential job functions. (p. 2)

The group recommends that FFDEs include a review of relevant background and collateral information; psychological testing; a comprehensive clinical interview and mental status examination; collateral interviews with relevant third parties, when applicable; and a referral to or consultation with a specialist, if necessary. Although the words *firearm* and *gun* are not included in the guidelines, we hypothesize that evaluators are much more likely to address firearm-specific issues when conducting FFDEs as compared to pre-employment evaluations. The question remains, however: How are these factors being addressed, specifically, and what is the relative weight placed upon them? What is clear is that officers' suitability to handle and carry guns safely and effectively is an inherent and fundamental aspect of their fitness to return to duty. For these reasons, the PF-10 may have utility in FFDEs as well, although further consideration and investigation is needed in this regard.

It is also important to note that law enforcement, correctional, and military positions can be quite stressful. In addition to often being associated with elevated levels of stress, they are also prone to traumatic exposures—directly and vicariously (e.g., criminality, accidents, complaints, altercations, death, periods of significant boredom followed by intense excitement, public and political pressures, interdepartmental problems, lawsuits, and rotating shifts). It comes as no surprise then that these positions are also linked to a wide range of problems that can develop—related to medical, mental health, substance misuse, domestic violence, and suicide. The professional literature on police stress is expansive and has steadily grown in decades. Indeed, the National Institute of Justice (NIJ) has noted that "for the law enforcement officer, the strains and tensions experienced at work are unique, often extreme, and sometimes unavoidable" (2000, p. 19), which led to the development of its Corrections and Law Enforcement Family Support program.

The literature related to negative outcomes for law enforcement, correctional, and military positions is longstanding and has remained concerning. For example, Hartley et al. (2011) found that officers over 40 years old had a higher 10-year risk of a heart attack compared to national standards; the majority of female officers and about half of male officers had higher cholesterol levels, pulse rates, and diastolic blood pressure levels than are recommended; and about one-quarter of officers reported more suicidal thoughts than the general population. Indeed, it has been suggested that police officers may take their own lives at a rate double that of officer deaths by felons (see Nanavaty, 2015). That said, national statistics are difficult to find in this regard because of reporting and related data-collection challenges; however, state-level numbers are often more easily accessible, and they reflect serious concerns. For instance, according to the New Jersey Police Suicide Task Force Report (2009), suicide rates are greater among all active male officers in the state between 25 and 64 years old compared to same-aged male civilians. In fact, when correctional officers are included in the analysis, the rate is 30% greater than that for civilians. Moreover, the analysis showed that officer suicides are "far more likely to be committed with a firearm than suicide among similarly aged males" (p. 8).

In addition to suicide-related concerns, DV is a significant problem among police populations (Cheema, 2016). In fact, the National Center for Women and Policing (n.d.) has noted research indicating that 24% to 40% of police officer families experience DV compared to 10% in the general population. There are also unique vulnerabilities inherent to police officer victims; namely, perpetrators have guns, they know the location of battered women's shelters, and they often know how to avoid penalty and blame.

Correctional officers have been found to have even higher levels of stress and DV-related problems than police officers (Summerlin et al., 2010). Moreover, substance misuse, divorce, and suicide rates are very high in correctional officer populations relative to the general public—and also compared to their police counterparts.

As for our active and retired military personnel, there are also many serious concerns we need to consider. In the largest study of mental health risk conducted among the U.S. military, Kessler et al. (2014) found that 25% of approximately 5,500 active-duty, non-deployed Army soldiers had some type of mental health disorder, 11% had more than one illness, and 13% reported severe role impairments. The rate of depression was five times greater than that for civilians, intermittent explosive disorder was six times greater, and PTSD was 15 times greater. In addition, 50% of soldiers with at least one internalizing disorder diagnosis (e.g., depression, anxiety, PTSD) reported onset prior to enlistment, whereas more than 80% of externalizing disorders (e.g., intermittent explosive, substance use) developed after enlistment. Per the U.S. Department of Veterans Affairs (VA; n.d.), SUDs co-occur with PTSD among veteran groups at problematic rates:

- More than two of 10 veterans with PTSD also have SUDs.
- War veterans with PTSD and alcohol problems tend to be binge drinkers. Binges may be in response to bad memories of combat trauma.
- Almost one out of every three veterans seeking treatment for an SUD also has PTSD.
- The number of veterans who smoke (nicotine) is almost double for those with PTSD (about six of 10) versus those without a PTSD diagnosis (three of 10).
- In the wars in Iraq and Afghanistan, about one in 10 returning soldiers seen in the VA system have a problem with alcohol or other drugs.

The VA has further indicated that female veterans and active-duty military personnel are more likely than their civilian counterparts to experience IPV. The Substance Abuse and Mental Health Services Administration has also set forth statistics that raise additional concerns for military personnel and their families (n.d.). Namely, the Army suicide rate reached an all-time high in 2012, which is consistent with 2014 statistics published by the VA indicating a rate of 20 veteran suicide deaths per day that year—a 21% greater rate than civilians—and accounting for 18% of all adult suicide deaths in the United States. Of particular note is that 66% of all veteran deaths were via firearm (VA Suicide Prevention Program, 2016).

In sum, the need to assess firearm-related risk factors when evaluating members of law enforcement, corrections, and military groups is clear. Therefore, there is a need to continue to develop firearm-specific assessment measures, guides, and frameworks (e.g., the PF-10) and investigate the utility of incorporating them into evaluations of law enforcement, correctional, and military personnel.

RECOMMENDED FURTHER READING

American Psychological Association. (2016, November 15). After decades of research, science is no better able to predict suicidal behaviors. https://www.apa.org/news/press/releases/2016/11/suicidal-behaviors

Gold, L. H., & Vanderpool, D. (2016). Relief from disabilities: Firearm rights restoration for persons under mental health prohibitions. In L. H. Gold & R. I. Simon (Eds.), *Gun violence and mental illness* (pp. 339–380). American Psychiatric Association.

Greenberg, S. A., & Shuman, D. W. (1997). Irreconcilable conflict between therapeutic and forensic roles. *Professional Psychology: Research and Practice, 28*(1), 50–57. https://doi.org/10.1037/0735-7028.28.1.50

Greenberg, S. A., & Shuman, D. W. (2007). When worlds collide: Therapeutic and forensic roles. *Professional Psychology: Research and Practice, 38*(2), 129–132. https://doi.org/10.1037/0735-7028.38.2.129

Meehl, P. E. (1954). *Clinical versus statistical prediction: A theoretical analysis and a review of the evidence.* University of Minnesota Press.

Melton, G. B., Petrila, J., Poythress, N. G., & Slobogin, C., Otto, R. K., Mossman, D., & Condie, L. O. (2018). *Psychological evaluations for the courts: A handbook for mental health professionals and lawyers* (4th ed.). Guilford Press.

Pirelli, G., Wechsler, H., & Cramer, R. (2015). Psychological evaluations for firearm ownership: Legal foundations, practice considerations, and a conceptual framework. *Professional Psychology: Research and Practice, 46*(4), 250–257.

Pirelli, G., Wechsler, H., & Cramer, R. (2019). *The behavioral science of firearms: A mental health perspective on guns, suicide, and violence.* Oxford University Press.

Van Orden, K. A., Witte, T. K., Cukrowicz, K. C., Braithwaite, S. R., Selby, E. A., & Joiner, T. E., Jr. (2010). The interpersonal theory of suicide. *Psychological Review, 117*(2), 575–600. https://doi.org/10.1037/a0018697

6

Ethical Considerations for Medical and Mental

Health Professionals

LEGAL AND ETHICAL considerations related to firearms are some of the most salient issues to address in clinical practice contexts. For many of us, even the mere mention of a gun by a client or potential client can raise concerns because, as we presented in the introduction at the start of the book, the vast majority of us are simply not trained to address firearm-specific issues in any real depth. Of course, some of us have had personal exposure to guns and particular firearm-related subcultures, which may provide a relative amount of comfort in dealing with these issues professionally. Yet, all of us are expected to be equipped to handle a fairly wide range of issues that could arise in our clinical practices vis-à-vis guns. Such high demand and stakes in relation to such low rates of professional and cultural competence is of great concern. Therefore, one word in particular is at the forefront of firearm-related issues in clinical practice: *liability*.

One of our central goals in writing this book is to better help you, as our colleagues, walk the risk-liability tightrope that we, as clinicians, must all walk at various timepoints in our work. Namely: Having clinical thresholds that are too high is associated with elevated *external* risk (i.e., to clients

Ψ Professional liability is correlated with clinical thresholds in both directions—external and internal. Having clinical thresholds that are too high is associated with elevated *external* risk (i.e., to clients and others), whereas having thresholds that are too low is associated with elevated *internal risk* (i.e., increased likelihood of professional liability concerns, such as ethics complaints and lawsuits).

and others), whereas having thresholds that are too low is associated with elevated *internal risk* (i.e., increased likelihood of professional liability concerns, such as ethics complaints and lawsuits). In other words, liability is correlated with our clinical thresholds in both directions—external and internal. This idea and writing of this book was primarily driven by the concept that proper education and training is one particularly useful way to manage both external and internal liability concerns. A main reason for this is that they are effective ways of mitigating bias in our decision-making (see the *Cognitive Bias and Professional Decision-Making* section later in this chapter).

While the entire book contributes to continued education efforts aimed at generally improving clinical decision-making and practice, this chapter is particularly focused on ethical considerations that we, as medical and mental health professionals, should account for when gun-related issues arise during the course of our work. To that end, we first present an overview of ethics codes associated with the practice areas of psychology, psychiatry, and counseling, respectively, followed by an outline of forensic psychology and psychiatry practice guidelines. In the second section of this chapter, we describe three ethical decision-making models that have been set forth in the context of forensic psychology but also have applicability across disciplines. We address four concepts in that section that are essential to consider in the context of ethical professional decision-making: hired guns, forensic identification, adversarial allegiance, and cognitive bias. In the third and final section of this chapter, we review five areas that are particularly important to know in relation to firearm-related issues in practice. These areas are reflected in ethical principles and professional guidelines across medical and mental health disciplines: identifying the client; dual roles and relationships, the "therefore" problem, and weapon focus; termination of services; cultural competence, and personal beliefs and experiences; and breaking confidentiality within the context of reporting requirements, such as duty to warn and protect, and releasing data. We also address contemporary considerations related to internet-based data in this final section.

ETHICS CODES AND PROFESSIONAL GUIDELINES

Before turning to specific ethics codes and professional guidelines, it is important to have a sense as to why they were developed in the first place and why they have evolved and persist. Therefore, let us first turn to a discussion of the purpose of professional ethics codes and guidelines.

Purpose

The main purposes for having an ethics code in place are to facilitate professional *objectivity*, to provide a foundation for (professional) *risk management and liability*, and to set a *standard of care* in a given area of practice. It is impossible for an ethics code to account for the endless possibilities of situations that could arise in clinical practice; therefore, a useful code is one that is sufficiently vague to capture the most important underlying principles in a particular context. It is for this reason that ethics codes, such as the American Psychological Association's Ethical Principles of Psychologists and Code of Conduct (EPPCC; American

> Ψ The main purposes for having an ethics code in place are to facilitate professional *objectivity*, to provide a foundation for (professional) *risk management and liability*, and to set a *standard of care* in a particular area of practice.

Psychological Association, 2017a), have actually become much more concise and focused over the years. Some areas are intended to be very black and white, leaving little room for interpretation and discretion, whereas others are written in a manner to be more broadly applied. Two examples from the EPPCC are illustrative:

> Before recording the voices or images of individuals to whom they provide services, psychologists obtain permission from all such persons or their legal representatives. (p. 7, Privacy and Confidentiality: 4.03 Recording)

> Psychologists administer, adapt, score, interpret, or use assessment techniques, interviews, tests, or instruments in a manner and for purposes that are appropriate in light of the research on or evidence of the usefulness and proper application of the techniques. (p. 13, Assessment: 9.02(a) Use of Assessments)

Although there can be nuances or exceptions present in a given case, the first standard presented here (4.03) is rather straightforward: Psychologists need to secure permission from people before recording them. However, the second principle presented (9.02(a)) is more subjective: Psychologists engage in assessments in a way that is "appropriate" given the extant research or evidence of their utility in particular contexts. In fact, this type of standard must be relatively vague, as it needs to account for research developments and other contemporary evidence related to employing certain evaluation techniques or measures for particular purposes. This latter principle reflects some of the real challenges of those who develop ethics codes and, of course, the potential dilemmas we may all encounter as clinicians. The term "appropriate" in and of itself is subjective and essentially equates to the concept of what a reasonable professional would believe. Indeed, ethics boards are made up of our peers, at least in part. Moreover, this particular standard indicates that appropriateness is to be considered in the context of research or evidence on the usefulness of the techniques in question. A discussion on what precisely constitutes "evidence-based" or "empirically based" is outside of the scope of this book; however, suffice to say that these terms are not as straightforward as they might appear at first glance.

Simply put: Many clinical techniques have not been empirically investigated across populations and contexts, and even those that have to a greater extent often have not been researched at methodologically rigorous or otherwise high-quality levels (e.g., randomized controlled trials [RCTs]; meta-analyses). This is not to say that mental health–related procedures do not have merit or utility or even should not be considered evidence-based. In fact, many mental health–related techniques have been found to outperform medical procedures (e.g., see Meyer et al., 2001). Still, we must recognize the limitations of our techniques, both generally and specifically in relation to a case at hand and proceed accordingly in a transparent manner. Nevertheless, remember that an ethics board may essentially have the final say as to the clinical appropriateness of a particular technique, whereas a judge would determine such in legal (forensic) matters, which may include via formal admissibility hearings.

A useful ethics code will facilitate *objectivity* by being sufficiently structured, yet appropriately vague. It will have clear requirements and prohibitions in some areas but will otherwise provide professionals with a road map of sorts to navigate potential ethical dilemmas. In addition to providing a framework to foster objectivity, a useful ethics code will also serve professional risk management needs. As clinicians practicing in the United States, we must all be very well aware of professional liability–related issues. To be clear: We cannot claim ignorance of professional ethics codes or guidelines—and, of course, of state regulations or laws. A good example is the American Psychological Association's *Specialty Guidelines for Forensic Psychologists* (SGFP; Committee on Ethical Guidelines for Forensic Psychologists, 1991), which was revised and is now titled the *Specialty Guidelines for Forensic Psychology* (American Psychological Association, 2013). The title change is subtle, yet substantive: from psychologists to psychology. The reason is because it does not matter what professionals call themselves; rather, it is the work in which they engage that defines them. As the Guidelines so eloquently indicate:

> Application of the Guidelines does not depend on the practitioner's typical areas of practice or expertise, but rather, on the service provided in the case at hand. (p. 7)

This is very important because some professionals may refer to themselves as forensic psychologists, but again, it is the service and not the self-bestowed title that matters. For instance, a clinician can provide therapy in a purely clinical context in the morning and conduct an adjudicative competency evaluation in the afternoon (on the same day). As such, she engaged in the practice of clinical psychology to start the day and subsequently and separately engaged in forensic psychology to end it. As such, she must be aware of and adhere to the guiding standards and principles of each, respectively. Consider another example, whereby a professional exclusively provides treatment services in clinical contexts and is by no means a forensic practitioner. However, an attorney reaches out and asks the clinician to

> Ψ It is the nature of the work in which we engage at a given moment that defines our practice, such as forensic psychology, not a label we decide to bestow upon ourselves (e.g., forensic psychologist). We could engage in clinical psychology in the morning and in forensic psychology in the afternoon.

conduct a legal capacity evaluation for his client. If the clinician decides to move forward, she cannot claim that she is "not forensic," because she becomes accountable for adhering to forensic considerations once she accepts and engages in a forensic role or service. Although professional guidelines are aspirational and not enforceable like ethics codes and state regulations, practicing within one's area of professional competence and remaining within the scope of particular roles are undoubtedly (enforceable) principles.

An additional point to highlight within the context of professional *risk management* considerations is that it is *bidirectional*. That is, our professional liability is associated with some combination of our actions and inactions, as both areas reflect our professional decision-making. Indeed, the decision not to act is a decision, nonetheless. Therefore, we must remain cognizant of our thresholds across situations. Imagine a client presents as a potential suicide risk. We must conduct a risk assessment in this regard and, ultimately, decide on what to do (and not do). Of course, there are processes we will need to set forth with numerous associated considerations, such as those we have outlined in Chapter 4—and, while we have stressed the critical importance of "process" throughout this book, here we are focusing on the ultimate decision we come to in a given matter. At some point,
based on our suicide risk assessment, we will need to decide if we will intervene further and, if so, how. For example, we may decide that a client's risk level is sufficiently elevated and warrants external reporting (e.g., opining that our duty to warn and protect is incurred). This is a very serious time in our professional relationship with our client, as we will

> Ψ Our professional liability is associated with some combination of our actions and inactions, as both areas reflect our professional decision-making. Indeed, the decision not to act is a decision, nonetheless.

be breaching confidentiality and putting certain wheels in motion that may very well lead to a scenario we do not anticipate or even intend. Even if we are justified and the decision is thought to be appropriate, unintended consequences are not necessarily uncommon.

This is true in other reporting contexts as well (e.g., child abuse). None of these remarks are made to deter clinicians from fulfilling their responsibilities, protecting others, and engaging in ethical and competent practice. To the contrary, the intention of highlighting these issues is to heighten awareness, so that we recognize the potential implications of our professional decisions in advance—to better inform our decision-making in the first place. Rarely can decisions be made in a vacuum; rarely are ethical situations so blatantly obvious, so black and white. This is particularly true when we are discussing risk assessment-related decisions. If we agree that we do not have a crystal ball and we should avoid trying to predict future behaviors, including those related to suicide, then we can agree that there is a certain level of unavoidable subjectivity in our ultimate clinical decisions. It is for these reasons professional risk management is bidirectional and managing our thresholds is so important. If too low, our false positives will rise; too high and our false negatives will increase. Put differently, if our bar is too low related to a client's risk, we may inappropriately flag him; if it is too high, we may fail to intervene appropriately. Either way, our professional liability risk elevates: Unnecessarily flagging people raises our risk of receiving complaints, whereas failing to do so with those who are actually at higher risk can potentially increase the likelihood of a negative outcome for the client and others (e.g., suicide).

A third reason for having a professional ethics code is to set the *standard of care* in a given area. Most importantly, we must recognize that standard of care is a legal rather than clinical term, which is particularly associated with cases in the medical malpractice and personal injury arenas. Per Cornell Law School's Legal Information Institute, standard of care is defined as follows:

> The degree of care (watchfulness, attention, caution, and prudence) that a reasonable person should exercise under the circumstances. If a person does not meet the standard of care, he or she may be liable to a third party for negligence. (Cornell Law School, n.d.)

On the other hand, a standard of practice may not rise to the level of a legally recognized standard of care; this is true for related terms, such as "best practices." While certain standards of practice and best practices may be promoted by leaders in a given area of practice, they are not actually (legally) enforceable. The American Psychological Association's *Specialty Guidelines for Forensic Psychology* (2013), which we previously noted, is an example of aspirational best practices, or even standards of practice. While it would likely behoove professionals to engage in forensic psychology practice that generally comports with these Guidelines, one cannot be held in violation of them. As such, primary concerns about professional liability are associated with standards of care and not necessarily standards of practice. One way to look at it is that best practices often correspond to optimal practice, whereas the standard of care pertains to minimal practice.

Ψ *Standard of care* is a legal rather than a clinical term, as compared to *standard of practice* or *best practices*, which may be recommended but not (legally) enforceable.

Professional Ethics Codes

In this section, we provide a brief overview of the ethics codes for psychologists, psychiatrists, and counselors, before turning to a review of two leading sets of professional guidelines in forensic psychology and psychiatry, respectively. Of course, there are very many other important medical and mental health disciplines we do not directly cover here (e.g., nursing). Such is not to exclude these other medical and mental health professionals from the conversation, but rather to be parsimonious and illustrative instead of being comprehensive vis-à-vis covering every set of professional standards. Various types of mental health and medical professionals, including but certainly not limited to nursing personnel, are often critically important players in firearm-involved violence and suicide prevention efforts. Indeed, many are literally leading the way—at both case and more general levels (e.g., as evaluators or administrators). While not exhaustive, the ethics codes presented here reflect the same types of principles and substantive areas covered by most, if not all, codes in medical and mental health.

Ethical Principles of Psychologists and Code of Conduct

Although the American Psychological Association was established in 1892, its first ethics code was not published until 1953. It has gone through numerous revisions over the last six-plus decades, with the 1992 revision being its most substantive. In response to issues related to the use of torture in governmental interrogations, it has been further amended since 2010 to make it clear that it can never be interpreted to justify the violation of human rights. Otherwise, the current EPPCC has the same general format and substantive areas it has had for many years. Namely, it begins with an introduction and preamble, followed by five general principles, which are aspirational and not enforceable:

1. Beneficence and nonmaleficence
2. Fidelity and responsibility
3. Integrity
4. Justice
5. Respect for people's rights and dignity.

The EPPCC subsequently contains 10 ethical standard areas, presented along with approximately 90 corresponding subsections. These reflect the enforceable part of the EPPCC. The overarching standards are as follows:

1. Resolving ethical issues
2. Competence
3. Human relations
4. Privacy and confidentiality
5. Advertising and other public statements
6. Recordkeeping and fees
7. Education and training
8. Research and publication
9. Assessment
10. Therapy.

A deeper dive into the EPPCC is outside of the scope of this book, but the interested reader is directed to the document itself as well as to books related to it (e.g., Bersoff, 2008; Pirelli et al., 2017).

Principles of Medical Ethics with Annotations Especially Applicable to Psychiatry

The first edition of *The Principles of Medical Ethics with Annotations Especially Applicable to Psychiatry* was published by the American Psychiatric Association in 1973 and various revisions have since been published. As these Principles make clear: "ALL PHYSICIANS should practice in accordance with the medical code of ethics set forth in the *Principles of Medical Ethics* of the American Medical Association" (p. 1). While the basic principles remain the same, this document addresses the particular ethical issues psychiatrists face in practice—distinct from other areas of medical practice. In this document, a preamble and nine sections are followed by the principles, with 43 annotations for psychiatry across areas. The nine sections are as follows:

1. A physician shall be dedicated to providing competent medical care, with compassion and respect for human dignity and rights.
2. A physician shall uphold the standards of professionalism, be honest in all professional interactions, and strive to report physicians deficient in character or competence, or engaging in fraud or deception, to appropriate entities.
3. A physician shall respect the law and also recognize a responsibility to seek changes in those requirements which are contrary to the best interests of the patient.
4. A physician shall respect the rights of patients, colleagues, and other health professionals, and shall safeguard patient confidences and privacy within the constraints of the law.
5. A physician shall continue to study, apply, and advance scientific knowledge, maintain a commitment to medical education, make relevant information available to patients, colleagues, and the public, obtain consultation, and use the talents of other health professionals when indicated.
6. A physician shall, in the provision of appropriate patient care, except in emergencies, be free to choose whom to serve, with whom to associate, and the environment in which to provide medical care.
7. A physician shall recognize a responsibility to participate in activities contributing to the improvement of the community and the betterment of public health.
8. A physician shall, while caring for a patient, regard responsibility to the patient as paramount.
9. A physician shall support access to medical care for all people.

American Counseling Association Code of Ethics

The American Counseling Association's (2014) ethics code contains initial sections outlining its preamble and purpose, followed by nine sections:

1. The counseling relationship
2. Confidentiality and privacy

3. Professional responsibility
4. Relationships with other professionals
5. Evaluation, assessment, and interpretation
6. Supervision, training, and teaching
7. Research and publication
8. Distance counseling, technology, and social media
9. Resolving ethical issues.

Consistent with the ideals of all professional ethics codes, the American Counseling Association code highlights two of its six main purposes: It "sets forth the ethical obligations of ACA members and provides guidance intended to inform the ethical practice of professional counselors" and its standards "serve as the basis for processing inquiries and ethics complaints concerning ACA members" (p. 3).

American Mental Health Counselors Association Code of Ethics

The ethics code of the American Mental Health Counselors Association (2015) consists of a preamble and six main sections, which have 14 corresponding subsections. The primary sections are as follows:

1. Commitment to clients
2. Commitment to other professionals
3. Commitment to students, supervisees, and employee relationships
4. Commitment to the profession
5. Commitment to the public
6. Resolution of ethical problems.

Consistent with other codes, this code indicates:

This code is a document intended as a guide to: assist members to make sound ethical decisions; to define ethical behaviors and best practices for Association members; to support the mission of the Association; and to educate members, students and the public at large regarding the ethical standards of mental health counselors. Mental health counselors are expected to utilize carefully considered ethical decision making processes when faced with ethical dilemmas. (p. 1)

To be clear, none of the ethics codes outlined here mention guns, firearms, or any language related to such. While this is not necessarily a surprising or unexpected observation, it is also not outside of the realm of possibility that firearm-specific concepts may be included in one or more of these codes in the future. Timely and pressing issues that affect our professions have certainly been included in revised versions of ethics codes in the past. As noted, the American Psychological Association has amended its code in recent years in the wake of concerns that arose vis-à-vis psychologists' involvement in torture-related interrogations enacted by the U.S. government. Moreover, codes of both the American Counseling Association and the American Mental Health Counselors Association have incorporated considerations related to social media, although others have yet to do so. These are examples of contemporary issues of significant relevance to clinicians across disciplines, and their inclusion in certain ethics codes demonstrates the iterative nature of professional standards. Their flexibility is evidenced by being appropriately vague to cover a range of potential scenarios and also their ability to be revised and otherwise updated to address particularly important areas warranting attention. Practice guidelines can be very useful to clinicians in this way as well, and by tapping into more nuanced practice considerations. We present two such guidelines in the following section pertaining to the practice of forensic psychology and psychiatry, respectively, which are well regarded and instructive.

Professional Guidelines for the Practice of Forensic Psychology and Psychiatry

Although aspirational and not enforceable, professional guidelines are important because they provide a framework for engaging in best practices rather than solely adequate practices. For something to be unethical or illegal, it essentially has to be below what is *minimally* required or expected in a given context. Professional guidelines seek to promote a higher level of practice. We can think of it in terms of the difference between passing a course versus earning an A. In this section, we outline forensic psychology and psychiatry guidelines, but it is also important to highlight the fact that even more nuanced guidelines exist. In fact, the American Psychological Association has set forth over 20 sets of practice guidelines in a number of areas over the years (see www.apa.org/practice/guidelines/). Some are related to psychological practice with particular groups, such as boys and men; girls and women; lesbian, gay, and bisexual clients; transgender and gender-nonconforming people; those with disabilities; and older adults. There are also a number of guidelines available for particular areas of psychology practice, such as occupationally mandated psychological evaluations, telepsychology, parenting coordination, and child custody evaluations. Moreover, guidelines have also been developed to address the treatment of particular clinical issues, such as posttraumatic stress disorder (PTSD), obesity, and depression. This wide range of guidelines reflects the significant level of nuance that exists in the practice of psychology alone. Of course, each discipline has its own set of guidelines across areas, and this also does not account for the myriad of publications and trainings that exist and arise daily, which can contribute to contemporary best practices. In the same way our ethics codes and laws set the stage for what can be thought of as minimally competent practice, our early education and training was a prerequisite to begin to engage in competent practice. Indeed, nearly every state now has continuing education requirements for psychologists, psychiatrists, and other mental health professionals. As such, it has been determined that even our early training and education is necessary, yet insufficient. Given the complexity of mental health–related issues and practice, professional guidelines can provide us with much-needed guidance in many respects. Now, let us look at two noteworthy examples.

Specialty Guidelines for Forensic Psychology

The Specialty Guidelines for Forensic Psychologists (1991) were originally published over 30 years ago and have been revised once since: the Specialty Guidelines for Forensic Psychology (American Psychological Association, 2013). The Specialty Guidelines are informed by and essentially supplement the American Psychological Association's ethics code (i.e., EPPCC). Like other guidelines, these are aspirational and advisory, not mandatory or enforceable; however, they provide useful guidance in a number of practice areas and contexts. While intentionally broad, they largely mirror the EPPCC. The Specialty Guidelines consist of 11 areas:

1. Responsibilities
2. Competence
3. Diligence
4. Relationships
5. Fees
6. Informed consent, notification, and assent
7. Conflicts in practice
8. Privacy, confidentiality, and privilege
9. Methods and procedures
10. Assessment
11. Professional and other public communications.

In total, there are over 50 subsections, subsumed in each of these areas. We will highlight some of them in the *Ethical Decision-Making Models* section that follows. The interested reader may also review one or more of the books that have been written on forensic psychology practice ethics, including our own (Pirelli et al., 2017) and two we review in the following section.

Ethics Guidelines for the Practice of Forensic Psychiatry

The Ethics Guidelines for the Practice of Forensic Psychology was adopted in 2005 by the American Academy of Psychiatry and the Law to supplement the "Annotations Especially Applicable to Psychiatry of the American Psychiatric Association to the Principles of Medical Ethics of the American Medical Association." It consists of a preamble and five primary areas: confidentiality, consent, honesty and striving for objectivity, qualifications, and procedures for handling complaints of unethical conduct.

ETHICAL DECISION-MAKING MODELS:
FORENSIC PSYCHOLOGY AS EXEMPLAR

There is a fairly expansive literature on professional ethics relevant to the medical and mental health arenas, and a review of such is well outside of the scope of this

> Ψ The primary reasons for using (and documenting our use of) an ethical decision-making framework is to ensure both our adherence to ethical principles *and* consistency across cases. In other words, doing so covers the critical content-based and procedural components of ethical decision-making in our work.

book and chapter. However, what is critical to point out and emphasize within this context is the importance of working from a particular decision-making model or framework. Although one that is overly structured or rigid can be stifling and, therefore, lack utility for us as clinicians, forgoing the use of one completely can be just as problematic. This consideration is akin to the unstructured, semi-structured, and structured risk assessment models and approaches we outlined in Chapter 5. In that same way, we recommend using a semi-structured approach to ethical decision-making in clinical practice—by either subscribing to a formal model or by at least incorporating the most salient features of one into your decision-making process. The primary reasons for using (and documenting our use of) an ethical decision-making framework is to ensure both our adherence to ethical principles *and* consistency across cases. Simply put, doing so covers the critical content-based and procedural components of ethical decision-making in our work.

For illustrative purposes, we present three ethical decision-making models that have been set forth within the context of the subfield of forensic psychology. Many clinicians across medical and mental health subdisciplines are likely to find their foundational components to have utility despite the fact they were not developed with those disciplines in mind per se. We encourage clinicians in other subdisciplines to seek out frameworks within their areas, regardless.

Bush, Connell, and Denney (2006)

The book authored by Bush and colleagues is an important work in the forensic psychology ethics arena, as it was essentially the first text of its kind. Its primary goal was to outline a systematic model for decision-making in various forensic practice contexts. Bush and colleagues expounded upon earlier models and set forth an eight-step model designed for forensic psychological practitioners:

1. Identify the problem
2. Consider the significance of the context or setting
3. Identify and use ethical and legal resources
4. Consider personal beliefs and values
5. Develop possible solutions to the problems
6. Consider the potential consequences of various solutions
7. Choose and implement a course of action
8. Assess the outcome and implement changes as needed

The authors proceed to apply these concepts to case examples related to six overarching stages and areas of practice: the referral; collection and review of information; the evaluation; documentation of findings and opinions; testimony and termination; and addressing ethical misconduct.

Otto (2015)

During a 2015 ethics panel at the annual conference of the American Psychology-Law Society (Division 41 of the American Psychological Association), Otto set forth a particularly useful and compelling framework to facilitate ethical decision-making in forensic work. Namely, he recommended we view professional actions within a lens of those that are *required*; *permitted/advisable*; *permitted/not advisable*; or *prohibited*. The utility of Otto's guidance is mainly in the bifurcation of the gray area—that is, what is permitted. Too often we think in black and white terms, but this simple reframing highlights that there are, in fact, four general choices before us rather than two. When a potential ethical issue arises, we can start at the ends, or anchor points; that is, we can decide if an action (or inaction) is required or prohibited. Such definitive parameters are likely to be found in our ethics codes as well as state regulations, as they reflect "the letter of the law." Recall the example we used early in this chapter from the American Psychological Association's ethics code, the EPPCC: "Before recording the voices or images of individuals to whom they provide services, psychologists obtain permission from all such persons or their legal representatives" (p. 7). State licensing regulations are typically much more concrete than professional ethics codes because they are the law and, therefore, are designed differently. As such, it is often much easier to discern what is prohibited and required in state regulations as compared to professional ethics codes.

Ψ We agree with Otto's (2015) recommendation to conceptualize professional actions within a lens of those that are *required*; *permitted/advisable*; *permitted/not advisable*; or *prohibited*. Generally speaking, we are permitted to do (and not do) quite a lot, but what often takes so much of our resources and energy is deciding what we *should* do rather than what we *could* do.

Nevertheless, this is an important starting point—to ask ourselves what, if anything, is required or prohibited by our state laws and professional ethics code in a particular situation. Once we properly determine that there are no clear prohibitions or requirements in a given context, Otto's next recommended step is prompted: Determine what is *advisable*. To reiterate his key distinction here, let us remember that, just because something is legally or ethically permitted does not mean it is advisable. Or, as U.S. Supreme Court Justice Potter Stewart has been quoted as saying: "Ethics is knowing the difference between what you have a right to do and what is right to do." This is, perhaps, the core of professional decision-making: navigating the gray area. Generally speaking, we are permitted to do (and not do) quite a lot, but what often takes so much of our resources and energy is deciding what we *should* do rather than what we *could* do. Indeed, facilitating sound professional decision-making is the purpose, the essence, of a clinical handbook like this.

Otto, Goldstein, and Heilbrun (2017)

The nine-step decision-making model set forth by Otto and colleagues (2017) was adapted from the Canadian Code of Ethics for Psychologists (Canadian Psychological Association, 2000) and is as follows:

1. Identify the individuals and groups who may be affected by any course of action (with particular attention to individuals and groups to whom one owes a duty or duties), their rights, and interests.
2. Identify the ethical issues and principles at hand.
3. Consider how personal biases, stresses, or self-interest might influence decision making in this matter.
4. Seek various sources of authority that address or provide guidance with respect to the issue at hand.
5. Consult with colleagues.
6. Identify various courses of action and likely outcomes of each, along with associated risks and benefits to the relevant individuals and groups.
7. Choose a course of action after careful consideration of relevant principles, values, standards, and guidelines.
8. Evaluate and assume responsibility for the outcome, and take steps to remedy any negative outcomes that occurred.
9. Take appropriate action, if indicated and possible, to prevent future occurrences of the dilemma (e.g., communication and problem solving with colleagues; changes in procedures and practices). (p. 8)

As Otto and colleagues articulated it:

After taking these steps, one should identify different courses of action, consider each in light of relevant sources of authority and consultation, and decide which course of action is the best to take. This highlights the *process* of ethical decision making and behavior: identifying, considering, weighing, deciding, then taking action. At a minimum, this will guarantee a decision that is prudently considered, and quite likely a good one. Assuming responsibility for the outcome and dealing with any remaining problems, the next step in this model, becomes more straightforward when one has confidence in the decision. If there are remaining steps to be taken to reduce the likelihood of a recurring problem, then such a decision should also provide guidance in taking these steps. (p. 10, emphasis in the original)

Applying Ethical Decision-Making Models to Firearm-Related Contexts

In addition to reviewing the aforementioned models and publications more closely, the interested reader may wish to review our casebook on the ethical practice of forensic psychology (Pirelli et al., 2017) as well as other seminal, albeit more general, texts that facilitate the navigation of ethical dilemmas in mental health practice (e.g., Bersoff, 2008). While we may be aware of reference texts in our respective disciplines, the reality is that the foundational principles of ethical clinical decision-making transcend the confines of any one of our particular specialty areas. There are nuances, indeed, and sometimes important ones to consider. However, our goal in writing this chapter and this book, more generally, is to point out the comparable areas and highlight their applicability when firearm-related issues arise in all types of medical and mental health practices. Too often we focus on our differences, but a real effort to reduce gun-involved suicide and violence in our society requires us to reach some level of consensus, followed by consistency in our work. There will always be some level of disagreement and debate, which should be welcomed. There is always more than one way to do something, but the question is: How many ways are there to do it *right*? Professional research and commentary are called for to get us closer to an answer in this regard.

Of additional importance is to address the fact that mental health is sometimes viewed as a pseudo-science and less than that of medicine. Let us first agree that professionals in *any* field can conduct research or practice pseudo-scientifically. If we agree, the main question then pertains to why social sciences, to include mental health, are often viewed in a different light than medical sciences. There are likely very many explanations, but one is particularly relevant to our discussion here: a relative lack of consensus and consistency—that is, the lack of consensus vis-à-vis operationally defining constructs and the lack of consistency in the corresponding practice associated with their measurement (and intervention). Perhaps an example used in our previous book on firearms (Pirelli et al., 2019) is most illustrative. Namely, the second endnote in Chapter 4 of that book reads:

We take the term *blood pressure* for granted today, but it is worth a brief look back to illustrate the point. The measurement of the pressure of the blood in the circulatory system, or *sphygmomanometry*, has its roots in the Egyptians' recognition of the palpitation of the pulse; however, the actual measurement of circulatory pressure began in the early to mid-18th century with the experiments of Stephen Hales (Booth, 1977). Incidentally, Hales' scientific research was first on tree and vegetable sap but progressed to the circulatory pressure in horses in 1733. His work was not extended until approximately one century later when the physician-physicist Jean Léonard Marie Poiseuille began studying the cardiovascular system with a mercury manometer in 1828, at which point he won the gold medal from the Royal Academy of Medicine for his doctoral dissertation on the instrument's use in measuring arterial blood pressure. Various innovations and advancements followed until the first sphygmomanometer was developed by Karl Vierordt in the 1850s. Of course, the instrument was cumbersome and invasive and not without significant criticism in the medical field; in fact, it was admonished by the *British Medical Journal* as an instrument that would actually *weaken* clinical accuracy. It was not until 1896 that an Italian medical doctor named Scipione Riva-Rocci developed the method upon which the present-day technique is based—namely, the compression of the arm around its full circumference to include a rubber bag, a cuff, a rubber bulb for inflation, and the traditional use of the mercury manometer. The most notable advancements came in the early 1900s from the Russian surgeon, N. C. Korotkoff, such as the use of a stethoscope over the brachial artery and other ways in which he ensured the accuracy and ease of measuring blood pressure that have essentially remained unchanged for the past century (Booth, 1977). Although seemingly tangential, it is important to acknowledge that the development of what is now considered a basic and routine medical measurement was met with fairly harsh criticism at the onset and ultimately took 175 years to perfect. This realization certainly puts social science constructs, such as violence, into perspective. (p. 509)

To reiterate, nearly *two centuries* elapsed before the measurement of blood pressure, as we know it today, gained acceptance in the medical field. It is also important to note that mental health assessment and treatment has been found to be on par with or even superior to various types of medical exams or treatments. For instance, Meyer and colleagues (2001) examined data from more than 125 meta-analyses on test validity and 800 samples examining multimethod assessment and found psychological test validity to be strong and compelling, overall, and comparable and even better in some instances as compared to certain medical tests. There has also been a fair amount of research indicating that psychotherapeutic interventions are preferred (and recommended) before pharmacological ones in some cases (see McHugh et al., 2013). None of this is to put down the medical field in any way. To the contrary, it is to say that those of us in the mental health arena need to learn from and largely embrace the medical model—particularly as such pertains to the consensus and consistency reflected in all areas of medicine (i.e., education, training, research, and practice). While doing so across all areas of mental health is an overwhelmingly large undertaking and one that is well outside of the scope of this book, we can move closer to doing so in the context of firearm-related issues in clinical practice—both medical and mental health.

Incorporating a model, such as one of those presented in the preceding subsections, can facilitate sound professional decision-making. As is clear, there is considerable overlap in useful ethical decision-making frameworks because they draw from the same types of foundational clinical principles. Some are fairly technical; therefore, it can often be useful to have more of a shorthand conceptualization in our minds, particularly when we need to think more quickly on our feet. Otto's (2015) framework is a good illustration, as it is not wordy or particularly complicated; it is easy to remember and apply and provides us as clinicians with a clear strategy for making challenging decisions in practice. Nevertheless, essentially all frameworks have the following recommendations in common: Think, anticipate, consult, decide, and act. These five general steps are woven into the aforementioned models, so we will not detail them here. However, we would add a critically important first step: *Stop*. Taken together, the six steps we recommend clinicians consider when engaging in ethical decision-making are as follows:

1. Stop.
2. Think.
3. Anticipate.
4. Consult.
5. Decide.
6. Act (or do not act).

The importance of identifying *"stop"* as the first step cannot be overstated. On its face, stopping as a first step is counterintuitive and somewhat paradoxical; indeed, stepping and stopping are essentially opposing actions. However, it is important to remember that sound professional decision-making is a process comprising planning, action, *and* inaction. Moreover, it is largely a cognitive process in our fields, as even our actions typically involve very little physical activity per se. We address considerations related to cognitive bias in the decision-making process in the following section, but let us first reiterate and emphasize the initial point related to stopping here.

> Ψ The importance of identifying *"stop"* as the first step cannot be overstated. On its face, stopping as a first step is counterintuitive and somewhat paradoxical; indeed, stepping and stopping are essentially opposing actions. However, it is important to remember that sound professional decision-making is a process comprising planning, action, *and* inaction.

Consider how many times you have heard the phrase "Stop *and* think." These are, in fact, two distinct steps. However, many if not most of the situations that pose ethical dilemmas can be anxiety-provoking and, therefore, may lead us to make quicker, more emotional decisions (see the relatively extensive literature on hot vs. cold cognition). For this reason, many of us wait to reply to emails, for example. All that said, sometimes we must make fairly quick decisions, although we would strongly contend that the vast majority of ethical dilemmas in which we find ourselves are actually not emergencies that require immediate decisions to be made. Generally, only those situations involving the potential for immediate harm necessitate such urgency, but even

> Ψ The vast majority of ethical dilemmas in which we find ourselves are not emergencies requiring immediate decisions to be made. Generally, only those situations involving the potential for immediate harm necessitate such urgency, but even they are on a continuum. Put simply: We must even distinguish between an *immediate* danger and one that is *imminent* when making decisions.

they are on a continuum. For instance, if a client is actively harming or attempting to harm himself or others, immediate decisions must be made. Contrast that with a client who poses even an imminent threat. Put simply: We must even distinguish between an *immediate* danger and one that is *imminent* when making decisions. If we can step back for a moment and reflect on the ethical dilemmas we have faced, we are likely to realize that there were opportunities to stop before proceeding with our decision-making processes in many if not most cases.

The other steps are self-explanatory, and a more involved discussion is not warranted here, but we would also point out the distinction between deciding and acting (or not acting). A key feature of what we have suggested is the delineation of steps that we may have otherwise tended to group together, particularly stop and think, think and anticipate, and decide and act. The intention is for the conceptual separation to lead us to engage in distinguishable steps, thereby facilitating sound professional decision-making.

Another useful, working framework is actually a visualization of sorts. Namely, imagine an ethics board overlooking one shoulder and a cross-examining attorney on the other. While forensic practitioners should work from this perspective essentially at all times, it behooves clinicians across subdisciplines to adopt this mentality—at least, in part. The reality is that we are in a litigious society, necessitating heightened attention to liability issues in our professional lives. Think of all of the policies and documentation we must attend to on a daily basis, for instance. Of course, part of it is for clinical purposes, but the other part is to cover our professional responsibilities in the context of liability concerns. One of the most obvious examples is getting licensed, which binds us to a whole host of legal regulations and requirements. Another example is business formation. Most clinicians are a part of a registered business, to include those who form LLCs to run their independent practices. Indeed, LLC stands for "limited *liability* company," and the primary purpose of a formal business registration is to protect individuals on a personal level. This is related to the legal concept of *piercing the corporate veil*.

The take-home message here is that all of us interface with the law at some level, at certain times. The danger is to think of ourselves as being either forensic practitioners or not. As we discussed in Chapter 5, clinical-forensic subfields undoubtedly reflect specialized practice areas with their own set of considerations. However, all types of medical and mental health practice inherently have legal components, ranging from areas that are subtler (e.g., licensure, continuing education, informed consent, recordkeeping) to those more obvious (e.g., forced medication, capacity to make decisions, duty to warn and protect, subpoenas). Therefore, when an ethical dilemma arises, it can be useful to employ the aforementioned visual of the ethics board and cross-examining attorney looking over our shoulders.[1] Of course, the next step is to walk through a theoretical explanation for the actions (and inactions) we are thinking

---

[1] This visual is akin to the so-called Policeman at the Elbow test in the context of criminal insanity, which has been applied to the concept "irresistible impulse." Namely, the test calls for consideration of whether a defendant would have engaged in the act in question if a policeman was standing next to him or her.

of taking in a given situation. After all, if we would not be able to explain our anticipated actions and inactions at this time, hypothetically, during a decision-making
process, how would we be able to do so
later to an actual ethics board or cross-
examining attorney? While this exercise
is not intended to replace consultation,
it is another potentially useful decision-
making tool.

> Ψ When an ethical dilemma arises, it
> can be useful to employ the visual of
> the ethics board and cross-examining
> attorney looking over our shoulders.

Biased Decision-Making: A Note on Hired Guns, Forensic Identification,
Adversarial Allegiance, and Cognitive Bias

In this section, we address the very important concept of biased professional decision-
making by outlining three areas of consideration related to such: hired guns, forensic
identification and adversarial allegiance, and cognitive bias. In most contexts, these
areas are presented in a different order, such that cognitive bias is addressed first and
then the other areas are addressed to exemplify different ways in which professional
bias is manifested. However, we have decided to begin with the most blatant, specific
types of bias and work backwards toward general considerations, as we are optimis-
tic that concepts such as "hired guns" do not require as much attention among our
readers.

Hired Guns

The term *hired gun* is a pejorative name for an expert witness who is willing to provide
an opinion in support of the retaining side's position essentially regardless of the data
available. In other words, the professional's opinions are for sale. What is critical to
remember is that expert witnesses are to be paid for their time, not their opinions
per se. Frankly, the presence of a hired gun tends to be fairly obvious, such as when
there is a blatant disconnect from the data available and the expert's opinion, or when
there is no effort to link them at all—as in the case of a *net opinion*. Of course, not all
net opinions are the result of hired guns; they may simply be reflective of inadequate
professional effort. The key point here, though, is that the distinguishing feature of
a hired gun is the *intentional* or willful
act of setting forth an expert opinion
for the primary purpose of supporting
the retaining party, regardless of the
data available to said expert. There are
certainly times when expert opinions
are biased for unintentional or, at least,
less intentional reasons. We address two
concepts in this regard in the following
subsection; namely, *forensic identification*
and *adversarial allegiance.*

> Ψ The distinguishing feature of a
> hired gun is the *intentional* or willful
> act of setting forth an expert opinion
> for the primary purpose of support-
> ing the retaining party, regardless of
> the data available to said expert (vs.
> the concepts of forensic identification
> and adversarial allegiance).

Forensic Identification and Adversarial Allegiance

A concept somewhat related to hired guns is that of *forensic identification*, which has been defined as "the subtle influence of adversarial proceedings on initially neutral witnesses" (Zusman & Simon, 1983, p. 1300). The more contemporary term associated with this issue is *adversarial allegiance*, which has been characterized as "the pull for forensic evaluators in adversarial proceedings to reach opinions that support the party who retained them" (Murrie et al., 2009, p. 23). Although the empirical literature related to adversarial allegiance is still developing, a number of studies have found support for the concept. What has been compelling, methodologically, about the extant research is that it has been conducted in both experimental and field study contexts, whereby the scoring of forensic assessment measures in actual cases has been investigated. Researchers conducting field studies have looked at various measures used in sex offender evaluations (see, e.g., Boccaccini et al., 2017; Murrie et al., 2009), and those conducting experimental studies have done so with samples of national experts (e.g., Murrie et al., 2013; McAuliff & Arter, 2016) as well as with potential, or venire, jurors (Scurich et al., 2015). Indeed, some researchers have found no evidence of adversarial allegiance in their samples, such as Edens and colleagues (2016), who investigated such in the context of a violence risk assessment measure called the Violence Risk Appraisal Guide. While a detailed review or deeper dive into the adversarial allegiance literature is outside of the scope of this chapter and this book, more generally, it is important to highlight because it serves as a conceptual springboard for the following discussion on cognitive bias and professional decision-making.

Cognitive Bias and Professional Decision-Making

While being a hired gun is wholly inappropriate and we should also take the necessary steps to avoid succumbing to a place of forensic identification or adversarial allegiance, the reality is that we all have biases. The question is not whether we have them, but rather, how they are manifested—namely, if they are explicit or implicit, and how they impact our clinical work in a given situation. To ultimately be able to manage our biases, we first need to be able to identify them. In other words, we need to put procedural safeguards in place that foster awareness and are subsequently linked to (both proactive and reactive) bias reduction strategies.

In the context of professional decision-making, the term *cognitive bias* is used throughout the literature. We have already outlined the more explicit types of biases, particularly as they relate to hired guns, but implicit bias

Ψ As Neal and Grisso have noted, there are three overarching types of cognitive bias in forensic assessment contexts: *representativeness, availability*, and *anchoring*. The first is related to two other known biases: conjunction fallacy and base rate neglect. The second is associated with confirmation bias and what is referred to as WYSIATI (What You See Is All There Is). The third is related to the bias of framing/context.

presents significant concerns for all of us because it is outside of our awareness—and, therefore, is not (consciously) intentional. As Neal and Grisso (2014) have noted, there are three overarching types of cognitive bias in forensic assessment contexts: *representativeness, availability,* and *anchoring.* They aptly point out that the first is related to two other known biases: conjunction fallacy and base rate neglect (see the discussion on local norms in Chapter 1, within the context of Case Example 1: Melissa Porter); the second is associated with confirmation bias and what is referred to as WYSIATI (What You See Is All There Is); and the third is related to the bias of framing/context. A full review of each is outside of the scope of this chapter and book, but the interested reader is encouraged to read Neal and Grisso's manuscript for a more detailed account of each concept and their scholarly origins.

Within the purview of our discussion here, though, it is important to address the concept of reducing bias in our decision-making processes. As Neal and Grisso (2014) pointed out, cognitive biases in this regard essentially reflect a *reliability* problem. This has become apparent from results of the types of studies noted in the preceding *Forensic Identification and Adversarial Allegiance* section. If we can agree that one way to improve professional decision-making is to reduce bias, then we must collectively take a closer look at what are referred to as *debiasing strategies.* In a subsequent paper, Neal and Brodsky (2016) provide a useful outline in this regard. Specifically, they distinguished between literature-identified *effective* debiasing strategies perceived as useful by forensic clinicians and literature-identified *ineffective* strategies (but still perceived as useful). Effective strategies included training and reading the professional literature; taking time to think about the assessment rather than immediately issuing a report; consulting with colleagues; using structured evaluation methods; and critically examining conclusions, to include exploring alternative hypotheses.

There are also debiasing strategies that clinicians perceive to be useful but are not. Perhaps the most notable example is *introspection.* In fact, Neal and Brodsky suggest that it "is not just a poor strategy for bias correction, but may actually exacerbate bias," as this "bias blind spot" may lead to false confidence (p. 72). Evidence of practitioners' blind spot biases and reliance upon introspection-based efforts to mitigate bias has continued to be found in forensic contexts, in particular (e.g., see Zapf et al., 2018; Zappala et al., 2018). Perhaps the title of Zappala et al.'s article is most illustrative of the issue at hand: "Anything You Can Do, I Can Do Better: Bias Awareness in Forensic Evaluators." As we indicated at the onset of this chapter, a main purpose of ethics codes and professional guidelines is to facilitate objectivity, or to mitigate biased professional decision-making. Now that we have introduced and reviewed these concepts, let us now turn to ethical principles and professional guidelines that are particularly relevant to consider in the context of firearm-related matters.

> Ψ There are debiasing strategies that clinicians perceive to be useful but are not. Perhaps the most notable is *introspection.*

ETHICAL PRINCIPLES AND PROFESSIONAL GUIDELINES RELEVANT
TO FIREARM-RELATED MATTERS

In this section, we present five overarching areas of ethical principles and professional guidelines that are particularly relevant to consider in relation to firearm-related issues and clinical practice:

1. Identifying the client
2. Dual roles and relationships, the "therefore" problem, and weapon focus
3. Termination of services
4. Cultural competence, and personal beliefs and experiences
5. Breaking confidentiality within the context of reporting requirements, such as duty to warn and protect, and releasing data.

Identifying the Client

An essential first step in the provision of medical and mental health services is the need to identify the client. In most treatment contexts, this is obvious because it is the person receiving the treatment. However, there can be multiple clients in evaluation contexts, particularly when engaging in forensic roles. As we outlined in Chapter 5, this was the first area presented by Greenberg and Shuman (1997, 2007) in their seminal work, whereby they distinguished between therapeutic and forensic roles. The need to identify the client at the onset is critical because it will set the stage for our services moving forward, including many associated professional responsibilities (e.g., confidentiality, payment). For these reasons, it is advisable to prioritize this issue by identifying the client at the time a referral is made, while also clarifying the referral question. Again, there may be multiple clients in a given matter—just as there may be multiple referral questions. For example, an examinee is certainly one of an evaluator's clients, but the person may have been referred (and mandated) by any number of sources, such as by schools, employers, attorneys, or courts. Identifying the client is a necessary yet insufficient step, as we must then ascertain our professional responsibilities within the context of a given referral. For instance, there may be very limited confidentiality with particular examinees, in general, and our evaluation reports may need to be issued directly to referral sources and not examinees.

This issue is addressed directly and indirectly in various professional ethics codes and guidelines. For example, according to Standard 3.07 of the American Psychological Association's EPPCC (2017a), titled *Third-Party Requests for Services*:

When psychologists agree to provide services to a person or entity at the request of a third party, psychologists attempt to clarify at the outset of the service the nature of the relationship with all individuals or organizations involved. This clarification includes the role of the psychologist (e.g., therapist, consultant, diagnostician, or expert witness), an identification of who is the client, the probable uses of the services provided or the information obtained, and the fact that there may be limits to confidentiality. (p. 6)

The Specialty Guidelines for Forensic Psychology (2013) also addresses this issue, particularly via Guideline 4.01: Responsibilities to Retaining Parties. As the American Academy of Psychiatry and the Law's Ethics Guidelines for the Practice of Forensic Psychiatry (2005) note with respect to confidentiality:

Psychiatrists should indicate for whom they are conducting the examination and what they will do with the information obtained. At the beginning of a forensic evaluation, care should be taken to explicitly inform the evaluee that the psychiatrist is not the evaluee's "doctor." (pp. 1–2)

Both the American Counseling Association and the American Mental Health Counselors Association have comparable standards in their respective codes of ethics. In sum, all leading professional organizations recognize the need to identify the client and address the corresponding implications. The issue for us here, though, is to highlight how these considerations might play out in firearm-related matters involving patients or examinees. Let us look at a vignette for an illustration of such within the context of treatment and evaluation roles.

CASE EXAMPLE 8: TERRANCE BLAIR (THERAPEUTIC AND FORENSIC PROFESSIONALS)

Ana Moreno, MD, is a psychiatrist at the University Hospital Wellness Clinic in the city center. Given that the intake coordinator at the clinic schedules the doctor's appointments, Dr. Moreno did not meet Terrance Blair (age 43) until he arrived for his first session. However, she was notified in advance that he was self-referred to address depressive symptoms related to his recent loss of employment. At the onset of the first session, Dr. Moreno reviewed informed consent procedures with Mr. Blair, to include the limits of confidentiality. Based on her intake assessment, Dr. Moreno diagnosed Mr. Blair with an adjustment disorder and recommended he begin taking a relatively low dose of Celexa to address his symptoms. She continued to treat him for the next 6 months with good results, such that his symptoms significantly dissipated, and he was effectively on a maintenance regimen, with the expectation that he could come off the medication in the coming months. By all accounts, he was functioning very well, having secured employment and a relationship.

Unexpectedly, Dr. Moreno was contacted by a sergeant in the city's police department, asking about Mr. Blair. The officer indicated that Mr. Blair applied for a firearm ownership permit and noted his ongoing mental health treatment with her. The screening officer stated that he simply needed to know if Mr. Blair was psychiatrically stable and if he was suitable to own and operate guns. Given that Dr. Moreno did not have a release to speak with the officer, she informed him that she would need to get back to him. She then contacted Mr. Blair and he confirmed that he, in fact, did apply and provided her contact information at that time. Dr. Moreno informed Mr. Blair that, with his expressed consent, she could provide a treatment summary to the officer, but she would not be able to speak to Mr. Blair's firearm ownership suitability, specifically. Mr. Blair understood and signed a release accordingly (see also Case Example 5: Tonya Sorenson in Chapter 4).

Dr. Moreno subsequently spoke to the sergeant, but he indicated that he would need a professional opinion regarding Mr. Blair's appropriateness to own and operate guns. As such, Mr. Blair retained a psychologist who specializes in forensic assessment and conducts firearm-specific evaluations: Anthony Hogan, PhD. In contrast to Dr. Moreno's role, Dr. Hogan was hired as a forensic expert and, therefore, provided more nuanced informed consent. Namely, he explained to Mr. Blair that he would need to be able to conduct a collateral interview with Dr. Moreno for a treatment summary. He also reminded Mr. Blair that the information gathered throughout the evaluation process would be shared with the police sergeant via a report, if requested.

Dual Roles and Relationships, the "Therefore" Problem, and Weapon Focus

Perhaps one of the most oft-cited, yet misunderstood ethical areas is that which pertains to dual or multiple roles and relationships with clients. First and foremost, it is essential to point out that such is not necessarily unethical or even inappropriate. In fact, sometimes there is no choice but to engage in multiple roles with certain clients for particular reasons. It should also be highlighted that the concept of multiple relationships also applies to our work with those closely associated with our clients, and even includes promises of future relationships with either party. Again, engaging in a multiple relationship is not necessarily inappropriate. The line is drawn when it could interfere with a professional's services or lead to exploitation of the client, or harm otherwise. The language in the American Psychological Association's ethics code (EPPCC Standard 3.05, Multiple Relationships) is instructive in this regard:

> A psychologist refrains from entering into a multiple relationship if the multiple relationship could reasonably be expected to impair the psychologist's objectivity, competence, or effectiveness in performing his or her functions as a psychologist, or otherwise risks exploitation or harm to the person with whom the professional relationship exists.
>
> Multiple relationships that would not reasonably be expected to cause impairment or risk exploitation or harm are not unethical. (p. 6)

The code then goes on to indicate that psychologists should take proper steps to resolve any unforeseen issues that arise in this context and, also, that professionals clarify issues of role expectations and confidentiality in advance when they are required by law or an institution to engage in multiple roles. The American Counseling Association addresses this issue in Section A of its code, The Counseling Relationship, particularly in Section A.6, Managing and Maintaining Boundaries and Professional

Relationships. The American Mental Health Counselors Association addresses it in its code as well: I.A.3. Dual/Multiple Relationships as well as I.A.4. Exploitive Relationships. Both of these codes largely mimic that of the American Psychological Association. The American Psychiatric Association's annotations of the Principles of Medical Ethics does not explicitly address the issue. However, the American Academy of Psychiatry and the Law specifically addresses it in its 2005 Ethics Guidelines for the Practice of Forensic Psychiatry. Namely, the Commentary part of Section IV, Honesty and Striving for Objectivity, reads, in part:

> Treating psychiatrists appearing as "fact" witnesses should be sensitive to the unnecessary disclosure of private information or the possible misinterpretation of testimony as "expert" opinion. In situations when the dual role is required or unavoidable (such as Workers' Compensation, disability evaluations, civil commitment, or guardianship hearings), sensitivity to differences between clinical and legal obligations remains important.
>
> When requirements of geography or related constraints dictate the conduct of a forensic evaluation by the treating psychiatrist, the dual role may also be unavoidable; otherwise, referral to another evaluator is preferable.

The reality is that it is not uncommon for medical and mental health professionals to serve multiple roles for a client, particularly in institutions. For example, psychiatrists in state hospitals often serve as both evaluating and treating doctors for the same patients. As a result, they often testify in courtrooms situated in the hospital. It is also the case that professionals working in certain states with the insanity defense testify in state superior courts and the like, in relation to insanity acquitees who are being followed under such a jurisdictional requirement. In theory, multiple relationships may be more avoidable at the independent practice level as compared to institutional settings. Still, potentially exploitive relationships must be avoided in all settings and contexts.

In the firearm context, the most likely dual role in which we might potentially engage would be serving as a treating professional and, subsequently, an evaluating professional specific to the question of firearm ownership. However, as we have addressed in the preceding section, *Identifying the Client*, and in Chapter 4, this is a problematic dual role that should be completely avoided. We must distinguish between the concept of multiple relationships and dual roles in this regard. Here, the dual role would not simply be functioning as both a treating and evaluating professional, but as a forensic evaluator. The issue arises when we are confronted with what we refer to as the "therefore" problem.

Namely, when we are functioning in a therapeutic role, we can certainly provide treatment summaries and related information when authorized to do so,

> Ψ In the firearm context, the most likely dual role in which we might potentially engage would be serving as a treating professional and, subsequently, an evaluating professional specific to the question of firearm ownership. However, this is a problematic dual role that should be completely avoided.

> Ψ The "therefore" problem arises when we find ourselves providing clinical, treatment-related information and come to a "therefore" statement associated with a legal question. Such is likely an indication to stop.

but we can run into trouble if we link such to a legal question—hence the "therefore" problem. If we find ourselves providing clinical, treatment-related information and coming to a "therefore" statement associated with a legal question, it is likely an indication to stop. A basic example of a conclusion from a treatment summary is as follows:

In conclusion, Mr. Martin's anxiety has remained well managed and he remains psychiatrically and behaviorally stable.

Now, let us look at the "therefore" problem in action:

In conclusion, Mr. Martin's anxiety has remained well managed and he remains psychiatrically and behaviorally stable. Therefore, he is suitable to own and operate firearms at this time.

Some may raise an additional concern with the second illustration: The ultimate issue is answered directly. That calls for a separate discussion, unrelated to our primary focus here, which is the second sentence—the "therefore" sentence. Although it may seem like a minor, semantic issue, by connecting our clinical findings to a legal issue in this manner, we are essentially entering a forensic role. Perhaps the best way to further illustrate the point is via what we refer to as *weapon focus*. Typically, weapon focus is a concept used in the eyewitness reliability arena, whereby it refers to the phenomenon of witnesses focusing on the weapon a perpetrator is holding rather than the perpetrator himself. In our context, we are referring to clinicians' alteration of procedures when firearm-related issues arise.

> Ψ Typically, *weapon focus* is a concept used in the eyewitness reliability arena, whereby it refers to the phenomenon of witnesses focusing on the weapon a perpetrator is holding rather than the perpetrator himself. In our context, we are referring to clinicians' alteration of procedures when firearm-related issues arise.

This effect may prompt action or inaction in either direction, be it in support of or against a patient's gun rights. In other words, some clinicians may answer the ultimate issue, thereby overstepping therapeutic roles and embracing forensic ones. Others may be repelled by firearms and become resistant to sharing information that is expected and well within patients' rights, such as the issuance of treatment summaries.

To counteract potential bias associated with this type of weapon focus, we advise colleagues to substitute the gun-related question with others to see how their procedures might differ. A more obvious example would be to ask ourselves if we should sign off on patients' appropriateness to fly planes, or even drive cars for that matter (e.g., for those with seizure or neurodevelopmental disorders). Other more common examples include but are certainly not limited to questions related to child custody, employment, and personal injury. We must ask ourselves if, as treatment providers, we should answer the ultimate questions in these contexts—for instance, within the context of a therapeutic role, addressing which parent should have custody of a child or what the proximate cause was in an employment harassment or personal injury matter. The answer is "no." In fact, child custody matters, in particular, are associated with a fair amount of substantiated ethics complaints for blurring therapeutic and forensic roles.

So, why is this so confusing and misunderstood in firearm-related contexts? One reason may be that police departments, prosecutors, and judges do not readily distinguish between therapeutic and forensic roles at the onset of a matter. Police departments, in particular, may simply be looking for a clearance—a brief letter or the like—as a formality. Indeed, this can be quickly written and shifts liability to the clinician and away from the actual decision-maker—at least, in part. We must ask ourselves as clinicians, though, why such a brief sentence holds so much weight. Perhaps it is not so basic after all. To the contrary, we have found in our work (anecdotally, in New Jersey, New York, and Pennsylvania) that even the most comprehensive treatment report will be insufficient if it does not include the magic words from the legal standard in question. For example, in New Jersey, there must be some verbiage akin to saying the issuance of a firearms purchaser identification card or gun permit is not contrary to the "public health, safety or welfare." Sometimes, other types of language are specifically requested, such as explicitly indicating a patient is appropriate to own and operate firearms. Once again, such a statement would need to be based on a firearm-specific, forensic assessment and not simply on data gathered within a therapeutic role.

Termination of Services

At first glance, the ethical issue of terminating services may appear peculiar in the context of firearm-related issues; however, situations can arise whereby clinicians are uncomfortable working with gun owners. Indeed, we have seen this first-hand, more than once. For example, one of us (G.P.) was in the process of conducting a firearm ownership suitability evaluation for a gun owner who applied for an additional handgun permit. He had been engaging in psychotherapy with a psychologist for just over 1 year and disclosed such on his (handgun permit) application. As a result, his residential police department asked him to provide supporting documentation about his suitability to own and operate guns. However, his therapist declined to address this specific question, prompting him to retain a forensic evaluator. As is typical, consent was secured to conduct a collateral interview with the treating doctor to serve as a collateral source as part of the evaluation. However, the applicant noted that the therapist became uncomfortable when she found out he was a gun owner, as it was her (personal) belief that "no one" other than those in law enforcement should have guns in the home. While the therapist initially agreed to engage in a collateral interview for the evaluation and did so at some length, she later attempted to block her statements from entering the corresponding report. While this was unsuccessful because the proper consent was in place and the therapist voluntarily provided information already, the therapist subsequently terminated services with this patient, whom she had treated for quite a while. This type of situation raises concerns of *patient abandonment*, but there are actually various issues at play. Let us unpack a few.

In contrast to the question of abandonment, the therapist could argue that one should not proceed with clinical services if there would be interference due to personal reasons, such as bias or the like. If we consult the American Psychiatric Association's Annotations to the Principles of Medical Ethics, Section 6 indicates: "A physician shall, in the provision of appropriate patient care, except in emergencies, be free to choose whom to serve, with whom to associate, and the environment in which to provide medical care" (p. 8). No additional clarification applicable to our scenario here is provided, but a counterpoint would be that cultural competence is a necessary component of professional competence, which we will address in greater detail in the following subsection: *Cultural Competence and Personal Beliefs and Experiences*.

The American Psychological Association's EPPCC explicitly addresses termination in its section titled Terminating Therapy (10.10). However, the reasons for termination listed pertain to when a patient is no longer in need of the service, when the patient is unlikely to benefit from it, or when there would be harm by continuing it. Psychologists may also terminate when threatened or endangered by the patient or a related party. This standard does not quite capture the issue at hand for us. There is another section of the ethics code that is ostensibly more relevant: 2.06, Personal Problems and Conflicts. In this section, the EPPCC indicates that psychologists should refrain from engaging in activities when it is likely that personal problems or conflicts would interfere with their ability to competently render services. Moreover, Standard 2.01 (Boundaries of Competence) notes that psychologists should only provide services "with populations and in areas only within the boundaries of their competence, based on their education, training, supervised experience, consultation, study, or professional experience" (p. 5). As such, the therapist could argue that she lacks the professional competence to work with a gun owner or that her personal views on guns would interfere with her ability to properly treat him.

Both arguments raise additional concerns, though, as we will outline the following subsection. Namely, we would contend that these stances effectively preclude providing most clinical services because all clinicians must be able to assess suicide and violence risk at some level—and assessing firearm-related risk is inherent to both. In addition, the patient in our example had already been treated by this therapist for quite some time and, therefore, would essentially be admitting to doing so incompetently. Of course, this situation begs the question of how much we need to know about a patient before agreeing to provide services in the first place. In theory, there may be very many aspects of our patients' lives that are either against our personal views or outside of our areas of professional competence. The main issue we are addressing here is that of termination.

The American Mental Health Counselors Association and American Counseling Association ethics codes are similar to that of the American Psychological Association's, such that they indicate termination should be based on concerns for the patient and not the clinician per se, although exceptions are noted. Still, Section 5 (Termination and Referral) of the American Mental Health Counselors Association Code of Ethics is clear: "Mental health counselors do not abandon or neglect their clients in counseling" (p. 9). The American Counseling Association goes a step further than all of the codes reviewed here, though, and uses particularly strong language in this regard:

> Counselors refrain from referring prospective and current clients based solely on the counselor's personally held values, attitudes, beliefs, and behaviors. Counselors respect the diversity of clients and seek training in areas in which they are at risk of imposing their values onto clients, especially when the counselor's values are inconsistent with the client's goals or are discriminatory in nature. (p. 6, A.11.b, Values Within Termination and Referral)

Still, the question of professional competence remains:

> If counselors lack the competence to be of professional assistance to clients, they avoid entering or continuing counseling relationships. Counselors are knowledgeable about culturally and clinically appropriate referral resources and suggest these alternatives. If clients decline the suggested referrals, counselors discontinue the relationship. (p. 6, A.11.a, Competence Within Termination and Referral)

Let us now turn to a more focused discussion on the concept of cultural competence within the overarching context of professional competence, particularly in relation to our personal beliefs and experiences.

Cultural Competence and Personal Beliefs and Experiences

The concept of cultural competence has become synonymous with professional competence for medical and mental health professionals. The most common characteristics discussed in the context of diversity and cultural considerations are those related to sex, gender, race, religion, ethnicity, and language. However, cultural identities go well beyond these areas. Indeed, the American Psychological Association adopted the following definition of culture in its *Guidelines on Multicultural Education, Training, Research, Practice, and Organizational Change for Psychologists* (2017b):

> "Culture" is defined as the belief systems and value orientations that influence customs, norms, practices, and social institutions, including psychological processes (language, care taking practices, media, educational systems) and organizations (media, educational systems; Fiske, Kitayama, Markus, & Nisbett, 1998). (p. 8)

Of note is that the fifth principle in the American Psychological Association's EPPCC actually lists the term "culture" separately from other areas throughout. For example:

Psychologists are aware of and respect cultural, individual, and role differences, including those based on age, gender, gender identity, race, ethnicity, culture, national origin, religion, sexual orientation, disability, language, and socioeconomic status, and consider these factors when working with members of such groups. (p. 4, Principle E: Respect for People's Rights and Dignity)

The EPPCC also notes the importance of recognizing cultural differences in four additional areas; namely, ethical standards related to boundaries of competence, human relations (discrimination and harassment), and interpreting assessment results. As we indicated in the preceding section, *Termination of Services*, psychologists are to provide services, teach, and conduct research only with populations for whom they have sufficient competence. However, the code also includes a section on discrimination:

In their work-related activities, psychologists do not engage in unfair discrimination based on age, gender, gender identity, race, ethnicity, culture, national origin, religion, sexual orientation, disability, socioeconomic status, or any basis proscribed by law. (p. 6, Standard 3.01, Unfair Discrimination)

The need to recognize what is often termed "individual differences" is a core competency of medical and mental health education and training, and the other ethics codes reviewed here also address these concerns. For instance, per the American Mental Health Counselors Association Code of Ethics:

Mental health counselors are aware of their own values, attitudes, beliefs and behaviors, as well as how these apply in a society with clients from diverse ethnic, social, cultural, religious, and economic backgrounds. (p. 6, I.A.4, Exploitive Relationships)
    Recognize the important need to be competent in regard to cultural diversity and are sensitive to the diversity of varying populations as well as to changes in cultural expectations and values over time. (p. 15, C.1, Competence)
    Mental health counselors do not condone or engage in any discrimination based on ability, age, color, culture, disability, ethnic group, gender, gender identity, race, religion, national origin, political beliefs, sexual orientation, marital status, or socioeconomic status. (pp. 15–16, 2, Non-discrimination)
    Mental health counselors have a responsibility to educate themselves about their own biases toward those of different races, creeds, identities, orientations, cultures, and physical and mental abilities; and then to seek consultation, supervision and or counseling in order to prevent those biases interfering with the counseling process. (p. 16, 2, Non-discrimination)

The issue of nondiscrimination is salient in each code across disciplines. Indeed, according to Section 1 of the Principles of Medical Ethics, "A psychiatrist should not be a party to any type of policy that excludes, segregates, or demeans the dignity of any patient because of ethnic origin, race, sex, creed, age, socioeconomic status, or sexual orientation" (p. 3).

In the American Counseling Association's code, the term *culture* is used over 50 times—also in areas related to boundaries of competence and nondiscrimination, comparable to the American Psychological Association and American Mental Health Counselors Association codes. Of particular note is that the American Counseling Association is the only group to explicitly define the term:

> Culture—membership in a socially constructed way of living, which incorporates collective values, beliefs, norms, boundaries, and lifestyles that are cocreated with others who share similar worldviews comprising biological, psychosocial, historical, psychological, and other factors. (p. 20)

In the firearm context, all of the areas delineated are potentially applicable for a given person, as clients may be a part of a group that employs certain collective values, beliefs, norms, boundaries, and lifestyles by virtue of some firearm-related association. This is consistent with the cultural framework we outlined in Chapter 1 in the sections *Firearm-Related Subcultures* and *Taking Steps to Develop Firearm-Related Cultural Competence*. The take-home message within the ethical context here is that we cannot (and should not) discriminate against clients or potential clients, and we need to be sufficiently competent to provide services for those across firearm-related subcultures.

The discrimination question is likely more complicated than most of us may think at first glance. For those of us practicing in so-called blue states, particularly those with low gun ownership, it is not necessarily uncommon for our colleagues to simply refuse to assist gun applicants or owners in securing permits and the like. When a firearm-specific evaluation is called for, this type of stepping away is necessary because of the forensic nature of the service. On the other hand, it would be improper to refuse to provide records to clients or to otherwise impede their efforts to secure firearm-related approvals. Of course, if risk-related concerns are present, we can and should certainly note them when applicable, but setting forth a client-specific, risk-related concern is wholeheartedly different than imposing our personal or even broad-based professional views in a given situation. For example, some of us may believe that no one other than those in law enforcement should own a gun. However, this worldview cannot be applied to every client who asks us for a treatment summary, which is what we can typically reasonably provide when functioning in a therapeutic role. Presumably, those willing to conduct forensic, firearm-specific evaluations are willing to indicate certain people are appropriate for gun ownership, so the bigger focus in that regard is ensuring personal views do not interfere with the procedures and ultimate opinions (as with all forensic assessments). Let us address treatment providers for a moment once again before moving on to the next section.

As we discussed in detail in Chapter 4, assessing firearm-related risk is a core component of suicide and violence risk assessment in therapeutic and other contexts. Moreover, gun owners make up roughly one-third of the U.S. population. Therefore, a rhetorical question is called for: Is it reasonable to recuse ourselves from having any involvement at all in gun-related matters, even in treatment contexts, particularly given that assessing this type of risk is a necessity when conducting suicide and violence risk assessments? To reiterate: It is appropriate and advisable to decline engaging in problematic dual roles (e.g., treatment provider and forensic evaluator) or to provide services outside of our areas of professional competence. However, if we do not recognize firearm-related education and training as an essential area of professional competence (see Pirelli & Gold, 2019), we would be conceding that we are unable to assess firearm-related risk at any level or engage with clients from firearm-related subcultures. This would effectively exclude our ability to work with very many clients across a wide range of contexts. This book is designed in large part to assist in navigating the countless nuances that may arise in our clinical practices. As such, it is essential to remember that overly broad exclusionary practices are just as ill advised as those that are completely inclusive, as our professional liabilities hang in the balance. Simply put, there are certain things we can and should do, and there are others we cannot and should not do. The key is developing the ability to distinguish between these paths. In fact, professional decision-making, to include that which is ethical, depends on it.

> Ψ If we do not recognize firearm-related education and training as an essential area of professional competence, we would be conceding that we are unable to assess firearm-related risk at any level or engage with clients from firearm-related subcultures. This would effectively exclude our ability to work with very many clients across a wide range of contexts.

Breaking Confidentiality: Reporting Requirements,
Duty to Warn and Protect, and Releasing Data

As we addressed in greater detail in Chapter 2, reporting laws are particularly relevant in firearm-related contexts because of the importance of violence and suicide risk assessment. At the same time, breaking clients' confidentiality warrants very close attention and serious consideration. We are required to do so in some situations, whereas we are prohibited from doing so in others. Of course, there are many situations wherein we are asked to do so and, therefore, we must use our discretion. Nevertheless, all situations call for sound professional decision-making based on not only our knowledge of legal and ethical requirements but also case-specific information.

Before we continue it is essential to preface our discussion here by reiterating that we must be aware of our state laws and regulations as well as the ethical standards from our respective disciplines. There is consensus across disciplines with regard to breaking confidentiality and related issues, but state laws can vary considerably and may change at any given time. Thus, it is incumbent upon us as clinicians to be well aware of our requirements related to confidentiality and to stay abreast of potential developments in this regard. These considerations are applicable to all areas of practice but are particularly worth emphasizing in this context.

> Ψ There is consensus across disciplines with regard to breaking confidentiality and related issues, but state laws can vary considerably and may change at any given time. We must be aware of our state laws and regulations as well as the ethical standards from our respective disciplines.

With the aforementioned caveats in mind, let us first address reporting requirements in relation to so-called duty to warn and protect regulations. The American Psychological Association's ethics code has a full section titled Privacy and Confidentiality, Section 4, which clearly indicates that disclosure of confidential information is done with the appropriate consent in place—and only without consent when such disclosure is mandated by law. The American Psychiatric Association's Principles of Medical Ethics is the same in this regard and notes that "Confidentiality is essential to psychiatric treatment" (p. 6). Furthermore, the ethics codes of the American Counseling Association and the American Mental Health Counselors Association both have sections solely dedicated to confidentiality. The American Counseling Association code notes: "Counselors recognize that trust is a cornerstone of the counseling relationship" (p. 6) and the American Mental Health Counselors Association indicates: "Mental health counselors have a primary obligation to safeguard information about individuals obtained in the course of practice, teaching, or research," adding that "Confidentiality is a right granted to all clients of mental health counseling services" (p. 2).

Indeed, maintaining confidentiality is regarded with the utmost importance across disciplines, as is reflected in their respective ethics codes. However, all of them also highlight exceptions, particularly associated with risk-related concerns. Namely, all four ethics codes reviewed here note that confidentiality can be broken when there are concerns of harm to self or others:

> Psychologists disclose confidential information without the consent of the individual only as mandated by law, or where permitted by law for a valid purpose such as to . . . (3) protect the client/patient, psychologist, or others from harm. (American Psychological Association's EPPCC, 4.05 Disclosures, p. 8)

> When, in the clinical judgment of the treating psychiatrist, the risk of danger is deemed to be significant, the psychiatrist may reveal confidential information disclosed by the patient. (American Psychiatric Association, Section 4, p. 7)

> The general requirement that counselors keep information confidential does not apply when disclosure is required to protect clients or identified others from serious and foreseeable harm or when legal requirements demand that

confidential information must be revealed. (American Counseling Association, B.2.a, Exceptions, Serious and Foreseeable Harm and Legal Requirements, p. 7)

The release of information without consent of the client may only take place under the most extreme circumstances: the protection of life (suicidality or homicidality), child abuse, and/or abuse of incompetent persons and elder abuse. Above all, mental health counselors are required to comply with state and federal statutes concerning mandated reporting. (American Mental Health Counselors Association, 2. Confidentiality, p. 2)

It is for this reason that states adopting firearm-related legislation that interferes with the therapeutic relationship, particularly in relation to confidentiality, have done so in direct contrast to recommendations made by leading mental health organizations and professionals. For instance, per the American Psychiatric Association's 2015 position statement on firearm-related issues:

Because privacy in mental health treatment is essential to encourage persons in need of treatment to seek care, laws designed to limit firearm possession that mandate reporting to law enforcement officials by psychiatrists and other mental health professionals of all patients who raise concerns about danger to themselves or others are likely to be counterproductive and should not be adopted. In contrast to long-standing rules allowing mental health professionals flexibility in acting to protect identifiable potential victims of patient violence, these statutes intrude into the clinical relationship and are unlikely to be effective in reducing rates of violence. (Pinals et al., 2015, p. 198)

Because we are obligated to adhere to state laws when engaging in our professional work as clinicians, those of us living in states that force such broader disclosures (e.g., New Jersey) must not only be cautious in our own right but must also highlight these types of nuanced issues in our informed consent processes. Remember: Providing proper informed consent information to our patients and examinees requires that we be fully informed, first and foremost.

> Ψ Remember: Providing proper informed consent information to our patients and examinees requires that we be fully informed, first and foremost.

An important point to highlight before moving on, though, is that duty to warn and/or protect laws are not based on the presence or absence of a firearm during an incident of potential concern. In fact, so-called red flag laws are not even based on such. Therefore, firearm ownership or easy access otherwise is a potential moderating risk factor and should be considered in the context of means restriction in cases wherein interventions are warranted. In other words, the presence of or easy access to a gun does not in and of itself place someone at a high risk of suicide or violence, but such is a great concern for those at elevated risk—particularly those at acute, elevated risk. It is for this reason that the concept of gun rights restoration exists (i.e., mental health statuses and associated risk levels can, and often do, change over time).

Ethics codes and state laws are often fairly straightforward in terms of the practical aspects of the actual reporting and releasing of confidential information, and all ethics codes defer to state laws in relation to confidentiality. What is much less clearly defined (and definable), however, is the process that leads us to the very important decision of breaking confidentiality. For example, some states with "red flag" laws (e.g., New Jersey) have lengthy procedures mapped out by their state attorney general's offices, which correspond to legislation in these contexts. However, these address what is to happen *after* reporting has taken place. Put differently, clinical discretion cannot be legislated (see Chapters 4 and 5 for discussions on risk assessment in both clinical and forensic contexts). The take-home message for us here is that we must look to our state laws for primary information on our reporting requirements, and to our respective ethics codes for general guidance in this regard, but to the contemporary professional literature for the more specific and applied practice standards and guidelines that will facilitate the best possible procedural decisions in a given case.

While disclosure of confidential information is, perhaps, most typically considered by clinicians in the context of risk-related scenarios (i.e., duty to warn and/or protect), the issue certainly arises in less imminently concerning contexts. Namely, records can be requested by patients or examinees for the sole reason of recordkeeping on their end. In other cases, treating professionals may wish to see the records to ensure effective continuity of care and communication. In others still, records may be requested by courts, attorneys, or other agencies—informally or via subpoena or even court order. To be clear, we must always comply with court orders. However, if there is an order that is inconsistent with our role or scope, or otherwise causes us concern or pause, we can seek clarification from the court. In these (usually rare) instances, we may want to consult with legal counsel, which is typically available through malpractice insurance carriers and professional agencies—aside from private attorneys.

Many of us work for agencies or institutions that have in-house counsel who would need to be consulted anyhow in these instances. Regardless of our potential resources, the take-home message here is: Never ignore a court order. That said, we should not ignore most other requests either; the idea is not to dismiss requests, but rather, to determine how to respond to them.

> Ψ Do not ignore requests for records, from court orders, subpoenas, or even less formal requests; rather, seek clarification and consultation as needed to determine the most appropriate responses.

For instance, while a subpoena may technically hold less weight than a court order per se, it still is a formal summons to provide records and/or appear for testimony, and failure to respond could result in legal sanctions. The question is not really whether we should respond, but instead, how and to what extent. Herein lies the endless possibilities and nuances. Let us start with what we should definitely not do, which is to simply respond immediately with everything requested. While we certainly cannot and will not attempt to offer legal advice, it is incumbent upon all of us as clinicians to ensure that requests are appropriate and that our adherence to them would not be problematic—legally or otherwise. A specific set of directions for handling a subpoena is outside of our scope here, but suffice to say that we should take proper and reasonable steps to ensure our responses to such requests are sound. For example, we may receive subpoenas seeking our patients' records from third parties of whom we have literally never heard. In most cases, it is appropriate to contact the party with whom we have established a professional relationship (e.g., patient, retaining attorney) and confirm the legitimacy of the request—to include confirmation that the patient or client in question signed the proper releases and the like. This is a very basic, initial step, and the reality is that the issue of responding to subpoenas can be rather complex. Take, for example, subpoenas that include requests for raw test data and even test materials, or that simply ask for all available records. In many cases, patients have never even seen their mental health treatment records, and we have a professional obligation to protect various types of information—especially if we believe it could be (psychologically) harmful to our clients. Given the potential complexities in any given subpoena, the concepts of seeking *clarification* and *consultation* cannot be overemphasized here, whereas avoidance is ill advised.

Requests via court orders and subpoenas can be anxiety-provoking, especially for those of us who do not interface with the legal system much, but less formal requests for records should not necessarily be treated less seriously. One particularly important concept to remember is that, in many instances, our patients are entitled to their records, the operative term being *their records*. As medical and mental health providers, we are required to engage in proper recordkeeping practices, but the records are not ours per se. At the risk of entering a complicated legal discussion on the issue, let us be clear that we are addressing this from a professional practice perspective. Of course, there are federal and state laws and regulations pertaining to recordkeeping, and many of us must navigate our employers' policies in this regard. In addition, each discipline has ethics codes and professional guidelines corresponding to recordkeeping do's and don'ts. While the nuances across the aforementioned sources are critically important to know and consider, they are outside of our particular scope here; rather, we want to focus on the general concept of less formal record requests for a moment (i.e., those not court-ordered or subpoenaed).

> Ψ One particularly important concept to remember is that, in many instances, our patients are entitled to their records, the operative term being *their records*.

As a rule, we should all be following predetermined procedures that are in line with federal and state laws and consistent with professional ethics and practice standards. This may seem like an obvious point to clinicians employed by established agencies or institutions. However, those of us in private, or independent, practices must also have procedures in place to properly handle record requests. Perhaps the best starting point in this context is to be very clear as to who is our client, as we discussed in some detail in the *Forensic Mental Health Assessment* section of Chapter 5. Remember that identifying the client and managing expectations should occur prior to engaging in services in the first place, and that patients, examinees, and other clients (e.g., retaining attorneys, judges) should be provided with informed consent–related information at the onset of such services. Proper informed consent procedures include an explanation of recordkeeping practices, such as how and what type of data will be gathered, generated, stored, and disbursed.

As with many issues in clinical practice, the informed consent process can prevent serious misunderstandings and related problems that can arise when a client requests records at a later point. For this main reason, to effectively manage expectations, the informed consent process should be sufficiently thorough and carefully conducted. Indeed, problems often come about when people's expectations are violated. Therefore, it is our job to ensure our clients' expectations are consistent with our actual practices rather than their assumptions. Keep in mind that medical, dental, and related clinical records are often readily available to people in this day and age. As such, clients are likely to assume mental health–related records are no different and they might be correct; we should not assume clients are not entitled to their records simply because relatively few people ask for them or our employers deter these types of requests.

> Ψ To effectively manage expectations, the informed consent process should be sufficiently thorough and carefully conducted. Proper informed consent procedures include an explanation of recordkeeping practices, such as how and what type of data will be gathered, generated, stored, and disbursed.

Denying or otherwise stalling a record request is essentially just as serious of a matter as readily complying with such. There are countless scenarios in which we might find ourselves with clients, but one thing is for certain: We should not decline record requests because we have *personal* opinions about what clients want to do with the records. The reader is encouraged to revisit the section in this chapter titled *Dual Roles and Relationships, the "Therefore" Problem, and Weapon Focus*, particularly as such relates to our concept of weapon focus. Of course, the previous section, *Cultural Competence and Personal Beliefs and Experiences*, is also directly related to the issue at hand. In a nutshell, as clinicians, we must have a *professional* rather than personal reason to decline a record request, usually based on either a practical or a clinical reason. For instance, a practical reason may simply be that the direct client is not the requesting party

> Ψ As clinicians, we must have *professional* rather than personal reasons to decline record requests; we should not decline record requests because we have *personal* opinions about what clients want to do with their records. Do not succumb to potential weapon focus. Rather, focus on the procedural aspects of the requests.

and, therefore, we need a release (e.g., an examinee request records, but the retaining party/direct client was another entity, such as a school, community agency, or court). A clinical reason could be we are concerned exposure to the documented material in question would be psychologically deleterious to a particular patient. The latter example is one that is likely most familiar to those of us who engage in treatment, or therapeutic, roles. Nevertheless, the central point for our purposes here is that records cannot be withheld simply because a client wants them for the purposes of (legally) securing firearms. Just as in other contexts, requests may entail sending records to clients and/or their designees (e.g., other clinicians or police departments), and laws and professional guidelines corresponding to the dissemination of records come into play just the same. The take-home message is: Do not succumb to potential weapon focus. Rather, focus on the procedural aspects of the requests—again, with attention to concerns based on professional-clinical reasons and not personal ones.

Considerations for Internet-Based Data

We would be remiss if we omitted a particularly timely and crucial area of consideration in contemporary medical and mental health practice; namely, that which pertains to internet-based data associated with patients and examinees. The literature related to using the internet to provide mental health services, variously called teletherapy, telepsychology, e-therapy, online counseling, cybertherapy, web counseling, and computer-mediated psychotherapy, has continued to develop over the last decade or so (see, e.g., Alleman, 2002; Drum & Littleton, 2014; Grajales et al., 2014; Heinlen et al., 2003; Manhal-Baugus, 2001; Midkiff & Wyatt, 2008; Wells et al., 2007; Zur et al., 2009). Of course, the COVID-19 pandemic forced us and our respective professional associations to quickly adapt and offer remote services on a much wider scale than we would have otherwise.

Indeed, the internet was created in 1983 and social media platforms like Facebook (2004), Twitter (2006), and Instagram (2010) were all created over 10 years prior to the onset of the pandemic in 2020. Yet, our professional associations and corresponding ethics codes remained largely silent on how to navigate internet-based issues in practice. The ethics codes of the American Counseling Association (2014) and the American Mental Health Counselors Association (2015) address internet- and social media–related considerations, although they do so rather briefly and in relation to teletherapy. The ethics codes for the American Psychological Association and American Psychiatric Association offer no guidance in this regard. Still, there is a fair amount of literature and professional guidance associated with virtual practice and internet-based data that is available to treatment providers at this point, especially since 2020.

The mental health assessment arena has yet to catch up, as the literature is still developing along with practical aspects of the field (e.g., remote administration of tests). The subdiscipline of forensic psychiatry has begun to address these types of issues at some level (e.g., see the practice guideline of the American Academy of Psychiatry and the Law, 2015; Metzner & Ash, 2010; Neimark et al., 2006; Recupero, 2008, 2010), as has neuropsychology (e.g., see Bilder et al., 2020; Thibodaux et al., 2021).

In 2016, we published considerations for using internet and social media data as a collateral source in forensic mental health evaluations, followed by an empirical investigation (Pirelli et al., 2016, 2018) that provided additional support for the five considerations we previously set forth:

1. Forensic practitioners who utilize internet data should conceptualize it as a type of collateral information.
2. Although searching for and using internet-based data is not prohibited by the EPPCC or forensic practice guidelines, forensic practitioners should consider conducting internet searches in evaluations on a case-by-case basis, weighing the potential utility versus the potentially prejudicial effects of such data.
3. With rare exceptions, forensic practitioners who gather and/or rely on internet-based data should discuss this practice during the retention and informed consent processes.
4. With rare exceptions, forensic practitioners should provide examinees with data gathered via the internet and allow them to address it.
5. Forensic practitioners should be explicit about their use of and reliance upon any data gathered via the internet in their reports and testimony.

More recently, Batastini and Vitacco (2020) published an edited book on the topic of conducting forensic mental health assessments in the digital age, which includes chapters on criminal responsibility, competency to stand trial, violence risk and threat assessment, sexually problematic behaviors, child custody litigation and parental fitness, pre-employment and fitness-for-duty evaluations in the law enforcement arena, and personal injury and disability. Contributions like this are instrumental in creating a solid foundation of guidance vis-à-vis remote practice and data generated online.

Internet-based considerations are particularly relevant to firearm-related concerns for patients and examinees because there are many instances whereby people post statements and images online that raise concerns. This is especially true in school-aged circles, including at the college and even graduate levels. Still, the striking proliferation of internet and social media use throughout the U.S. population (and the world) has made it so that almost everyone is producing some level of data online, directly or indirectly. Approximately three-quarters of the U.S. population uses at least one social media platform and, at this point, usage rates are comparable across age groups between 18 and 65 (Pew Research Center, 2021). That said, even 45% of the age group of 65+ reports social media usage. Moreover, there are essentially no differences in rate of usage across races, genders, income levels, education levels, or community settings (i.e., urban, suburban, rural). As a result, we should assume the vast majority of our patients and examinees are directly producing data online or, at the very least, others are doing so in relation to them—even in ways such as a photo on Facebook. While certain posts may seem benign, even the simplest of images, statements, memes, and the like can lead others to raise flags. As forensic evaluators, we are routinely called to evaluate risk because of concerns prompted by internet-based data, often but not always from schools and employment settings. Still, all of us—medical and mental health treatment and evaluating professionals alike—must be attuned to the realities of how our digital world interfaces with practice, and recognize that firearm-related issues require additional, important considerations.

RECOMMENDED FURTHER READING

American Academy of Psychiatry and the Law. (2005). Ethics guidelines for the practice of forensic psychiatry. https://www.aapl.org/ethics.htm

American Academy of Psychiatry and the Law. (2015). AAPL practice guideline for the forensic assessment. *Journal of the American Academy of Psychiatry and the Law*, 43(2 Supplement), S3–S53.

American Counseling Association. (2014). 2014 ACA code of ethics. https://www.counseling. org/docs/default-source/default-document-library/2014-code-of-ethics-finaladdress.pdf

American Mental Health Counselors Association. (2015, October). AMHCA code of ethics. https://www.amhca.org/HigherLogic/System/DownloadDocumentFile.ashx?Document FileKey=5ff5bc94-e534-091e-c7c1-e3ea45cf943e%26forceDialog=0

American Psychiatric Association. (2013). *The principles of medical ethics with annotations especially applicable to psychiatry.* https://www.psychiatry.org/File%20Library/Psychiatrists/ Practice/Ethics/principles-medical-ethics.pdf

American Psychological Association. (2013). Specialty guidelines for forensic psychology. *American Psychologist*, 68(1), 7–19. https://doi.org/10.1037/a0029889

American Psychological Association. (2017). Ethical principles of psychologists and code of conduct. https://www.apa.org/ethics/code/ethics-code-2017.pdf

Neal, T. M. S., & Grisso, T. (2014). The cognitive underpinnings of bias in forensic mental health evaluations. *Psychology, Public Policy, and Law*, 20(2), 200–211.

Otto, R. K., Goldstein, A. M., & Heilbrun, K. (2017). *Ethics in forensic psychology practice.* Wiley.

Pirelli, G., Beattey, R. A., & Zapf, P. A. (2017). *The ethical practice of forensic psychology: A casebook.* Oxford University Press.

Pirelli, G., & Gold, L. (2019). Leaving Lake Wobegon: Firearm-related education and training for medical and mental health professionals is an essential competence. *Journal of Aggression, Conflict and Peace Research*, 11(2), 78–87.

GLOSSARY OF FIREARM-RELATED TERMS

ACP Automatic Colt pistol, a type of ammunition.

Action The mechanism of a firearm involved with presenting the cartridge for firing, removing the spent casing, and introducing a fresh cartridge.

Airsoft Gun A firearm pressurized by air to shoot non-metal projectiles.

Ammunition A supply or quantity of bullets and shells that are fired from a firearm.

AR-15 ArmaLite Rifle, a semiautomatic firearm that is gas-operated.

Assault Weapon An automatic firearm with a detachable magazine and a pistol grip, often a type of rifle typically for military use.

Automatic A firearm that continues to fire as long as the trigger remains depressed.

Backstrap The rear of two gripstraps on a handgun, which lies beneath the heel of the hand when gripping the gun.

Ball A military term for standard, full metal–jacketed ammunition.

Ballistics The science of cartridge discharge and the bullet's flight.

Barrel The barrel serves the purpose of providing direction and velocity to the bullet; it is long and in the shape of a tube (cylinder).

BB Gun A firearm that fires small pellets (BBs) using pressurized air.

Blowback The backpressure in an internal combustion when firing a firearm.

Bluing The chemical process of artificial oxidation (rusting) applied to gun parts so that the metal attains a dark blue or nearly black appearance.

Bore The interior of a gun barrel.

Bore Diameter The diameter of the inside of the barrel. The land-to-land diameter.

Breech That portion of the gun that contains the rear chamber of the barrel; the action, trigger, or firing mechanism; and the magazine.

Breechblock The part of the weapon that seals the rear of the chamber and supports the casehead when the cartridge is fired.

Bull Barrel A heavier, thicker-than-normal barrel with little or no narrowing toward the end.

Bullet The metal projectile, typically in the shape of a pointed cylinder, expelled from the mouth of a firing cartridge.

Butt The part of a firearm that is held or shouldered, where the firing mechanism and barrel are connected.

Caliber The diameter of the bore of a barrel measured from land to land, usually measured in tenths of an inch or in millimeters. It does not designate the actual diameter of a bullet.

Cannelure A groove or indention around the circumference of a bullet.

Cartridge In modern terms, a round of ammunition consisting of casing, primer, powder, and projectile. In the "percussion-cap" era, the cartridge consisted of the projectile and powder in a paper packet, with the primer cap separate.

Casing A cylindrical tube closed at one end that holds the primer and powder of a cartridge. The cartridge bullet is crimped into the open end of the casing. They are typically made from brass but can be steel, aluminum, or even plastic.

Centerfire A cartridge in which the primer or primer assembly is seated in a pocket or recess in the center of the base of the casing (the casing head). Also refers to a firearm that uses centerfire cartridges.

Chamber The part of the firearm at the rear of the barrel that is reamed out so that it can contain a cartridge for firing.

Charger A device typically made from stamped metal that holds a group of cartridges for easy and virtually simultaneous loading.

Choke To keep the shotgun pellets in a tighter group, there is a constriction of the shotgun bore at the muzzle.

Clip This term is often used when referring to a detachable magazine, but, in fact, it is a device, usually of stamped metal similar to a charger, that holds a group of cartridges and is inserted along with the cartridges into certain magazines. It is expelled after the last round in the magazine is spent.

Cock The term referring to the action of manually drawing the hammer back against its spring until it becomes latched against the sear, or sometimes the trigger itself, arming the hammer to be released by a subsequent pull of the trigger.

Concealed Carry To carry a firearm on one's person that cannot be seen by the public.

Constitutional Carry To carry a firearm in public that does not need to be concealed without a government permit.

Cylinder A rotating cartridge holder in a revolver. The cylinder also contains the chamber portion of the revolver. Cartridges are held, and fired, within the cylinder. Cartridge chambers are evenly placed around the axis of the cylinder. The cylinder has a linkage to the firing mechanism, which rotates each chamber into alignment with the barrel prior to each firing.

Cylinder Stop On a revolver, a spring-activated device housed in the bottom of the frame beneath the cylinder that engages alignment notches in the cylinder. It stops the cylinder's rotation and holds it in place each time a chamber in the cylinder is in alignment with the barrel.

Double-Action (DA) A revolver or pistol on which a long trigger pull can both cock and release the hammer to fire the weapon. In a revolver this action also rotates the cylinder to the next chambered round. DA also implies a single-action stage that can cock the gun separately, alternately called double-action/single-action, or DA/SA.

Double-Action Only Typically on striker-fired pistols and spurless-hammer revolvers and referring to a trigger where the firing mechanism cannot be cocked in a single-action stage. Firing always occurs as a double-action sequence where pulling the trigger both cocks and then fires the gun.

Double Barrel Two barrels that are side by side or one on top of the other, which bullets are shot through, typically on a shotgun.

Dovetail A flaring machined or hand-cut slot that is also slightly tapered toward one end. Cut into the upper surface of barrels and sometimes actions, the dovetail accepts a corresponding part on which the sight is mounted.

Ears Hearing protection.

Ejector The part on the firearm whose function is to throw a spent casing from the gun after firing.

Ejector Star On a revolver, the collective ejector, manually operated through the center of an opened cylinder; when activated, clears all chambers at once.

Extractor On a pistol, a part attached to the breechblock, which withdraws the spent casing from the chamber.

Eyes Eye protection (safety glasses).

Firearms Identification Card A permit issued by a state or local government allowing the sale, purchase, or ownership of a firearm.

Firing Pin In a hammer-fired gun, this is a hardened pin housed in the breechblock, centered directly behind the primer cap of a chambered cartridge. When struck by the hammer it impacts the primer cap of the cartridge, discharging the weapon.

Frame The common part of a handgun to which the action, barrel, and grip are connected.

Front Strap The part of a revolver or pistol grip frame that faces forward and often joins with the trigger guard.

Full Metal Jacket A round of ammo where each bullet is encased in a stronger/ harder metal.

GAP Glock auto pistol, a type of ammunition.

Gauge The amount of lead balls you can make from one pound of lead of equal diameter to a shotgun's barrel.

Grip The handle used to hold a handgun. Often refers to the side panels of the handle.

Gripstraps The exposed portion of a handgun's frame, the frontstrap and backstrap, that provides the foundation for the handgun's grip.

Grooves Spiral cuts made in the bore of a barrel that give the bullet its spin or rotation as it moves down the barrel.

Gunpowder A propellant explosive.

Half Cock The position of the hammer in a hammer-activated firing mechanism that acts as a manual safety.

Hammer That part of a revolver or pistol that impacts the firing pin or the cartridge directly, discharging the weapon. Its movement is rotational around its axis, which is fixed to the frame.

Hammerless This general term can refer to either (1) revolver or pistol designs that actually have hammers that are fully encased inside the frames, (2) hammer designs where the spurs have been removed for concealment, or (3) striker-fired pistols that are truly hammerless.

Hammer Spur The thumb piece on the top rear of the hammer that enables it to be manually drawn back to full cock.

Handgun A firearm, typically a pistol or revolver, that can be fired and held with one hand.

Handloading The process of loading a firearm with cartridges assembled from the individual components (primer, shell casing, gunpowder, and bullet).

HMR Hornady Magnum Rimfire, a type of ammunition.

Holster A case (usually made of leather or fabric) that is on a person (typically on the hip) used to carry a firearm.

Ignition The way gunpowder is lit.

Jacket The casing surrounding a bullet.

Laser A laser is used for accurately aiming a firearm in a quick manner.

LC Long Colt, a type of ammunition.

Long Recoil A semiautomatic pistol in which the barrel and breechblock are locked together for the full distance of rearward recoil travel, after which the barrel returns forward, while the breechblock is held back. After the barrel has fully returned, the breechblock is released to fly forward, chambering a fresh round in the process.

LR Long rifle, a type of ammunition.

Machine Gun A firearm where a single pull of the trigger fires multiple shots; an automatic weapon.

Magazine A container, either fixed to a pistol's frame or detachable, that holds cartridges under spring pressure to be fed into the gun's chamber.

Magnum A modern cartridge with a higher-velocity load or heavier projectile than standard.

Mainspring Term often used for the hammer spring.

Master Marksman A person who has mastered the use of a weapon.

Match Grade When a modification is made to a firearm to increase accuracy.

Misfeed Entering a round into a chamber incorrectly.

Misfire A condition when firing a gun in which the cartridge fails to discharge.

Muzzle The forward end of the barrel where the projectile exits.

Muzzle Velocity The speed of the bullet, measured in feet per second or meters per second, as it leaves the barrel.

Neck The constricted forward section of a bottle-necked cartridge casing—the portion that grips the bullet.

NICS (National Instant Criminal Background Check System) Used by Federal Firearms License holders for determining whether it is legal to sell a firearm to a prospective purchaser.

Ogive A type of curve represented by the curved section of a bullet between its bearing surface and its tip.

Open Carry To carry a firearm that is not concealed from the public.

Open Frame Refers to a revolver frame that has no topstrap over the cylinder.

Pellet Gun A firearm that fires a skirted pellet using pressurized air (CO_2).

Pistol Refers generally to any handgun that is not a revolver. This includes self-loaders, manual repeaters, single-shots, double- or multiple-barrel pistols, and derringers.

Plinking Shooting at inanimate objects, typically to practice shooting.

Polygonal Rifling without hard-edged lands or grooves, typically consisting of flat surfaces that meet at angles around the bore.

Powder A chemical that is ignited in order for a bullet to be fired.

Primer A small detonating cap fitted in the head of a centerfire cartridge casing that, when struck by a firing pin, ignites the powder charge.

Primer Pocket The counter bore in the center of the base of a centerfire cartridge casing in which the primer assembly is seated.

Primer Ring Refers to a visible dark ring created by the primers in centerfire ammunition around the firing pin hole in the frame after much use.

Receiver In handguns, this refers to the frame.

Recoil-Operated Refers to a semiautomatic pistol whose barrel and breechblock both recoil rearward in reaction to the discharging bullet.

Revolver A handgun that has revolving cylinder chambers that hold several cartridges, allowing several shots to be fired without reloading.

Rifle A long gun with a grooved barrel, fired from shoulder level, that causes a bullet to spin for an increase in accuracy.

Rifling Typically, a series of spiral grooves cut into the bore of the barrel. Rifling stabilizes the bullet in flight by causing it to spin. Rifling may rotate to the right or left. See *twist*.

Rimfire A self-contained metallic cartridge where the primer is contained inside the hollow rim of the cartridge case. The primer is detonated by the firing pin striking the outside edge of the rim, crushing the rim against the rear face of the barrel.

Rimless Refers to a cartridge in which the base diameter is the same as the body diameter. The casing will normally have an extraction groove machined around it near the base, creating a "rim" at the base that is the same diameter as the body diameter.

Round A unit of ammunition consisting of the primer, casing, propellant, and bullet; a cartridge.

Safety A mechanical device built into a weapon intended to prevent accidental discharge. It may be either manually operated or automatic.

Sawed-Off Shotgun A shotgun that has a shorter barrel (usually under 18 inches) than a standard shotgun.

Sear A pivoting part of the firing mechanism of a gun, either part of the trigger or an intermediate piece, that catches and holds the hammer or striker at full cock. Pressure on the trigger causes the sear to release the hammer or striker, allowing it to strike the firing pin and discharge the weapon.

Self-Loader Another term for semiautomatic; more commonly refers to early designs of semiautomatic pistols.

Semiautomatic A pistol that is loaded manually for the first round. Upon pulling the trigger, the gun fires. Energy from the discharging bullet is used to eject the fired round, cock the firing mechanism, and feed a fresh round from the magazine. The trigger must be released after each shot and pulled again to fire the next round.

Shell An empty ammunition case.

Shotgun A long gun with smoothbore barrels that usually fires shotshells. Shotshell cartridges contain numerous pellets that spread when fired.

Sight A device on top of a barrel that allows a gun to be aimed accurately.

Silencer A device placed over the muzzle of a firearm used to reduce/muffle the sound of gunfire.

Single-Action (SA) A pistol or revolver, in which the trigger is only used for firing the weapon and cannot be used to cock the firing mechanism. On SA revolvers, the hammer must be manually drawn back to full cock for each shot. On pistols, the recoil action will automatically recock the hammer for the second and subsequent shots.

Skeet A shooting sport in which a clay target (pigeon) is thrown to simulate the flight of a bird.

Slide The upper portion of a semiautomatic pistol that houses the barrel and contains the breechblock and portions of the firing mechanism. As its name states, it slides along tracks in the top of the frame during the recoil process, providing the linkage between the breechblock and barrel.

Slide Lever Typically refers to a lever either on the left or right side of a pistol's frame that is used to release the slide for removal, maintenance, and cleaning.

Small Arms Portable firearms.

Solid Frame Refers to a revolver in which the cylinder window is cut into a single solid piece of frame stock. The construction is neither break-open nor open frame. This type of revolver is loaded by the cylinder flipping out of the solid frame or by feeding individual rounds into exposed chambers that are rotated out to the side of the frame.

Speed Loader In revolvers in which the entire rear of the cylinder can be exposed for loading, the speed loader is a circular device or clip that holds a complete set of cartridges aligned to insert into all chambers of the cylinder simultaneously.

Stock A frame that holds the action and barrel of a firearm that is held against one's shoulder when firing the gun.

Straw Purchase A criminal act in which a person who is prohibited from buying firearms uses another person to buy a gun on his or her behalf, often related to a person wanting to remain unidentified.

Striker In a handgun that does not have a hammer, the striker is a linearly driven, spring-loaded cylindrical part that strikes the primer of a chambered cartridge. The striker replaces both the hammer and firing pin found in hammer-driven pistols.

Topstrap The part of a revolver frame that extends over the top of the cylinder and connects the top of the standing breech with the forward portion of the frame into which the barrel is mounted.

Trajectory The arc described by a projectile traveling from the muzzle to the point of impact.

Trigger Refers to the release device in the firing system that initiates the cartridge discharge. Usually a curved, grooved, or serrated piece that is pulled rearward by the shooter's finger, which then activates the hammer or striker.

Trigger Guard Usually a circular or oval band of metal, horn, or plastic that goes around the trigger to provide both protection and safety in shooting circumstances.

Twist The rate at which rifling grooves arc around the core of the barrel, measured in calibers, inches, or centimeters. Twists can arc from left to right or from right to left from the rear of the barrel. This is described as either a right-hand or a left-hand twist.

WCF Winchester Centerfire, a type of ammunition.

WMR Winchester Magnum Rimfire, a type of ammunition.

GLOSSARY OF FIREARM-RELATED LAW AND LEGAL CASES

Armed Career Criminal Act of 1984 A federal law that increases penalties, through sentence enhancements, for individuals found in possession of firearms who are not qualified to own them (such as felons with three or more "violent felonies" and/or "serious drug offenses"). The law has since been revised numerous times as various terms were vague and difficult to interpret.

Brady Handgun Violence Prevention Act Also referred to as the "Brady Act" or the "Brady Bill." This law mandated a 5-day wait period before the purchase of a handgun (until the National Instant Criminal Background Check System [NICS] system was implemented in 1998). It also requires local law enforcement to conduct federal background checks on individuals attempting to purchase a handgun.

***Caetano v. Massachusetts*, 136 S.Ct. 1027 (2016)** The U.S. Supreme Court sought to expound upon the meaning of the right "to keep and bear arms." Massachusetts had flatly banned stun guns from use by anyone other than law enforcement and military personnel. In this case, a woman threatened to use a stun gun against her ex-boyfriend, who had repeatedly assaulted her. The police found her in possession of the stun gun, however, and she was prosecuted. The Supreme Court came to a unanimous opinion to vacate Massachusetts's highest state court's upholding of the flat ban on possessing stun guns for personal self-defense.

***Commonwealth v. McGowan*, 464 Mass. 232 (2013)** A law that required firearms to be secured in a locked container or equipped with a safety device that would make the firearm inoperable by anyone other than the owner or an authorized user, when not carried by or under the control of the owner or other authorized user. The court stated the law exists to prevent accidents, violence, and suicide by those unlicensed to possess or carry a firearm.

Crime Control Act of 1990 (Public Law 101-647) Enacted to ban semiautomatic weapon production and importation into the United States. This law also encourages authorities to post "Gun-Free Zone" signs in school zones and increases the penalties for individuals found in possession of firearms in federal court facilities.

***District of Columbia v. Heller*, 554 US 570 (2008)** A landmark case in which the U.S. Supreme Court held in a 5–4 decision that the Second Amendment to the U.S. Constitution applies to federal enclaves and protects an individual's right to possess a firearm for traditionally lawful purposes, such as self-defense within the home. The decision did not address the question of whether the Second Amendment extends beyond federal enclaves to the states, which was addressed later by *McDonald v. Chicago* (2010). It was the first Supreme Court case to decide whether the Second Amendment protects an individual's right to keep and bear arms for self-defense.

Firearms Owners Protection Act (Public Law 99-308) A law that revised many of the provisions of the Gun Control Act of 1968. This law relaxed some of the restrictions on gun and ammunitions sales, while also establishing mandatory penalties for individuals who are in possession of a firearm during the commission of a crime. Some of the loosened restrictions included a limited reopening of the interstate sale of long guns, legalizing the shipping of ammunition through the U.S. Postal Service, removal of the requirement to keep records on the sale of non–armor-piercing ammunition, and federal protection of individuals transporting firearms through states where firearm possession is illegal. The list of circumstances by which individuals would be prohibited from owning firearms was also modified.

Gun Control Act of 1968 This act, passed after the assassinations of John F. Kennedy, Robert Kennedy, and Dr. Martin Luther King, Jr., aimed to regulate interstate and foreign commerce of firearms. In an effort to impose stricter licensing and regulation of firearms, the Gun Control Act mandated the licensing of individuals and companies who sell firearms, established a new category of firearms offenses, and also prohibited the sale of firearms to certain persons, such as felons. The act required all newly manufactured firearms to bear a serial number. Finally, Congress reorganized the Alcohol Tax Unit and created the Alcohol and Tobacco Tax Division, which would provide enforcement.

Law Enforcement Officers Protection Act (Public Law 99-408) A law that bans the possession, manufacture, and import of bullets that can penetrate bulletproof clothing, also known as "cop killer" bullets (with minor exceptions). If someone is found in possession of armor-piercing ammunition during the commission of a violent crime, an additional mandatory sentence of no less than 5 years is imposed.

***McDonald v. City of Chicago*, 561 US 742 (2010)** After *District of Columbia v. Heller*, there was uncertainty regarding the scope of gun rights as they applied to the states. While the *Heller* case reasoned that the Second Amendment was applicable since the original Chicago firearm ban was enacted under the authority of the federal government, the *McDonald* case argued that the Second Amendment should also apply to state and local governments. Essentially, the U.S. Supreme Court ruled that the Fourteenth Amendment included the Second Amendment and applied it to the states, thereby finding Chicago's firearm ban to be unconstitutional. Thus, the individual rights perspective (the individual right to possess and use firearms for lawful purposes is a fundamental American right) is the prevailing view at this time, at least in the higher courts.

***New York State Rifle & Pistol Association Inc. v. Bruen* (2022)** In June 2022, the U.S. Supreme Court set forth another major 2A ruling via *Bruen*. In November 2021, the Court heard arguments proposing a challenge to New York State's law that currently requires those applying for a license to carry a concealed, loaded firearm outside the home to demonstrate "proper cause." This was based on the assertion that carrying a gun outside the home is a constitutional right and not a situation that should require demonstration of need. By way of a 6-3 vote, Justice Clarence Thomas wrote the majority opinion, indicating New York's proper-cause requirement violates the Fourteenth Amendment by precluding law-abiding citizens to exercise their self-defense needs vis-à-vis their Second Amendment right to keep and bear arms in public. Time will show the full impact of the *Bruen* ruling, but certain effects were immediately seen, such as in the removal of similar provisions "may-issue" jurisdictions (e.g., New Jersey's removal of their "justifiable need" requirement to carry).

NICS Improvement Act of 2007 This act set out to revise the National Instant Criminal Background Check System (NICS) after the Virginia Tech shootings. The law's intention was to address loopholes that allowed the Virginia Tech shooter, Seung-Hui Cho, to buy firearms even though he was previously deemed a danger to himself by a Virginia court. However, because the Commonwealth of Virginia had not submitted his disqualifying mental health adjudication to the NICS (which was all too common across the country), Seung-Hui Cho was able to complete the sale. The law enhanced the requirements that federal departments and agencies provide relevant information to the NICS, through implementation assistance to states and penalties for noncompliance, among other things.

***Presser v. Illinois*, 116 US 252 (1886)** In 1886, Herman Presser was part of an armed citizen militia group of over 400 German workers associated with the Socialist Labor Party who were charged with parading in the streets of Chicago on horseback and the like. They had no license to do so, nor were they a recognized organization permitted to engage in such by the government. Presser claimed that his Second Amendment rights were violated, but the U.S. Supreme Court held that forbidding armed bodies of people to gather, drill, or parade did not violate an individual right to keep and bear arms.

***Printz v. United States*, 521 US 898 (1997)** The Brady Act required state and local law enforcement officials to conduct background checks on a temporary basis (until the national background check system was computerized). According to this law, Congress cannot compel state or local governments to implement or administer federal regulatory programs under Tenth Amendment protections.

***Redford v. US Dept. of Treasury, Bur. of Alcohol, Tobacco and Firearms*, 691 F.2d 471 (1982)** A man challenged the seizure of his arsenal of firearms due to a previous not guilty by reason of insanity (NGRI) determination, stating that the statutory prohibition against possession of firearms by individuals adjudicated as mentally incompetent was sufficiently vague (and perhaps would not include a finding of NGRI). But the court upheld the seizure, citing the belief that people of common intelligence would recognize that individuals found NGRI for a criminal charge would fall under the same category as those deemed mentally incompetent.

***Tyler v. Hillsdale County Sheriff's Department*, 775 F.3d 308 (2014)** Twenty-eight years before this case, Tyler had been involuntarily hospitalized due to suicide risk following an especially difficult divorce. Many years later, he wanted to own a gun and argued that he was not mentally ill and, thus, should not be precluded from owning a firearm. Congress had previously created a program that would allow individuals who were otherwise restricted from owning firearms to seek relief so that they may regain their firearm rights.

Tyler's state (Michigan) did not have a relief program in place; thus, he was unable to regain his Second Amendment right. The court held that Tyler should be able to exercise the right to bear arms in any state he chooses to live, regardless of whether the state has chosen to accept federal grant money to fund a relief program. The court further stated that Congress designed the law to enforce prohibitions only during periods in which the person is deemed dangerous, which does not necessarily equal a lifelong prohibition. Ultimately, the court did not order that Tyler's rights be restored immediately but provided him with the opportunity to prove that he had regained mental stability and that his mental illness did not pose a risk to himself or others.

United States v. Chamberlain, **159 F.3d 656 (1st Cir. 1998)** The court found that while a 5-day emergency detention is considered a "commitment" because it implies the potential for harm to self or others, the court realized that there is a possibility of someone being mistakenly committed in such a fashion under other circumstances. The court noted that there are procedures in place that would allow an individual to seek relief from the firearms ban.

United States v. Cruikshank, **92 US 542 (1875)** This was the first case in which the U.S. Supreme Court interpreted the Second Amendment. In 1873, an armed White militia attacked and killed over 100 African American Republican freedman who gathered at a Colfax, Louisiana, courthouse to prevent a Democratic takeover. Some of the White mob members were charged under the Enforcement Act of 1870 and part of the indictment suggested a conspiracy to prevent Blacks from exercising their civil rights, including bearing arms lawfully. The Court ultimately held that the Second Amendment only ensures that Congress will not infringe upon the right of gun ownership—it does not specifically set forth a right to own guns. Moreover, the Court cited that the Fourteenth Amendment protected individuals from the state and not from other individuals per se (i.e., the State Action Doctrine).

United States v. Dorsch, **363 F.3d 784 (2004)** Dorsch was indicted after having been found in possession of firearms following an involuntary commitment to a psychiatric center. Dorsch argued that his commitment did not meet the statutory criteria according to the Gun Control Act, stating that his commitment was for observation only and not treatment. As such, he argued that the results of his case should be similar to the results of *United States v. Hansel*. The court found that since Dorsch had the opportunity to appeal his commitment (and raise his inability to possess a firearm according to the Gun Control Act) but did not take advantage of the opportunity, his due process rights were not violated.

United States v. Giardina, **861 F.2d 1334 (5th Cir. 1988)** Giardina was committed to a hospital in New Orleans for 2 weeks of treatment following the issuance of a physician's emergency certificate and a coroner's emergency certificate. After his release, he required no further treatment. Upon procuring two firearms, he signed federal paperwork stating he had never been committed to a mental institution (as he believed this particular hospital did not count as a mental institution). He was consequently indicted on two counts of receiving and possessing a firearm after having been committed to a mental institution. The Fifth Circuit Court of Appeals held that admission by emergency certificate did not constitute a commitment for the purposes of the Gun Control Act, stating that "[t]emporary, emergency detentions for treatment of mental disorders or difficulties, which do not lead to formal commitments under state law, do not constitute the commitment envisioned" (ref. 17, p. 1337).

United States v. Hansel, 474 F.2d 1120 (8th Cir. 1973) Hansel was involuntarily committed for formal observation but not by judicial or administrative proceedings. In fact, after receiving a firearm following being committed to a mental institution and subsequently being convicted of two counts of violating the Gun Control Act of 1968, the examining physician testified at trial that Hansel did not have a serious mental illness, nor was he in need of hospitalization. Therefore, the appeals court found that Hansel was not committed for the purposes of the Gun Control Act. As such, the Gun Control Act's firearm restrictions would not apply to him.

United States v. Miller, 307 US 174 (1939) This is a unique case wherein the U.S. Supreme Court had the opportunity to apply the Second Amendment to a federal firearms statute. Namely, this involved a criminal prosecution under the National Firearms Act of 1934, which passed subsequent to the St. Valentine's Day Massacre. The Act, in part, banned fully automatic guns and short-barreled rifles and shotguns. In this case, Miller challenged certain aspects of the Act as a violation of his Second Amendment rights, but the U.S. Supreme Court ultimately held that banning a shotgun having a barrel less than 18 inches was not because it did not have any relation to a well-regulated militia or ordinary military equipment. Therefore, the Second Amendment would not guarantee a civilian's right to keep and bear such a firearm.

United States v. Portillo-Munoz, 643 F.3d 437 (5th Cir. 2011) Portillo-Munoz, an undocumented immigrant, was arrested after he was found in possession of a handgun, which he stated was to protect chickens from coyotes on the ranch where he was employed. He was convicted of unlawfully possessing a weapon and sentenced to 10 months in prison. He appealed, and a Fifth Circuit panel held that the Second Amendment does not provide undocumented immigrants currently in the United States the individual right to bear arms. The panel noted that these undocumented immigrants are not among "the people" referred to in the Second Amendment.

United States v. Rehlander, 666 F.3d 45 (1st Cir. 2012) A court case where Rehlander argued that a temporary hospitalization under an ex parte proceeding should not disqualify him from purchasing or possessing firearms under *Heller* as an ex parte proceeding does not qualify as a commitment for federal purposes. The court ultimately concluded that *Heller* did not apply to a temporary hospitalization, although this might be a different case if the Gun Control Act provided for a *temporary* prohibition from possessing firearms.

United States v. Waters, 23 F.3d 29, 30 (2d Cir. 1994) Waters was indicted by a federal grand jury for illegally possessing a firearm following his commitment to a mental institution. Waters moved to dismiss the indictment on the grounds that there was no formal judicial order of commitment to the psychiatric hospital, especially as the federal gun control statute had not defined the term *commitment*. His motion was rejected by the court, which stated that Waters's commitment to the hospital (under New York State law) was sufficient under federal policy. This case set the precedent that while the question of whether an admission constitutes a commitment to a mental institution is a matter of federal law, the court reviewing such cases may seek guidance from state laws.

Violent Crime Control and Law Enforcement Act of 1994 A law that banned the manufacture of 19 military-style assault weapons, as well as certain high-capacity ammunition magazines. The law also established a firearm prohibition for individuals subject to family violence restraining orders and strengthened licensing standards for firearms dealers. Finally, the law created new crimes or penalties for drive-by shootings and the use of semiautomatic weapons.

***Wollschlaeger v. Farmer*, 814 F.Supp.2d 1367, 1384 (S.D.Fla. 2011)** The petitioners argued that various provisions of the Firearm Owners Privacy Act, which barred physicians both from asking questions related to firearm possession and ownership and from entering related information into patients' medical records, violate the First and Fourteenth Amendments of the U.S. Constitution. In this matter, the plaintiffs stated that the act violated the First Amendment by preventing open communication with their patients about ways to reduce the safety risks posed by firearms. The court, in this case, issued a *preliminary* injunction against the provisions of the act, stating that they violated the First Amendment right of free speech.

***Wollschlaeger v. Farmer*, 880 F.Supp.2d 1251, 1267–69 (S.D.Fla. 2012)** The court issued a *permanent* injunction against the provisions of the Firearm Owners Privacy Act (i.e., inquiry, recordkeeping, discrimination, harassment) due to infringement upon doctors' free speech rights according to the First Amendment.

***Wollschlaeger v. Governor of Florida*, 760 F.3d 1195 (11th Cir. 2014)** Dr. Wollschlaeger, other medical professionals, and various Florida chapters of medical organizations sued the governor of Florida and the state (officials) for setting forth the Firearm Owners Privacy Act. The Eleventh Circuit vacated the injunction and upheld the Firearm Owners Privacy Act, which banned medical doctors from asking their patients questions about firearm ownership. According to the court, because the law only restricts speech uttered in doctors' examination rooms, it is exempt from First Amendment scrutiny, which otherwise allows freedom of speech.

KNOW, ASK, DO (KAD) MODEL FOR MEDICAL AND MENTAL
HEALTH PROFESSIONALS

GUN CULTURE, SAFETY, AND LAWS

Cultural Competence

Develop an awareness of:

- Gun-related language, terms, and definitions
- Clinicians' own potential biases related to patients' views on guns and ownership status
- Firearm-related subgroups, and identify which, if any, patients belong to—include patients' gun ownership status and/or level of access, including any changes to either
- Local norms (e.g., rates of gun ownership, public sentiment and practices, violence and suicide rates—with and without guns, legal regulations)

Gun Safety Principles

Gain an understanding of:

- Clinicians' and patients' knowledge of and adherence to gun safety principles, including patients' storage, transportation, handling, and gun use practices.

Gun-Related Laws

Identify clinicians' and patients' knowledge of:

- State laws on confidentiality and reporting (i.e., duty to warn and/or protect)
- Federal and state laws generally related to prohibited persons, firearms, ammunition, and magazine capacity, background checks, Castle doctrine ("stand your ground"), right to carry, transportation and storage (including child access prevention), transportation, and hunting

WHEN AND HOW TO ASK ABOUT GUNS

Local Laws and Policies

- Develop knowledge and a process for:
  - Clinicians' state- and institutional-level requirements regarding asking or counseling patients about guns
  - Clinicians' options when patients do not want to discuss/report guns or gun access
- In non-crisis situations, give patients the option to discuss/report their gun ownership status and/or level of access; maintain an open stance and invitation.
- For patients who decline, seek clarification as to why.
- For those who are agreeable, inquire about family support and assistance and/or other storage options for firearms should a risk management plan be needed in the future.

Professional Ethics and Standards of Practice

- Ensure patients understand the limits of confidentiality.
- Exhibit a professional and cultural competence–based approach to prioritize and facilitate rapport-building and to ensure the highest quality of care, to include consistency in procedures across patients and services versus arbitrary or casual inquiries. Avoid confirmation bias and knee-jerk reactions.
- Ask questions that seek to gain a clinical appreciation of both patients' group levels of acculturation and their individual differences.
- Know limits of professional competence and when to refer out, especially understanding therapeutic versus forensic roles.

HOW TO ASSESS RISK

General Violence and Suicide Risk Assessment Models and Principles

When applicable:

- Assess violence and/or suicide risk using questions from a step-wise, semi-structured, prevention-based framework. Avoid prediction-based approaches.
- Include questions related to nomothetic and idiographic (case-specific) factors.

Firearm-Specific Risk

When applicable:

- Inquire about the nature and extent of likely (or "easy") gun access.
- Assess for the presence of firearm-specific risk factors to distinguish patients who are likely to engage in firearm-involved violence and suicide from those who are not.

INTERVENTION OPTIONS

1. Remember: If a case extends beyond one's professional competence, seek consultation and/or refer out for further evaluation and/or treatment
2. Develop an emergency plan in advance, to include options for peer consultation as well as awareness of local firearm storage options and emergency care, or crisis, services.
3. Be prepared to provide general counseling in matters that do not reach a higher risk threshold, which may include psychoeducational materials regarding risk factors, warning signs, and preventive and emergency response measures.
4. When a concerning risk threshold is reached, attempt to collaborate on a risk management plan with the patient unless it is a crisis or a duty to warn and/or protect is prompted.
   - Updated inquiries about family support and assistance in this regard and/or other storage options for firearms
   - Is an emergency risk protection order or red flag order an option for the clinician or family?
5. Document relevant information, assessment, and procedural data.
6. Recognize when no particular action is clinically warranted.

Appendix D

PIRELLI FIREARM-10 (PF-10) CONCEPTUAL MODEL
AND DOMAINS

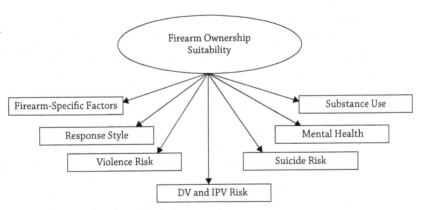

1. Reason for seeking licensure/reinstatement
2. Exposure to firearms
3. Knowledge of and perspectives on firearm safety precautions and relevant firearm regulations
4. Firearm use: experience, intent for use, storage, and continued education
5. Response style
6. Violence risk
7. Domestic and intimate partner violence risk
8. Suicide risk
9. Mental health
10. Substance use

REFERENCES

ABOUT THE AUTHORS

Pirelli, G., & Gold, L. (2019). Leaving Lake Wobegon: Firearm-related education and training for medical and mental health professionals is an essential competence. *Journal of Aggression, Conflict and Peace Research*, 11(2), 78–87.

Pirelli, G., & Witt, P. H. (2017). Firearms and cultural competence: Considerations for mental health practitioners. *Journal of Aggression, Conflict and Peace Research*, 10(1), 61–70. https://doi.org/10.1108/JACPR-01-2017-0268

Pirelli, G., Schrantz, K., & Wechsler, H. (2020). The emerging role of psychology in shaping gun policy in the United States. In M. K. Miller & B. H. Bornstein (Eds.), *Advances in psychology and law* (vol. 5, pp. 373–411). Springer.

Pirelli, G., Wechsler, H., & Cramer, R. (2019). *The behavioral science of firearms: A mental health perspective on guns, suicide, and violence.* Oxford University Press.

Pirelli, G., Wechsler, H., & Cramer, R. (2015). Psychological evaluations for firearm ownership: Legal foundations, practice considerations, and a conceptual framework. *Professional Psychology: Research and Practice*, 46(4), 250–257.

Wechsler, H., Struble, C., Pirelli, G., & Cramer, R. (2015, August). Firearm ownership evaluations: A local norms perspective. Presented at the 2015 Annual American Psychological Association (APA) Convention, Toronto, Canada.

PREFACE

Pirelli, G., & Gold, L. (2019). Leaving Lake Wobegon: Firearm-related education and training for medical and mental health professionals is an essential competence. *Journal of Aggression, Conflict and Peace Research*, 11(2), 78–87.

217

Pirelli, G., Wechsler, H., & Cramer, R. (2019). *The behavioral science of firearms: A mental health perspective on guns, suicide, and violence*. Oxford University Press.

INTRODUCTION

American Psychological Association. (2013). Gun violence: Prediction, prevention, and policy. http://www.apa.org/pubs/info/reports/gun-violence-prevention.aspx

Barry, C. L., McGinty, E. E., Vernick, J. S., & Webster, D. W. (2013). After Newtown—public opinion on gun policy and mental illness. *New England Journal of Medicine, 368*, 1077–1081.

Carney, C. P., Allen, J., & Doebbeling, B. N. (2002). Receipt of clinical preventive medical services among psychiatric patients. *Psychiatric Services, 53*(8), 1028–1030.

Centers for Disease Control and Prevention. (n.d.). Rates of homicide, suicide, and firearm-related death among children—26 industrialized countries. https://www.cdc.gov/mmwr/preview/mmwrhtml/00046149.htm

Centers for Disease Control and Prevention. (2021, January 7). Stats of the states—firearm mortality. https://www.cdc.gov/nchs/pressroom/sosmap/firearm_mortality/firearm.htm

Consortium for Risk-Based Firearm Policy. (2013a). *Guns, public health, and mental illness: An evidence-based approach for federal policy*. https://efsgv.org/wp-content/uploads/2014/10/Final-Federal-Report.pdf

Consortium for Risk-Based Firearm Policy. (2013b). *Guns, public health, and mental illness: An evidence-based approach for state policy*. https://efsgv.org/wp-content/uploads/2014/10/Final-State-Report.pdf

Dahlberg, L., Ikeda, R., & Kresnow, M. (2004). Guns in the home and risk of a violent death in the home: Findings from a national study. *American Journal of Epidemiology, 160*(10), 929–936.

Degutis, L. C., & Spivak, M. H. R. (2021). *Gun violence prevention: A public health approach*. American Public Health Association Press.

Desmarais, S. L., Van Dorn, R. A., Johnson, K. L., Grimm, K. J., Douglas, K. S., & Swartz, M. S. (2014). Community violence perpetration and victimization among adults with mental illness. *American Journal of Public Health, 104*(12), 2342–2349.

End the gun epidemic in America. (2015, December 4). *New York Times*. www.nytimes.com/2015/12/05/opinion/end-the-gun-epidemic-in-america.html?_r=0

Fact sheet: New executive actions to reduce gun violence and make our communities safer. (2016, January 4). https://obamawhitehouse.archives.gov/the-press-office/2016/01/04/fact-sheet-new-executive-actions-reduce-gun-violence-and-make-our

Gold, L. H., & Simon, R. I. (2016). *Gun violence and mental illness*. American Psychiatric Association.

Greenberg, D. (2016, June 13). APHA mourns Orlando shootings. https://www.apha.org/news-and-media/news-releases/apha-news-releases/2019/apha-mourns-gun-violence

Jenson, J. M. (2007). Aggression and violence in the United States: Reflections on the Virginia Tech shootings. *Social Work Research, 31*(3), 131–134. https://doi.org/10.1093/swr/31.3.131

McGinty, E. E., Frattaroli, S., Appelbaum, P. S., Bonnie, R. J., Grilley, A., Horwitz, J., Swanson, J. W., & Webster, D. W. (2014). Using research evidence to reframe the policy debate around mental illness and guns: Process and recommendations. *American Journal of Public Health, 104*(11), e22–e26.

McGinty, E. E., Webster, D. W., & Barry, C. L. (2013). Effects of news media messages about mass shootings on attitudes toward persons with serious mental illness and public support for gun control policies. *American Journal of Psychiatry, 170*(5), 494–501.

Merica, D. (2017, November 6). Trump points to mental health after shootings, but action has been minimal. CNN. www.cnn.com/2017/11/06/politics/trump-guns-mental-health-texas-shooting/index.html

Miller, M., Barber, C., White, R. A., Azrael, D. (2013). Firearms and suicide in the United States: Is risk independent of underlying suicidal behavior? *American Journal of Epidemiology, 178*(6), 946–945.

Nagle, M. E., Joshi, K. G., Frierson, R. L., Durkin, M. W., & Karydi, A. (2021). Knowledge and attitudes of psychiatrists about the gun rights of persons with mental illness. *Journal of the American Academy of Psychiatry and the Law, 49*(1), 28–37.

Pew Research Center. (2013, May 9). *Why own a gun? Protection is now top reason.* https://www.pewresearch.org/fact-tank/2013/05/09/why-own-a-gun-protection-is-now-top-reason/

Pinals, D. A., Appelbaum, P. S., Bonnie, R., Fisher, C. E., Gold, L. H., & Lee, L. (2015a). American Psychiatric Association: Position statement on firearm access, acts of violence and the relationship to mental illness and mental health services. *Behavioral Sciences and the Law, 33*(2/3), 195–198.

Pinals, D. A., Appelbaum, P. S., Bonnie, R. J., Fisher, C. E., Gold, L. H., & Lee, L. (2015b). Resource document on access to firearms by people with mental disorders. *Behavioral Sciences and the Law, 33*(2/3), 186–194.

Pirelli, G., & Gold, L. H. (2019). Leaving Lake Wobegon: Firearm-related education and training for medical and mental health professionals is an essential competence. *Journal of Aggression, Conflict and Peace Research, 11*(2), 78–87.

Pirelli, G., Schrantz, K., & Wechsler, H. (2020). The emerging role of psychology in shaping gun policy in the United States. In M. K. Miller & B. H. Bornstein (Eds.), *Advances in psychology and law* (vol. 5, pp. 373–411). Springer.

Pirelli, G., Wechsler, H., & Cramer, R. (2019). *The behavioral science of firearms: A mental health perspective on guns, suicide, and violence.* Oxford University Press.

Price, J. H., Kinnison, A., Dake, J. A., Thompson, A. J., & Price, J. A. (2007). Psychiatrists' practices and perceptions regarding anticipatory guidance on firearms. *American Journal of Preventive Medicine, 33*(5), 370–373. https://doi.org/10.1016/j.amepre.2007.07.021

Price, J., Mrdjenovich, A. J., Thompson, A., & Dake, J. A. (2009). College counselors' perceptions and practices regarding anticipatory guidance on firearms. *Journal of American College Health, 58*(2), 133–139.

Price, J. H., Thompson, A. J., Khubchandani, J., Mrdjenovich, A. J., & Price, J. A. (2010). Firearm anticipatory guidance training in psychiatric residency programs. *Academic Psychiatry, 34*(6), 417–423. https://doi.org/10.1176/appi.ap.34.6.417

Roy, L., Crocker, A. G., Nicholls, T. L., Latimer, E. A., & Ayllon, A. R. (2014). Criminal behavior and victimization among homeless individuals with severe mental illness: A systematic review. *Psychiatric Services, 65*(6), 739–750. https://doi.org/10.1176/appi.ps.201200515

Saad, L. (2015). Americans fault mental health system most for gun violence. Gallup. www.gallup.com/poll/164507/americans-fault-mental-health-system-gun-violence.aspx

Simpson, J. R. (2021). The need for systematic training on gun rights and mental illness for forensic psychiatrists. *Journal of the American Academy of Psychiatry and the Law, 49*(1), 38–41.

Slovak, K., Brewer, T. W., & Carlson, K. (2008). Client firearm assessment and safety counseling: The role of social workers. *Social Work, 53*(4), 358–366.

Steadman, H. J., Monahan, J., Pinals, D. A., Vesselinov, R., & Robbins, P. C. (2015). Gun violence and victimization of strangers by persons with a mental illness: Data from the MacArthur violence risk assessment study. *Psychiatric Services*, 66(11), 1238–1241. https://doi.org/10.1176/appi.ps.201400512

Swanson, J. W., Holzer, C. E., Ganju, V. K., & Jono, R. T. (1990). Violence and psychiatric disorder in the community: Evidence from the Epidemiologic Catchment Area surveys. *Hospital & Community Psychiatry*, 41(7), 761–770.

Swanson, J. W., McGinty, E. E., Fazel, S., & Mays, V. M. (2015). Mental illness and reduction of gun violence and suicide: Bringing epidemiologic research to policy. *Annals of Epidemiology*, 25(5), 366–376. https://doi.org/10.1016/j.annepidem.2014.03.004

Traylor, A., Price, J. H., Telljohann, S. K., King, K., & Thompson, A. (2010). Clinical psychologists' firearm risk management perceptions and practices. *Journal of Community Health*, 35(1), 60–67.

Yip, P. S., Caine, E., Yousef, S., Chang, S-S., Wu, K. C-C., & Chen, Y-Y. (2012). Means restriction for suicide prevention. *Lancet*, 379(9834), 2393–2399.

CHAPTER 1

Advanced Law Enforcement Rapid Response Training (ALERRT) Center at Texas State University & the Federal Bureau of Investigation. (2018, April). Active shooter incidents in the United States in 2016 and 2017. U.S. Department of Justice. https://www.fbi.gov/file-repository/active-shooter-incidents-us-2016-2017.pdf/view

American Psychological Association. (2017a). Multicultural guidelines: An ecological approach to context, identity, and intersectionality. http://www.apa.org/about/policy/multicultural-guidelines.pdf

American Psychological Association. (2017b). *Ethical principles of psychologists and code of conduct* (2002, amended effective June 1, 2010, and January 1, 2017). https://www.apa.org/ethics/code/ethics-code-2017.pdf

Barry, C. L., McGinty, E. E., Vernick, J. S., & Webster, D. W. (2013). After Newtown—Public opinion on gun policy and mental illness. *New England Journal of Medicine*, 368(12), 1077–1081. https://doi.org/10.1056/NEJMp1300512

Betz, M. E., & Wintemute, G. J. (2015). Physician counseling on firearm safety: A new kind of cultural competence. *Journal of the American Medical Association*, 314(5), 449–450. https://doi.org/10.1001/jama.2015.7055

Blair, J. P., Schwieit, K. W., & Federal Bureau of Investigation. (2014). A study of active shooter incidents in the United States between 2000 and 2013. U.S. Department of Justice. https://www.fbi.gov/file-repository/active-shooter-study-2000-2013-1.pdf

Bureau of Alcohol, Tobacco, Firearms and Explosives. (2009). ATF national firearms act handbook. https://www.atf.gov/firearms/docs/guide/atf-national-firearms-act-handbook-atf-p-53208/download

Capatides, C. (2015, December 4). How heavily armed is your state? CBS News. www.cbsnews.com/pictures/most-heavily-armed-states-in-america/4/

Ciyou, B. L. (2018). *2018 edition: Gun laws by state. Reciprocity and gun laws quick reference guide*. Peritus Holdings.

Czajkowski, E. (2016, May 12). Comedians come together to make it clear that gun violence is no joke. *The Guardian*. https://www.theguardian.com/stage/2016/may/12/amy-schumer-gun-control-brady-comics-benefit-show

District of Columbia v. Heller, 554 US 570 (2008).

Guns 101. (n.d.). The firearms guide. www.thefirearms.guide/guns/guns-101

Herschberger, K. (2017, February 16). 15 superheroes whose powers are basically just guns. Comic Book Resources (CBR). https://www.cbr.com/15-superheroes-whose-powers-areguns

Holly, C., Porter, S., Kamienski, M., & Lim, A. (2019). School-based and community-based guns afety educational strategies for injury prevention. *Health Promotion Practice*, 20(1), 38–47. https://doi.org/10.1177/1524839918774571

"Hollywood & Guns." (2013, June 4). Hollywood & guns: Weapons still prevalent in pop culture. HuffPost. https://www.huffpost.com/entry/hollywood-guns-weapons-revalent-pop-culture_n_3489996

Hunts, G. (2020, January 25). Hunting age requirements for each state. *Got Hunts*. https://gothunts.com/hunting-age-requirements/

Jacquemin, B. (2016, April 26). Increase in suicide in the United States, 1999–2014 (Data Brief No. 241). National Center for Health Statistics. https://www.nj.gov/health/chs/documents/suicide_nj1999-2014.pdf

Jacquemin, B. (2017, September 12). Suicide in New Jersey. New Jersey Department of Health. https://www.nj.gov/health/chs/documents/DMHAS%20Suicide%20Prevention%20Event%202017.pdf

Jones, J. M. (2018, March 14). US preference for stricter gun laws highest since 1993. Gallup. https://news.gallup.com/poll/229562/preference-stricter-gun-laws-highest-1993.aspx

Kappas, J. S. (2021). *2021 traveler's guide to the firearm laws of the fifty states*. Traveler's Guide.

Luciano, J. (2015). *Guns the right way: Introducing kids to firearm safety and shooting*. Gun Digest Books.

McGinty, E. E., Webster, D. W., & Barry, C. L. (2013). Effects of news media messages about mass shootings on attitudes toward persons with serious mental illness and public support for gun control policies. *American Journal of Psychiatry*, 170(5), 494–501.

McNab, C. (2009). *Guns: A visual history*. DK Publishing.

Merriam-Webster. (n.d.). Culture. In Merriam-Webster.com dictionary. https://www.merriam-webster.com/dictionary/culture

National Rifle Association. (n.d.). Gun safety rules. https://gunsafetyrules.nra.org/

National Shooting Sports Foundation. (n.d.). Firearms safety—10 rules of safe gun handling. https://www.nssf.org/safety/rules-firearms-safety/

Parham-Payne, W. (2014). The role of the media in the disparate response to gun violence in America. *Journal of Black Studies*, 45(8), 752–768. doi:10.1177/0021934714555185

Pirelli, G., & Witt, P. H. (2018). Firearms and cultural competence: Considerations for mental health practitioners. *Journal of Aggression, Conflict and Peace Research*, 10(1), 61–70.

Schildkraut, J., & Muschert, G. W. (2014). Media salience and the framing of mass murder in schools: A comparison of the columbine and Sandy Hook massacres. *Homicide Studies*, 18(1), 23–43. doi:10.1177/1088767913511458

Scole. (2016, August 15). Superheroes and super villains who use guns. *The Artifice*. https://the-artifice.com/superheroes-super-villains-guns

Swanson, J. W. (1994). Mental disorder, substance abuse, and community violence: An epidemiological approach. In J. Monahan & H. J. Steadman (Eds.), *Violence and mental disorder: Developments in risk assessment* (pp. 101–136). University of Chicago Press.

Supica, J. (n.d.). A brief history of firearms. National Rifle Association. https://www.nramuseum.org/gun-info-research/a-brief-history-of-firearms.aspx

U.S. Department of Justice, Federal Bureau of Investigation. (2017, September). Crime in the United States, 2016. https://ucr.fbi.gov/crime-in-the-u.s/2016/crime-in-the-US-2016/tab les/expanded-homicide-data-table-4.xls

United States v. Cruikshank, 92 US 542 (1875).

CHAPTER 2

42 USC. § 3796gg-4 (2012).

430 Ill. Comp. Stat. 65/1.1 (n.d.).

American Academy of Psychiatry and the Law. (2005). Ethics guidelines for the practice of forensic psychiatry. https://www.aapl.org/ethics.htm

Bailey, J. E., Kellermann, A. L., Somes, G. W., Banton, J. G., Rivara, F. P., & Rushforth, N. P. (1997). Risk factors for violent death of women in the home. *Archives of Internal Medicine*, 157 (7), 777–782.

Cal. Welf. & Inst. Code §§ 8100(a), 8103(a), (b), (d), (e), (d), (g) (2016).

Campbell, J. C., Webster, D., Koziol-McLain, J., Block, C., Campbell, D., Curry, M. A., Gary, F., Glass, N., McFarlane, J., Sachs, C., Sharps, P., Ulrich, Y., Wilt, S., Manganello, J., Xu, X., Schollenberger, J., Frye, V., & Laughon, K. (2003). Risk factors for femicide in abusive relationships: Results from a multisite case control study. *American Journal of Public Health*, 93(7), 1089–1097.

Commerce in Firearms and Ammunition, 27 C.F.R. § 478 (2019). https://www.ecfr.gov/curr ent/title-27/chapter-II/subchapter-B/part-478

Consortium for Risk-Based Firearm Policy. (2013). Guns, public health, and mental illness: An evidence-based approach for state policy. Educational Fund to Stop Gun Violence. https:// efsgv.org/wp-content/uploads/2014/10/Final-State-Report.pdf

District of Columbia v. Heller, 554 US 570 (2008).

Elbogen, E. B., & Johnson, S. C. (2009). The intricate link between violence and mental dis-order: Results from the national epidemiologic survey on alcohol and related conditions. *Archives of General Psychiatry*, 66(2), 152–161. https://doi.org/10.1001/archgenpsychia try.2008.537

Farr, K. A. (2002). Battered women who were "being killed and survived it": Straight talk from survivors. *Violence and Victims*, 17(3), 267–281.

Gius, M. (2015). The impact of minimum age and child access prevention laws on firearm-related youth suicides and unintentional deaths. *Social Science Journal*, 52(2), 168–175. https://doi.org/10.1016/j.soscij.2015.01.003

Gold, L. H., & Vanderpool, D. (2018a). Legal regulation of restoration of firearms rights after mental health prohibition. *Journal of the American Academy of Psychiatry and the Law*, 46(3), 298–308.

Gold, L. H., & Vanderpool, D. (2018b). Psychiatric evidence and due process in firearms rights restoration. *Journal of the American Academy of Psychiatry and the Law*, 46(3), 309–321.

Gorshkalova, O., & Munakomi, S. (2020). Duty to warn. In *StatPearls*. StatPearls Publishing.

Grossman, D. C., Mueller, B. A., Riedy, C., Dowd, M. D., Villaveces, A., Prodzinski, J., Nakagawara, J., Howard, J., Thiersch, N., & Harruff, R. (2005). Gun storage practices and risk of youth suicide and unintentional firearm injuries. *Journal of the American Medical Association*, 293(6), 707–714. https://doi.org/10.1001/jama.293.6.707

Gun Control Act of 1968, 18 USC. § 921 et sq. (1968).

Haw. Rev. Stat. § 134-7 (2019).

Johnson, J. A., Lutz, V. L., & Websdale, N. (2000). Death by intimacy: Risk factors for domestic violence. *Pace Law Review, 20*(2), 263.

Kellermann, A. L., Rivara, F. P., Rushforth, N. B., Banton, J. G., Reay, D. T., Francisco, J. T., Locci, A. B., Prodzinski, J., Hackman, B. B., & Somes, G. (1993). Gun ownership as a risk factor for homicide in the home. *New England Journal of Medicine, 329*(15), 1084–1091. https://doi.org/10.1056/NEJM199310073291506

Lautenberg Amendment, 18 USC. § 922(g)(9) (1996).

McDonald v. Chicago, 561 US 742 (2010).

McGinty, E. E., & Webster, D. W. (2016). Gun violence and serious mental illness. In L. H. Gold & R. I. Simon (Eds.), *Gun violence and mental illness.* (pp. 3–30). American Psychiatric Association.

McGinty, E. E., Webster, D. W., & Barry, C. L. (2014). Gun policy and serious mental illness: Priorities for future research and policy. *Psychiatric Services, 65*(1), 50–58. https://doi.org/10.1176/appi.ps.201300141

Md. Code Ann., Pub. Safety § 5-1330 (2003).

Mich. Comp. Laws § 28.435 (1927).

Miller, M., Azrael, D., Hemenway, D., & Vriniotis, M. (2005). Firearm storage practices and rates of unintentional firearm deaths in the United States. *Accident Analysis and Prevention, 37*(4), 661–667. https://doi.org/10.1016/j.aap.2005.02.003

NICS Improvement Amendments Act of 2007, Pub. L. No. 110-180, 121 Stat. 2559 (2007). https://www.govinfo.gov/content/pkg/STATUTE-121/pdf/STATUTE-121-Pg2559.pdf

N.J. Rev. Stat. § 2A:62A-16 (2020).

N.J. Stat. Ann. § 2C:58-2a(5)(d),(e) (2009).

New York State Rifle & Pistol Association, Inc. v. Bruen, 597 U.S. (2022).

Office for Civil Rights. (2013). HIPAA administrative simplification regulation text. U.S. Department of Health and Human Services. https://www.hhs.gov/sites/default/files/hipaa-simplification-201303.pdf

Pinals, D. A., Appelbaum, P. S., Bonnie, R. J., Fisher, C. E., Gold, L. H., & Lee, L. (2015). Resource document on access to firearms by people with mental disorders. *Behavioral Sciences & the Law, 33*(2/3), 186–194. https://doi.org/10.1002/bsl.2181

Pirelli, G., Wechsler, H., & Cramer, R. (2019). *The behavioral science of firearms: A mental health perspective on guns, suicide, and violence.* Oxford University Press.

Presser v. Illinois, 116 US 542 (1886).

Price, M., & Norris, D. M. (2010). Firearm laws: A primer for psychiatrists. *Harvard Review of Psychiatry, 18*(6), 326–335. https://doi.org/10.3109/10673229.2010.527520

Prickett, K. C., Martin-Storey, A., & Crosnoe, R. (2014). State firearm laws, firearm ownership, and safety practices among families of preschool-aged children. *American Journal of Public Health, 104*(6), 1080–1086. https://doi.org/10.2105/AJPH.2014.301928

Protection of Human Subjects, 45 C.F.R. § 46 (2009). https://www.hhs.gov/ohrp/sites/default/files/ohrp/policy/ohrpregulations.pdf

Sorenson, S. B. (2006). Firearm use in intimate partner violence: A brief overview. *Evaluation Review, 30*(3), 229–236. https://doi.org/10.1177/0193841X06287220

Swanson, J. W., Holzer, C. E., Ganju, V. K., & Jono, R. T. (1990). Violence and psychiatric disorder in the community: Evidence from the Epidemiologic Catchment Area surveys. *Hospital & Community Psychiatry, 41*(7), 761–770.

Swanson, J. W., McGinty, E. E., Fazel, S., & Mays, V. M. (2015). Mental illness and reduction of gun violence and suicide: Bringing epidemiologic research to policy. *Annals of Epidemiology, 25*(5), 366–376. https://doi.org/10.1016/j.annepidem.2014.03.004

Swanson, J. W., Robertson, A. G., Frisman, L. K., Norko, M., Lin, H. J., Swartz, M. S., & Cook, P. J. (2013). Preventing gun violence involving people with serious mental illness. In D. W. Webster & J. S. Vernick (Eds.), *Reducing gun violence in America: Informing policy with evidence and analysis* (pp. 33–51). Johns Hopkins University Press.

Tarasoff v. Regents of University of California, *551 P.2d 334 (1976)*.

Truman, J. L., & Morgan, R. E. (2014). Nonfatal domestic violence, 2003–2012. U.S. Department of Justice. https://bjs.ojp.gov/content/pub/pdf/ndvo312.pdf

Tyler v. Hillsdale County Sheriff's Department, *837 F.3d 678 (6th Cir. 2016)*.

United States v. Cruikshank, *92 US 542 (1875)*.

United States v. Miller, *307 US 174 (1939)*.

Vest, J. R., Catlin, T. K., Chen, J. J., & Brownson, R. C. (2002). Multistate analysis of factors associated with intimate partner violence. *American Journal of Preventive Medicine, 22*(3), 156–164.

Violence Against Women Act, 42 USC. § 13981 (1994).

Violent Crime Control and Law Enforcement Act, 18 USC § 922[g][8].

Wintemute, G. J., Wright, M. A., Drake, C. M., & Beaumont, J. J. (2001). Subsequent criminal activity among violent misdemeanants who seek to purchase handguns. *Journal of the American Medical Association, 285*(8), 1019. https://doi.org/10.1001/jama.285.8.1019

Wollschlaeger v. Governor of Fla., 760 F.3d 1195 (11th Cir. 2014).

CHAPTER 3

American Psychiatric Association. (2013). *Diagnostic and statistical manual of mental disorders* (5th ed.). American Psychiatric Publishing.

Arsenault-Lapierre, C. K., & Turecki, G. (2004). Psychiatric diagnoses in 3275 suicides: A meta-analysis. *BMC Psychiatry, 4*(37), 37–48. https://doi.org/10.1186/1471-244X-4-37

Banks, L., Crandall, C., Sklar, D., & Bauer, M. (2008). A comparison of intimate partner homicide to intimate partner homicide-suicide: One hundred and twenty-four New Mexico cases. *Violence Against Women, 14*(9), 1065–1078. https://doi.org/10.1177/1077801208321983

Baumann, M. L., & Teasdale, B. (2018). Severe mental illness and firearm access: Is violence really the danger? *International Journal of Law and Psychiatry, 56*, 44–49. https://doi.org/10.1016/j.ijlp.2017.11.003

Betz, M. E., Barber, C., & Miller, M. (2011). Suicidal behavior and firearm access: Results from the second injury control and risk survey. *Suicide and Life-Threatening Behavior, 41*(4), 384–391.

Buchanan, L., Keller, J., Oppel, R., & Victor, D. (2018, February 16). How they got their guns. *New York Times.* www.nytimes.com/interactive/2015/10/03/us/how-mass-shooters-got-their-guns.html?_r=1

Bushman, B. J., Newman, K., Calvert, S. L., Downey, G., Dredze, M., Gottfredson, M., Jablonski, N. G., Masten, A. S., Morrill, C., Neill, D. B., Romer, D., & Webster, D. W. (2016). Youth violence: What we know and what we need to know. *American Psychologist, 71*(1), 17–39. https://doi.org/10.1037/a0039687

Campbell, J. C., Webster, D., Koziol-McLain, J., Block, C., Campbell, D., Curry, M. A., Gary, F., Glass, N., McFarlane, J., Sachs, C., Sharps, P., Ulrich, Y., Wilt, S. A., Manganello, J., Xu, X., Schollenberger, J., Frye, V., & Laughon, K. (2003). Risk factors for femicide in abusive relationships: Results from a multisite case control study. *American Journal of Public Health, 93*(7), 1089–1097. https://doi.org/10.2105/AJPH.93.7.1089

Carney, C. P., Allen, J., & Doebbeling, B. N. (2002). Receipt of clinical preventive medical services among psychiatric patients. *Psychiatric Services*, 53(8), 1028–1030.

Chermack, S. T., & Giancola, P. R. (1997). The relation between alcohol and aggression: An integrated biopsychosocial conceptualization. *Clinical Psychology Review*, 17(6), 621–649. https://doi.org/10.1016/S0272-7358(97)00038-X

Conwell, Y., Duberstein, P. R., Connor, K., Eberly, S., Cox, C., & Caine, E. D. (2002). Access to firearms and risk for suicide in middle-aged and older adults. *American Journal of Geriatric Psychiatry*, 10(4), 407–416. https://doi.org/10.1176/appi.ajgp.10.4.407

Cornell, D. (2018). *Comprehensive school threat assessment guidelines*. School Threat Assessment Consultants LLC.

Corrigan, P. W., & Watson, A. C. (2005). Findings from the national comorbidity survey on the frequency of violent behavior in individuals with psychiatric disorders. *Psychiatry Research*, 136(2–3), 153–162. https://doi.org/10.1016/j.psychres.2005.06.005

Dahlberg, L. L., Ikeda, R. M., & Kresnow, M. J. (2004). Guns in the home and risk of a violent death in the home: Findings from a national study. *American Journal of Epidemiology*, 160(10), 929–936. doi:10.1093/aje/kwh309

Douglas, K. S., Guy, L. S., & Hart, S. D. (2009). Psychosis as a risk factor for violence to others: A meta-analysis. *Psychological Bulletin*, 135(5), 679–706. https://doi.org/10.1037/a0016311

Elbogen, E. B., & Johnson, S. C. (2009). The intricate link between violence and mental disorder: Results from the national epidemiologic survey on alcohol and related conditions. *Archives of General Psychiatry*, 66(2), 152–161. https://doi.org/10.1001/archgenpsychiatry.2008.537

Farr, K. A. (2002). Battered women who were "being killed and survived it": Straight talk from survivors. *Violence and Victims*, 17(3), 267–281. https://doi.org/10.1891/vivi.17.3.267.33660

Fowler, K. A., Dahlberg, L. L., Haileyesus, T., & Annest, J. L. (2015). Firearm injuries in the United States. *Preventive Medicine*, 79, 5–14. https://doi.org/10.1016/j.ypmed.2015.06.002

Fox, J. A., & DeLateur, M. J. (2014). Mass shootings in America: Moving beyond Newtown. *Homicide Studies*, 18(1), 125–145. https://doi.org/10.1177/1088767913510297

Harford, T. C., Yi, H., & Grant, B. F. (2013). Other- and self-directed forms of violence and their relationships to DSM-IV substance use and other psychiatric disorders in a national survey of adults. *Comprehensive Psychiatry*, 54(7), 731–739. https://doi.org/10.1016/j.comppsych.2013.02.003

Harter, S., Low, S. M., & Whitesell, N. R. (2003). What have we learned from Columbine: The impact of the self-system on suicidal and violent ideation among adolescents. *Journal of School Violence*, 2(3), 3–26.

Ilgen, M. A., Zivin, K., McCammon, R. J., & Valenstein, M. (2008). Mental illness, previous suicidality, and access to guns in the United States. *Psychiatric Services*, 59(2), 198–200. https://doi.org/10.1176/appi.ps.59.2.198

Kachadourian, L. K., Homish, G. G., Quigley, B. M., & Leonard, K. E. (2012). Alcohol expectancies, alcohol use, and hostility as longitudinal predictors of alcohol-related aggression. *Psychology of Addictive Behaviors*, 26(3), 414–422. https://doi.org/10.1037/a0025842

Klinoff, V. A., Van Hasselt, V. B., & Black, R. A. (2015). Homicide-suicide in police families: An analysis of cases from 2007–2014. *Journal of Forensic Practice*, 17(2), 101–116. https://doi.org/10.1108/JFP-07-2014-0019

Knoll, J. L., IV, & Annas, G. D. (2016). Mass shootings and mental illness. In L. H. Gold & R. I. Simon (Eds.), *Gun violence and mental illness* (pp. 81–104). American Psychiatric Association.

Langman, P. (2009). Rampage school shooters: A typology. *Aggression and Violent Behavior*, 14(1), 79–86. https://doi.org/10.1016/j.avb.2008.10.003

McGinty, E. E., & Webster, D. W. (2016). Gun violence and serious mental illness. In L. H. Gold & R. I. Simon (Eds.), *Gun violence and mental illness* (pp. 3–30). American Psychiatric Association.

Miller, M., Barber, C., Azrael, D., Hemenway, D., & Molnar, B. E. (2009). Recent psychopathology, suicidal thoughts and suicide attempts in households with and without firearms: Findings from the national comorbidity study replication. *Injury Prevention*, 15(3), 183–187.

Moberg, T., Stenbacka, M., Jönsson, E. G., Nordström, P., Åsberg, M., & Jokinen, J. (2014). Risk factors for adult interpersonal violence in suicide attempters. *BMC Psychiatry*, 14, Article number 195. https://doi.org/10.1186/1471-244X-14-195

Nagle, M. E., Joshi, K. G., Frierson, R. L., Durkin, M. W., & Karydi, A. (2021). Knowledge and attitudes of psychiatrists about the gun rights of persons with mental illness. *Journal of the American Academy of Psychiatry and the Law*, 49(1), 28–37. https://doi.org/10.29158/JAAPL.200050-20

Pirelli, G., Wechsler, H., & Cramer, R. (2019). *The behavioral science of firearms: A mental health perspective on guns, suicide, and violence*. Oxford University Press.

Posner, K., Brent, D., Lucas, C., Gould, M., Stanley, B., Brown, G., Fisher, P., Zelazny, J., Burke, A., Oquendo, M., & Mann, J. (2009). Columbia Suicide Severity Rating Scale (C-SSRS). Columbia Lighthouse Project. https://cssrs.columbia.edu/wp-content/uploads/C-SSRS-Screening_AU5.1_eng-USori.pdf

Powell, K. E., Kresnow, M., Mercy, J. A., Potter, L. B., Swann, A. C., Frankowski, R. F., Lee, R. K., & Bayer, T. L. (2001). Alcohol consumption and nearly lethal suicide attempts. *Suicide and Life-Threatening Behavior*, 32(Suppl), 30–41. https://doi.org/10.1521/suli.32.1.5.30.24208

Price, J. H., Kinnison, A., Dake, J. A., Thompson, A. J., & Price, J. A. (2007). Psychiatrists' practices and perceptions regarding anticipatory guidance on firearms. *American Journal of Preventive Medicine*, 33(5), 370–373. https://doi.org/10.1016/j.amepre.2007.07.021

Price, J., Mrdjenovich, A. J., Thompson, A., & Dake, J. A. (2009). College counselors' perceptions and practices regarding anticipatory guidance on firearms. *Journal of American College Health*, 58(2), 133–139.

Price, J. H., Thompson, A. J., Khubchandani, J., Mrdjenovich, A. J., & Price, J. A. (2010). Firearm anticipatory guidance training in psychiatric residency programs. *Academic Psychiatry*, 34(6), 417–423. https://doi.org/10.1176/appi.ap.34.6.417

Rocque, M. (2012). Exploring school rampage shootings: Research, theory, and policy. *Social Science Journal*, 49(3), 304–313. https://doi.org/10.1016/j.soscij.2011.11.001

Simon, T. R., Swann, A. C., Powell, K. E., Potter, L. B., Kresnow, M., & O'Carroll, P. W. (2001). Characteristics of impulsive suicide attempts and attempters. *Suicide and Life-Threatening Behavior*, 32(Suppl), 49–59. https://doi.org/10.1521/suli.32.1.5.49.24212

Simpson, J. R. (2021). The need for systematic training on gun rights and mental illness for forensic psychiatrists. *Journal of the American Academy of Psychiatry and the Law*, 49(1), 38–41.

Slovak, K., Brewer, T. W., & Carlson, K. (2008). Client firearm assessment and safety counseling: The role of social workers. *Social Work*, 53(4), 358–366.

Sorenson, S. B. (2006). Firearm use in intimate partner violence: A brief overview. *Evaluation Review*, 30(3), 229–236. https://doi.org/10.1177/0193841X06287220

Sorenson, S. B., & Vittes, K. A. (2008). Mental health and firearms in community-based surveys: Implications for suicide prevention. *Evaluation Review*, 32(3), 239–256.

Spencer, C. M., & Stith, S. M. (2020). Risk factors for male perpetration and female victimization of intimate partner homicide: A meta-analysis. *Trauma, Violence, & Abuse*, 21(3), 527–540. https://doi.org/10.1177/1524838018781101

Steadman, H. J., Monahan, J., Pinals, D. A., Vesselinov, R., & Robbins, P. C. (2015). Gun violence and victimization of strangers by persons with a mental illness: Data from the MacArthur violence risk assessment study. *Psychiatric Services*, 66(11), 1238–1241. https://doi.org/10.1176/appi.ps.201400512

Steadman, H. J., Mulvey, E. P., Monahan, J., Robbins, P. C., Appelbaum, P. S., Grisso, T., Roth, L. H., & Silver, E. (1998). Violence by people discharged from acute psychiatric inpatient facilities and by others in the same neighborhoods. *Archives of General Psychiatry*, 55(5), 393–401. https://doi.org/10.1001/archpsyc.55.5.393

Swanson, J. W., Holzer, C. E., Ganju, V. K., & Jono, R. T. (1990). Violence and psychiatric disorder in the community: Evidence from the epidemiologic catchment area surveys. *Hospital & Community Psychiatry*, 41(7), 761–770.

Swanson, J. W., McGinty, E. E., Fazel, S., & Mays, V. M. (2015). Mental illness and reduction of gun violence and suicide: Bringing epidemiologic research to policy. *Annals of Epidemiology*, 25(5), 366–376. https://doi.org/10.1016/j.annepidem.2014.03.004

Swedler, D. I., Simmons, M. M., Dominici, F., & Hemenway, D. (2015). Firearm prevalence and homicides of law enforcement officers in the United States. *American Journal of Public Health*, 105(10), 2042–2048. https://doi.org/10.2105/AJPH.2015.302749

Too, L. S., Spittal, M. J., Bugeja, L., Reifels, L., Butterworth, P., & Pirkis, J. (2019). The association between mental disorders and suicide: A systematic review and meta-analysis of record linkage studies. *Journal of Affective Disorders*, 259, 302–313. https://doi.org/10.1016/j.jad.2019.08.054

Traylor, A., Price, J. H., Telljohann, S. K., King, K., & Thompson, A. (2010). Clinical psychologists' firearm risk management perceptions and practices. *Journal of Community Health*, 35(1), 60–67.

Trestman, R. L., Volkmar, F. R., & Gold, L. H. (2016). Accessing mental health care. In L. H. Gold & R. I. Simon (Eds.), *Gun violence and mental illness* (pp. 185–217). American Psychiatric Association.

Truman, J. L., & Morgan, R. E. (2014, April). Nonfatal domestic violence, 2003–2012 (NCJ Number 244697). U.S. Department of Justice, Bureau of Justice Statistics. https://bjs.ojp.gov/content/pub/pdf/ndv0312.pdf

Tyler v. Hillsdale County Sheriff's Department, 775 F.3d 308 (6th Cir. 2014).

Violanti, J. M., Hartley, T. A., Mnatsakanova, A., Andrew, M. E., & Burchfiel, C. M. (2012). Police suicide in small departments: A comparative analysis. *International Journal of Emergency Mental Health*, 14(3), 157–162.

Vossekuil, B., Fein, R. A., Reddy, M., Borum, R., & Modzeleski, W. (2004, June). The final report and findings of the Safe School Initiative: Implications for the prevention of school attacks in the United States (NCJ Number 195287). U.S. Secret Service, U.S. Department of Education. https://www2.ed.gov/admins/lead/safety/preventingattacksreport.pdf

Wintemute, G. J. (2015). Alcohol misuse, firearm violence perpetration, and public policy in the United States. *Preventive Medicine*, 79, 15–21. https://doi.org/10.1016/j.ypmed.2015.04.015

World Health Organization. (2002). World report on violence and health: Summary. https://www.who.int/violence_injury_prevention/violence/world_report/en/summary_en.pdf

Yip, P. S., Caine, E., Yousef, S., Chang, S-S., Wu, K. C-C., & Chen, Y-Y. (2012). Means restriction for suicide prevention. *Lancet*, 379(9834), 2393–2399.

CHAPTER 4

Allow doctors to talk about gun safety. (2017, March 10). *The Republic*. www.therepublic.com/2017/03/11/allow-doctors-to-talk-about-gun-safety/

American Civil Liberties Union. (2017, February). *Wollschlaeger v. Governor of Florida*. https://www.aclufl.org/en/cases/clone-stone-et-al-v-city-fort-lauderdale-0

American Psychological Association. (2013). Gun violence: Prediction, prevention, and policy. www.apa.org/pubs/info/reports/gun-violence-prevention.aspx

Appelbaum, P. S. (2017a). Does the Second Amendment protect the gun rights of persons with mental illness? *Psychiatric Services*, 68(1), 3–5.

Appelbaum, P. S. (2017b). "Docs vs. Glocks" and the regulation of physicians' speech. *Psychiatric Services*, 68(7), 647–649.

Ballenger, J. F., Best, S. R., Metzler, T. J., Wasserman, D. A., Mohr, D. C., Liberman, A., Delucchi, K., Weiss, D. S., Fagan, J. A., Waldrop, A. E., & Marmar, C. R. (2011). Patterns and predictors of alcohol use in male and female urban police officers. *American Journal on Addictions*, 20, 21–29.

Centers for Disease Control and Prevention. (2021). Risk and protective factors. https://www.cdc.gov/suicide/factors/index.html?CDC_AA_refVal=https%3A%2F%2Fw ww.cdc.gov%2Fv iolenceprevention%2Fsuicide%2Friskprotectivefactors.html

Cheema, R. (2016). Black and blue bloods: Protecting police officer families from domestic violence. *Family Court Review*, 54(3), 487–500. https://doi.org/10.1111/fcre.12226

Columbia Lighthouse Project. (n.d.). A unique suicide risk assessment tool. https://cssrs.columbia.edu/the-columbia-scale-c-ssrs/about-the-scale/

Counseling Center. (n.d.). A definition of pastoral counseling. https://counselingcenter.org/a-definition-of-pastoral-counseling/

Daniel, A. E. (2007). Care of the mentally ill in prisons: Challenges and solutions. *Journal of the American Academy of Psychiatry and the Law*, 35(4), 406–410.

Diurba, S., Johnson, R. L., Siry, B. J., Knoepke, C. E., Suresh, K., Simpson, S. A., Azrael, D., Ranney, M. L., Wintemute, G. J., & Betz, M. E. (2020). Lethal means assessment and counseling in the emergency department: Differences by provider type and personal home firearms. *Suicide and Life-Threatening Behavior*, 50(5), 1054–1064.

Edwards, T. M., Stern, A., Clarke, D. D., Ivbijaro, G., & Kasney, L. M. (2010). The treatment of patients with medically unexplained symptoms in primary care: A review of the literature. *Mental Health in Family Medicine*, 7(4), 209–221.

Galatzer-Levy, I. R., & Bryant, R. A. (2013). 636,120 ways to have posttraumatic stress disorder. *Perspectives on Psychological Science*, 8(6), 651–662.

Gilligan, J. (2001). The last mental hospital. *Psychiatric Quarterly*, 72(1), 45–61. https://doi.org/10.1023/A:1004810120032

Gold, L. H., & Simon, R. I. (Eds.). (2016). *Gun violence and mental illness*. American Psychiatric Association.

Greenberg, S. A., & Shuman, D. W. (1997). Irreconcilable conflict between therapeutic and forensic roles. *Professional Psychology: Research and Practice*, 28(1), 50–57.

Johnson, R. R. (2008). Officer firearms assaults at domestic violence calls: A descriptive analysis. *Police Journal*, 81(1), 25–45.

Kessler, R. C., Heeringa, S. G., Stein, M. B., Colpe, L. J., Fullerton, C. S., Hwang, I., Naifeh, J. A., Nock, M. K., Petukhova, M., Sampson, N. A., Schoenbaum, M., Zaslavsky, A. M., & Ursano, R. J.; Army STARRS Collaborators. (2014). Thirty-day prevalence of DSM-IV mental disorders among nondeployed soldiers in the US Army. Results from the Army Study to Assess Risk and Resilience in Service Members (Army STARRS). *JAMA Psychiatry*, 71(5), 504–513. https://doi.org/10.1001/jamapsychiatry.2014.28

Kirschman, E. (2006). *I love a cop: What police families need to know* (rev. ed.). Guilford Press.

Loftus, E. F., Loftus, G. R., & Messo, J. (1987). Some facts about weapon focus. *Law and Human Behavior*, 11, 55–62.

McGinty, E. E., Frattaroli, S., Appelbaum, P. S., Bonnie, R. J., Grilley, A., Horwitz, J., Swanson, J. W., & Webster, D. W. (2014). Using research evidence to reframe the policy debate around mental illness and guns: Process and recommendations. *American Journal of Public Health*, 104(11), e22–e26. https://doi.org/10.2105/AJPH.2014.302171

Missouri Rev. Stat. § 571.012, 2015.

Munsey, C. (2008). At least one in 10 Americans are prescribed psychotropics. *Monitor on Psychology*, 39(2), 52.

National Center for Women and Policing. (n.d.). Police family violence fact sheet. https://vaw net.org/material/police-family-violence-fact-sheet

Pickel, K. L. (1998). Unusualness and threat as possible causes of "weapon focus." *Memory*, 6, 277–295.

Pinals, D. A., Appelbaum, P. S., Bonnie, R., Fisher, C. E., Gold, L. H., & Lee, L. (2015a). American Psychiatric Association: Position statement on firearm access, acts of violence and the relationship to mental illness and mental health services. *Behavioral Sciences and the Law*, 33(2/3), 195–198.

Pinals, D. A., Appelbaum, P. S., Bonnie, R. J., Fisher, C. E., Gold, L. H., & Lee, L. (2015b). Resource document on access to firearms by people with mental disorders. *Behavioral Sciences and the Law*, 33(2/3), 186–194.

Pirelli, G., & Gold, L. (2019). Leaving Lake Wobegon: Firearm-related education and training for medical and mental health professionals is an essential competence. *Journal of Aggression, Conflict and Peace Research*, 11(2), 78–87. https://doi.org/10.1108/JACPR-11-2018-0391

Robinson, J. (2013, May 22). Three-quarters of your doctor bills are because of this. *HuffPost*. http://m.huffpost.com/us/entry/3313606

Sharp, J. (2016, August 15). As Alabama shuts down psychiatric hospitals, one jail is expanding to house mentally ill. www.al.com/news/mobile/index.ssf/2016/08/one_alabama_cou nty_looks_to_ex.html

Summerlin, Z., Oehme, K., Stern, N., & Valentine, C. (2010). Disparate levels of stress in police and correctional officers: Preliminary evidence from a pilot study on domestic violence. *Journal of Human Behavior in the Social Environment*, 20(6), 762–777. https://doi.org/10.1080/10911351003749169

Swanson, J. W., Holzer, C. E., Ganju, V. K., & Jono, R. T. (1990). Violence and psychiatric disorder in the community: Evidence from the Epidemiologic Catchment Area surveys. *Hospital and Community Psychiatry*, 41(7), 761–770.

Swanson, J. W., McGinty, E. E., Fazel, S., & Mays, V. M. (2015). Mental illness and reduction of gun violence and suicide: Bringing epidemiologic research to policy. *Annals of Epidemiology*, 25(5), 366–376. https://doi.org/10.1016/j.annepidem.2014.03.004

Swatt, M. L., Gibson, C. L., & Piquero, N. L. (2007). Exploring the utility of general strain theory in explaining problematic alcohol consumption by police officers. *Journal of Criminal Justice*, 35(6), 596–611.

Torrey, E. F. (1997). *Out of the shadows: Confronting America's mental illness crisis*. John Wiley & Sons.

Torrey, E. F. (1999, Autumn). Reinventing mental health care. *City Journal*. https://www.city-journal.org/html/reinventing-mental-health-care-11915.html

Torrey, E. F., Kennard, A. D., Eslinger, D., Lamb, R., & Pavle, J. (2010). More mentally ill persons are in jails and prisons than hospitals: A survey of the states. Treatment Advocacy Center.https://www.treatmentadvocacycenter.org/storage/documents/final_jails_v_hospitals_study.pdf

Torrey, E. F., Stieber, J., Ezekiel, J., Wolfe, S. M., Sharfstein, J., Noble, J. H., & Flynn, L. M. (1992). *Criminalizing the seriously mentally ill: The abuse of jails as mental hospitals*. Diane Pub. Co.

Treatment Advocacy Center. (2014). State standards for assisted treatment: Civil commitment criteria for inpatient or outpatient psychiatric treatment. www.treatmentadvocacycenter.org/storage/documents/Standards_-_The_Text-_June_2011.pdf

Tyler v. Hillsdale County Sheriff's Department, 775 F.3d 308 (2014). https://cite.case.law/f3d/775/308/

U.S. Department of Veterans Affairs. (n.d.). PTSD and substance abuse in veterans. https://www.ptsd.va.gov/understand/related/substance_abuse_vet.asp

VA Suicide Prevention Program. (2018, June). Facts about veteran suicide. https://www.mentalhealth.va.gov/docs/OMHSP_Suicide_Prevention_Fact_Sheet_Updated_June_2018_508.pdf

Violanti, J. M. (1999). Alcohol abuse in policing: Prevention strategies. *FBI Law Enforcement Bulletin, 68*(1), 16–18.

Violanti, J. M., Burchfiel, C. M., Miller, D. B., Andrew, M. E., Dorn, J., Wactawski-Wende, J., Beighley, C. M., Pierino, K., Joseph, P. N., Vena, J. E., Sharp, D. S., & Trevisan, M. (2006). The Buffalo Cardio-Metabolic Occupational Police Stress (BCOPS) pilot study: Methods and participant characteristics. *Annals of Epidemiology, 16*(2), 148–156. https://doi.org/10.1016/j.annepidem.2005.07.054

Yates, R. (2016, October 8). With Pennsylvania mental hospitals full, jails become way stations. *Morning Call*. https://www.mcall.com/news/local/mc-pa-long-waits-at-state-mental-hospitals-incompetency-20161008-story.html

CHAPTER 5

American Academy of Psychiatry and the Law. (2005, May). Ethics guidelines for the practice of forensic psychiatry. https://www.aapl.org/guidelines-and-practice-resources

American Psychiatric Association (2022). *Diagnostic and statistical manual of mental disorders* (5th ed., text revision). https://doi.org/10.1176/appi.books.9780890425787

American Psychiatric Association. (2013). *Diagnostic and statistical manual of mental disorders* (5th ed.). https://doi.org/10.1176/appi.books.9780890425596

American Psychological Association. (2013). Specialty guidelines for forensic psychology. *American Psychologist, 68*(1), 7–19. https://doi.org/10.1037/a0029889

American Psychological Association. (2016, November 15). After decades of research, science is no better able to predict suicidal behaviors. https://www.apa.org/news/press/releases/2016/11/suicidal-behaviors

Americans With Disabilities Act of 1990, 42 USC. § 12101 *et seq.* (1990). https://www.ada.gov/pubs/adastatute08.htm

Americans with Disabilities Act Amendments Act of 2008, Pub. L. No. 110-325, 122 Stat 3553 (2008).

Andrews, D. A., Bonta, J., & Wormith, J. S. (2006). The recent past and near future of risk and/or need assessment. *Crime & Delinquency*, 52(1), 7–27. https://doi.org/10.1177/0011128705281756

Application for Relief, 30 N.J.S.A. § 4-80.8 (2009). https://lis.njleg.state.nj.us/nxt/gateway.dll?f=templates&fn=default.htm&vid=Publish:10.1048/Enu

Basile, K. C., Hertz, M. F., & Back, S. E. (2007). *Intimate partner violence and sexual violence victimization assessment instruments for use in healthcare settings, version 1.* Centers for Disease Control and Prevention, National Center for Injury Prevention and Control.

Baumeister, R. F., & Leary, M. R. (1995). The need to belong: Desire for interpersonal attachments as a fundamental human motivation. *Psychological Bulletin*, 117(3), 497–529.

Bone, D. (2010). The *Heller* promise versus the *Heller* reality: Will statutes prohibiting the possession of firearms by ex-felons be upheld after *Britt v. State*? *Journal of Criminal Law & Criminology*, 100(4), 1633–1658.

Bonta, J. (2002). Offender risk assessment: Guidelines for selection and use. *Criminal Justice and Behavior*, 29(4), 355–379. https://doi.org/10.1177/0093854802029004002

Bonta, J., & Andrews, D. A. (2007). Risk–need–responsivity model for offender assessment and rehabilitation. *Rehabilitation*, 6(1), 1–22.

Brodsky, S. L., & Lichtenstein, B. (1999). Don't ask questions: A psychotherapeutic strategy for treatment of involuntary clients. *American Journal of Psychotherapy*, 53, 215–220.

Brodsky, S. L., & Wilson, J. K. (2013). Empathy in forensic evaluations: A systematic reconsideration. *Behavioral Sciences & the Law*, 31, 192–202.

Cheema, R. (2016). Black and blue bloods: Protecting police officer families from domestic violence. *Family Court Review*, 54(3), 487–500. https://doi.org/10.1111/fcre.12226

Columbia Lighthouse Project. (n.d.). A unique suicide risk assessment tool. https://cssrs.columbia.edu/the-columbia-scale-c-ssrs/about-the-scale/

Columbia Lighthouse Project. (2020). The Columbia Suicide Severity Rating Scale (C-SSRS): Supporting evidence. https://cssrs.columbia.edu/wp-content/uploads/CSSRS_Supporting-Evidence_Book_2020-01-14.pdf

Consortium for Risk-Based Firearm Policy. (2013a). *Guns, public health, and mental illness: An evidence-based approach for federal policy.* Johns Hopkins Center for Gun Policy and Research.

Consortium for Risk-Based Firearm Policy. (2013b). *Guns, public health, and mental illness: An evidence-based approach for state policy.* Johns Hopkins Center for Gun Policy and Research.

Cornell, D. (2018). *Comprehensive school threat assessment guidelines.* School Threat Assessment Consultants LLC.

Douglas, K. S., Hart, S. D., Webster, C. D., & Belfrage, H. (2013). *HCR-20 V3: Assessing risk for violence—User guide.* Mental Health, Law, and Policy Institute, Simon Fraser University.

Federal Bureau of Investigation (FBI) Behavioral Analysis Unit—National Center for the Analysis of Violent Crime. (2016). Making prevention a reality: Identifying, assessing, and managing the threat of targeted attacks. https://www.fbi.gov/file-repository/making-prevention-a-reality.pdf/view

Federal legislation passed: The Crystal Judson domestic violence protocol program. (n.d.). https://www.lanejudson.com/4_Brame_tragedy_spurs_federal_dv_program.htm

Firearms and Weapons, 13 N.J.A.C. § 54 (2002). https://www.state.nj.us/njsp/info/pdf/firearms/njac-title13-ch54.pdf

Franklin, J. C., Ribeiro, J. D., Fox, K. R., Bentley, K. H., Kleiman, E. M., Huang, X., Musacchio, K. M., Jaroszewski, A. C., Chang, B. P., & Nock, M. K. (2017). Risk factors for suicidal thoughts and behaviors: A meta-analysis of 50 years of research. *Psychological Bulletin, 143*(2), 187–232. https://doi.org/10.1037/bul0000084

Frye, V., Manganello, J., Campbell, J. C., Walton-Moss, B., & Wilt, S. (2006). The distribution of and factors associated with intimate terrorism and situational couple violence among a population-based sample of urban women in the United States. *Journal of Interpersonal Violence, 21* (10), 1286–1313.

Galatzer-Levy, I. R., & Bryant, R. A. (2013). 636,120 ways to have posttraumatic stress disorder. *Perspectives on Psychological Science, 8*(6), 651–662. https://doi.org/10.1177/1745691613504115

Gold, L. H., & Vanderpool, D. (2016). Relief from disabilities: Firearm rights restoration for persons under mental health prohibitions. In L. H. Gold & R. I. Simon (Eds.), *Gun violence and mental illness* (pp. 339–380). American Psychiatric Association.

Goldstein, A. M. (2001). *Handbook of psychology: Forensic psychology* (Vol. 11). John Wiley & Sons Inc.

Goldstein, A. M. (2007). *Forensic psychology: Emerging topics and expanding roles.* John Wiley & Sons, Inc.

Goldstein, D. G., & Gigerenzer, G. (2009). Fast and frugal forecasting. *International Journal of Forecasting, 25*(4), 760–772.

Greenberg, S. A., & Shuman, D. W. (1997). Irreconcilable conflict between therapeutic and forensic roles. *Professional Psychology: Research and Practice, 28*(1), 50–57. https://doi.org/10.1037/0735-7028.28.1.50

Greenberg, S. A., & Shuman, D. W. (2007). When worlds collide: Therapeutic and forensic roles. *Professional Psychology: Research and Practice, 38*(2), 129–132. https://doi.org/10.1037/0735-7028.38.2.129

Grisso, T. (1986). *Evaluating competencies: Forensic assessments and instruments.* Plenum Press.

Grisso, T. (2003). *Evaluating competencies: Forensic assessments and instruments* (2nd ed.). Kluwer Academic/Plenum Publishers.

Grove, W. M., Zald, D. H., Lebow, B. S., Snitz, B. E., & Nelson, C. (2000). Clinical versus mechanical prediction: A meta-analysis. *Psychological Assessment, 12*(1), 19–30.

Harris, G. T., Rice, M. E., & Quinsey, V. L. (1993). Violent recidivism of mentally disordered offenders: The development of a statistical prediction instrument. *Criminal Justice and Behavior, 20*(4), 315–335. https://doi.org/10.1177/0093854893020004001

Hart, S. D., Douglas, K. S., & Guy, L. S. (2016). The structured professional judgment approach to violence risk assessment: Origins, nature, and advances. In L. Craig & M. Rettenberger (Eds.), *The Wiley handbook on the theories, assessment and treatment of sexual offending: Assessment* (vol. 2, pp. 643–666). Wiley Blackwell.

Hartley, T. A., Burchfiel, C. M., Fekedulegn, D., Andrew, M. E., & Violanti, J. M. (2011). Health disparities in police officers: Comparisons to the US general population. *International Journal of Emergency Mental Health, 13*(4), 211–220.

Health care professionals, immunity from civil liability; duty to warn and protect, 2A N.J.S.A. § 62A-16 (2019). https://lis.njleg.state.nj.us/nxt/gateway.dll?f=templates&fn=default.htm&vid=Publish:10.1048/Enu

Health Insurance Portability and Accountability Act. Pub. L. No. 104-191, § 264, 110 Stat.1936.

Heilbrun, K. (2001). *Principles of forensic mental health assessment.* Kluwer Academic/Plenum Press.

Heilbrun, K. (2009). *Evaluation for risk of violence in adults.* Oxford University Press.

Heilbrun, K., DeMatteo, D., Brooks Holliday, S., & LaDuke, C. (2014). *Forensic mental health assessment: A casebook* (2nd ed.). Oxford University Press.

Heilbrun, K., Grisso, T., & Goldstein, A. M. (2009). *Foundations of forensic mental health assessment*. Oxford University Press.

Hilton, N. Z., Harris, G. T., Rice, M. E., Houghton, R. E., & Eke, A. W. (2008). An in-depth actuarial assessment for wife assault recidivism: The domestic violence risk appraisal guide. *Law and Human Behavior, 32*(2), 150–163. https://doi.org/10.1007/s10979-007-9088-6

International Association of Chiefs of Police. (2013). Psychological fitness-for-duty evaluation guidelines. https://www.theiacp.org/portals/0/documents/pdfs/psych-fitnessfordutyevaluation.pdf

International Association of Chiefs of Police. (2014). Preemployment psychological evaluation guidelines. https://www.theiacp.org/portals/0/documents/pdfs/psych-preemploymentpsycheval.pdf

Johnson, J. A., Lutz, V. L., & Websdale, N. (1999). Death by intimacy: Risk factors for domestic violence. *Pace Law Review, 20,* 263.

Kessler, R. C., Heeringa, S. G., Stein, M. B., Colpe, L. J., Fullerton, C. S., Hwang, I., Naifeh, J. A., Nock, M. K., Petukhova, M., Sampson, N. A., Schoenbaum, M., Zaslavsky, A. M., & Ursano, R. J.; Army STARRS Collaborators. (2014). Thirty-day prevalence of DSM-IV mental disorders among nondeployed soldiers in the US Army. Results from the Army Study to Assess Risk and Resilience in Service Members (Army STARRS). *JAMA Psychiatry, 71* (5), 504–513. https://doi.org/10.1001/jamapsychiatry.2014.28

Kropp, P. R., & Hart, S. D. (2015). *SARA-V3: User manual for version 3 of the Spousal Assault Risk Assessment Guide*. Proactive Resolutions.

Lieberman, J. D., & Krauss, D. A. (2009). *Psychology in the courtroom*. Ashgate Publishers.

Lisitsina, D. (2015, May 20). "Prison guards can never be weak": The hidden PTSD crisis in America's jails. *The Guardian*. https://www.theguardian.com/us-news/2015/may/20/corrections-officers-ptsd-american-prisons

Lopez, O. (2014, May 27). Prison officers need help, but they won't ask for it. *Newsweek*.https://www.newsweek.com/2014/06/06/prison-officers-need-help-they-wont-ask-it-252439.html

Meehl, P. E. (1954). *Clinical versus statistical prediction: A theoretical analysis and a review of the evidence*. University of Minnesota Press.

Melton, G. B., Petrila, J., Poythress, N. G., & Slobogin, C., Otto, R. K., Mossman, D., & Condie, L. O. (2018). *Psychological evaluations for the courts: A handbook for mental health professionals and lawyers* (4th ed.). Guilford Press.

Nanavaty, B. R. (2015, September 8). Addressing officer crisis and suicide: Improving officer wellness. *FBI Law Enforcement Bulletin*. https://leb.fbi.gov/2015/september/addressing-officer-crisis-and-suicide-improving-officer-wellness

National Center for Women and Policing. (n.d.). Police family violence fact sheet. http://womenandpolicing.com/violenceFS.asp#notes

National Institute of Justice. (2000). On-the-job stress in policing—Reducing it, preventing it. NCJ Publication No. 180079. https://www.ncjrs.gov/pdffiles1/jr000242d.pdf

New Jersey State Police. (2009, September). New Jersey application for firearms purchaser identification card and/or handgun purchase permit. https://www.njsp.org/firearms/pdf/sts-033.pdf

Nock, M. K., Park, J. M., Finn, C. T., Deliberto, T. L., Dour, H. J., & Banaji, M. R. (2010). Measuring the suicidal mind: Implicit cognition predicts suicidal behavior. *Psychological Science, 21*(4), 511–517.

Osman, A., Bagge, C. L., Gutierrez, P. M., Konick, L. C., Kopper, B. A., & Barrios, F. X. (2001). The Suicidal Behaviors Questionnaire—Revised (SBQ-R): Validation with clinical and non-clinical samples. *Assessment*, 8(4), 443–454. https://doi.org/10.1177/107319110100800409

Otto, R. K., DeMeier, R., L., & Boccaccini, M. T. (2014). *Forensic reports and testimony: A guide to effective communication for psychologists and psychiatrists*. Wiley.

Pinals, D. A., Appelbaum, P. S., Bonnie, R., Fisher, C. E., Gold, L. H., & Lee, L. (2015a). American Psychiatric Association: Position statement on firearm access, acts of violence and the relationship to mental illness and mental health services. *Behavioral Sciences and the Law*, 33(2–3), 195–198. doi:10.1002/bsl.2180

Pinals, D. A., Appelbaum, P. S., Bonnie, R. J., Fisher, C. E., Gold, L. H., & Lee, L. (2015b). Resource document on access to firearms by people with mental disorders. *Behavioral Sciences and the Law*, 33(2–3), 186–194. https://doi.org/10.1002/bsl.2181

Pirelli, G., Wechsler, H., & Cramer, R. (2015). Psychological evaluations for firearm ownership: Legal foundations, practice considerations, and a conceptual framework. *Professional Psychology: Research and Practice*, 46(4), 250–257.

Pirelli, G., Wechsler, H., & Cramer, R. (2019). *The behavioral science of firearms: A mental health perspective on guns, suicide, and violence*. Oxford University Press.

Pirelli, G., & Witt, P. (2015). Psychological evaluations for civilian firearm ownership in New Jersey. *New Jersey Psychologist*, 65(1), 7–9.

Pirelli, G., & Witt, P. H. (2017). Firearms and cultural competence: Considerations for mental health practitioners. *Journal of Aggression, Conflict and Peace Research*, 10(1), 61–70. https://doi.org/10.1108/JACPR-01-2017-0268

Posner, K., Brown, G. K., Stanley, B., Brent, D. A., Yershova, K. V., Oquendo, M. A., Currier, G. W., Melvin, G. A., Greenhill, L., Shen, S., & Mann, J. J. (2011). The Columbia-Suicide Severity Rating Scale: Initial validity and internal consistency findings from three multi-site studies with adolescents and adults. *American Journal of Psychiatry*, 168(12), 1266–1277. https://doi.org/10.1176/appi.ajp.2011.10111704

Quinsey, V. L., Harris, G. T., Rice, M. E., & Cormier, C. A. (1998). *Violent offenders: Appraising and managing risk*. American Psychological Association.

Rice, M. E. (1997). Violent offender research and implications for the criminal justice system. *American Psychologist*, 52, 414–423.

Rogers, R., & Bender, S. D. (Eds.). (2018). *Clinical assessment of malingering and deception* (4th ed.). Guilford Press.

Shneidman, E. S. (1985). *Definition of suicide*. John Wiley & Sons Inc.

Shneidman, E. S. (1987). A psychological approach to suicide. In G. R. VandenBos & B. K. Bryant (Eds.), *Cataclysms, crises, and catastrophes: Psychology in action* (pp. 147–183). American Psychological Association. https://doi.org/10.1037/11106-004

Shneidman, E. S. (1998). Perspectives on suicidology: Further reflections on suicide and psychache. *Suicide and Life-Threatening Behavior*, 28(3), 245–250.

Skeem, L., & Monahan, J. (2011). Current directions in violence risk assessment. *Current Directions in Psychological Science*, 20(1), 38–42. https://doi.org/10.1177/0963721410397271

Stack, S. J., & Tsoudis, O. (1997). Suicide risk among correctional officers. A logistic regression analysis. *Archives of Suicide Research*, 3, 183. https://doi.org/10.1023/A:1009677102357

State of New Jersey. (2009, January 30). New Jersey police suicide task force report. https://www.nj.gov/oag/library/NJPoliceSuicideTaskForceReport-January-30-2009-Final(r2.3.09).pdf

Stuart, H. (2008). Suicidality among police. *Current Opinion in Psychiatry, 21*(5), 505–509. https://doi.org/10.1097/YCO.0b013e328305e4c1

Substance Abuse and Mental Health Services Administration. (n.d.). Veterans and military families. https://www.samhsa.gov/veterans-military-families

Summerlin, Z., Oehme, K., Stern, N., & Valentine, C. (2010). Disparate levels of stress in police and correctional officers: Preliminary evidence from a pilot study on domestic violence. *Journal of Human Behavior in the Social Environment, 20*(6), 762–777. https://doi.org/10.1080/10911351003749169

Tarasoff v. Regents of the University of California, 131 *Cal. Rptr. 14 (Cal. 1976).*

U.S. Department of Justice. (2000). Addressing correctional officer stress: Programs and strategies. NCJ Publication No. 183474. https://www.ncjrs.gov/pdffiles1/nij/183474.pdf

U.S. Department of Veterans Affairs. (n.d.). PTSD and substance abuse in veterans. https://www.ptsd.va.gov/understand/related/substance_abuse_vet.asp

U.S. Secret Service. (2021). Averting targeted school violence. https://www.secretservice.gov/protection/ntac

Van Orden, K. A., Witte, T. K., Cukrowicz, K. C., Braithwaite, S. R., Selby, E. A., & Joiner, T. E., Jr. (2010). The interpersonal theory of suicide. *Psychological Review, 117*(2), 575–600. https://doi.org/10.1037/a0018697

VA Suicide Prevention Program. (2016, July). Facts about veteran suicide. https://www.va.gov/opa/publications/factsheets/suicide_prevention_factsheet_new_va_stats_070616_1400.pdf

Vera, L. M., Boccaccini, M. T., Laxton, K., Bryson, C., Pennington, C., Ridge, B., & Murrie, D. C. (2019). How does evaluator empathy impact a forensic interview? *Law and Human Behavior, 43*, 56–68. https://doi.org/10.1037/lhb0000310

Wechsler, H., Pirelli, G., & Cramer, R. (2014, May). Conducting forensic mental health assessments for firearm ownership. Presented at the 26th Annual Convention of the Association for Psychological Science (APS), San Francisco, CA.

Wechsler, H., Struble, C., Pirelli, G., & Cramer, R. (2015, August). Firearm ownership evaluations: A local norms perspective. Presented at the 2015 Annual American Psychological Association Convention, Toronto, Canada.

Weiner, I. B., & Otto, R. K. (2013). *Handbook of forensic psychology* (4th ed.). John Wiley & Sons.

Westen, D., & Weinberger, J. (2004). When clinical description becomes statistical prediction. *American Psychologist, 59*(7), 595–613. https://doi.org/10.1037/0003-066X.59.7.595

CHAPTER 6

Alleman, J. R. (2002). Online counseling: The Internet and mental health treatment. *Psychotherapy: Theory, Research, Practice, Training, 39*, 199–209. https://doi.org/10.1037/0033-3204.39.2.199

American Academy of Psychiatry and the Law. (2005). Ethics guidelines for the practice of forensic psychiatry. https://www.aapl.org/ethics.htm

American Academy of Psychiatry and the Law. (2015). AAPL practice guideline for the forensic assessment. *Journal of the American Academy of Psychiatry and the Law, 43*(2 Suppl.), S3–S53.

American Counseling Association. (2014). 2014 ACA code of ethics. https://www.counseling.org/docs/default-source/default-document-library/2014-code-of-ethics-finaladdress.pdf

American Mental Health Counselors Association. (2015, October). AMHCA code of ethics. https://www.amhca.org/HigherLogic/System/DownloadDocumentFile.ashx?Document FileKey=5ff5bc94-e534-091e-c7c1-e3ea45cf943e%26forceDialog=0

American Psychiatric Association. (2013). The principles of medical ethics with annotations especially applicable to psychiatry. https://www.psychiatry.org/File%20Library/Psychiatri sts/Practice/Ethics/principles-medical-ethics.pdf

American Psychological Association. (2013). Specialty guidelines for forensic psychology. *American Psychologist, 68*(1), 7–19. https://doi.org/10.1037/a0029889

American Psychological Association. (2017a). Ethical principles of psychologists and code of conduct. https://www.apa.org/ethics/code/ethics-code-2017.pdf

American Psychological Association. (2017b). Multicultural guidelines: An ecological approach to context, identity, and intersectionality. http://www.apa.org/about/policy/multicultural-guidelines.pdf

Batastini, A. B., & Vitacco, M. J. (Eds.). (2020). *Forensic mental health evaluations in the digital age: A practitioner's guide to using internet-based data.* Springer Nature.

Bersoff, D. N. (2008). Some contrarian concerns about law, psychology, and public policy. In D. N. Bersoff (Ed.), *Ethical conflicts in psychology* (4th ed., pp. 523–525). American Psychological Association.

Bilder, R. M., Postal, K. S., Barisa, M., Aase, D. M., Cullum, C. M., Gillaspy, S. R., Harder, L., Kanter, G., Lanca, M., Lechuga, D. M., Morgan, J. M., Most, R., Puente, A. E., Salinas, C. M., & Woodhouse, J. (2020). Inter-Organization Practice Committee recommendations/ guidance for teleneuropsychology (TeleNP) in response to the COVID-19 pandemic. *Clinical Neuropsychologist, 34*(7–8), 1314–1334. https://doi.org/10.1080/13854046.2020.1767214

Boccaccini, M. T., Chevalier, C. S., Murrie, D. C., & Varela, J. G. (2017). Psychopathy Checklist—Revised use and reporting practices in sexually violent predator evaluations. *Sexual Abuse: Journal of Research and Treatment, 29*(6), 592–614.

Bush, S. S., Connell, M. A., & Denney, R. L. (2006). *Ethical practice in forensic psychology: A systematic model for decision making.* American Psychological Association. https://doi.org/ 10.1037/11469-000

Canadian Psychological Association. (2017). *Canadian code of ethics for psychologists* (4th ed.). https://cpa.ca/docs/File/Ethics/CPA_Code_2017_4thEd.pdf

Committee on Ethical Guidelines for Forensic Psychologists. (1991). Specialty guidelines for forensic psychologists. *Law and Human Behavior, 15*, 655–665.

Cornell Law School. (n.d.). Standard of care. In *Wex legal dictionary.* https://www.law.cornell. edu/wex/standard_of_care

Drum, K. B., & Littleton, H. L. (2014). Therapeutic boundaries in telepsychology: Unique issues and best practice recommendations. *Professional Psychology: Research and Practice, 45*, 309–315. https://doi.org/10.1037/a0036127

Edens, J. F., Penson, B. N., Ruchensky, J. R., Cox, J., & Smith, S. T. (2016). Interrater reli-ability of Violence Risk Appraisal Guide scores provided in Canadian criminal proceedings. *Psychological Assessment, 28*(12), 1543–1549.

Grajales, F. J., 3rd, Sheps, S., Ho, K., Novak-Lauscher, H., & Eysenbach, G. (2014). Social media: A review and tutorial of applications in medicine and health care. *Journal of Medical Internet Research, 16*, e13. https://doi.org/10.2196/jmir.2912.

Greenberg, S. A., & Shuman, D. W. (1997). Irreconcilable conflict between therapeutic and forensic roles. *Professional Psychology: Research and Practice, 28*(1), 50–57. doi:10.1037/ 0735-7028.28.1.50

Greenberg, S. A., & Shuman, D. W. (2007). When worlds collide: Therapeutic and forensic roles. *Professional Psychology: Research and Practice, 38*(2), 129–132. doi:10.1037/0735-7028.38.2.129

Heinlen, K. T., Welfel, E. R., Richmond, E. N., & O'Donnell, M. S. (2003). The nature, scope, and ethics of psychologists' e-therapy Web sites: What consumers find when surfing the web. *Psychotherapy: Theory, Research, Practice, Training, 40*, 112–124. doi:10.1037/0033-3204.40.1-2.112

Manhal-Baugus, M. (2001). E-therapy: Practical, ethical, and legal issues. *Cyberpsychology & Behavior, 4*, 551–563. https://doi.org/10.1089/109493101753235142

McAuliff, B. D., & Arter, J. L. (2016). Adversarial allegiance: The devil is in the evidence details, not just on the witness stand. *Law and Human Behavior, 40*(5), 524–535.

McHugh, R. K., Whitton, S. W., Peckham, A. D., Welge, J. A., & Otto, M. W. (2013). Patient preference for psychological vs. pharmacologic treatment of psychiatric disorders: A meta-analytic review. *Journal of Clinical Psychiatry, 74*(6), 595–602.

Metzner, J. L., & Ash, P. (2010). Commentary: The mental status examination in the age of the internet—challenges and opportunities. *Journal of the American Academy of Psychiatry and the Law, 38*, 27–31.

Meyer, G. J., Finn, S. E., Eyde, L. D., Kay, G. G., Moreland, K. L., Dies, R. R., Eisman, E. J., Kubiszyn, T. W., & Reed, G. M. (2001). Psychological testing and psychological assessment: A review of evidence and issues. *American Psychologist, 56*(2), 128–165.

Midkiff, D. M., & Wyatt, W. J. (2008). Ethical issues in the provision of online mental health services (e-therapy). *Journal of Technology in Human Services, 26*, 310–332. https://doi.org/10.1080/15228830802096994

Murrie, D. C., Boccaccini, M. T., Guarnera, L. A., & Rufino, K. A. (2013). Are forensic experts biased by the side that retained them? *Psychological Science, 24*(10), 1889–1897.

Murrie, D. C., Boccaccini, M. T., Turner, D. B., Meeks, M., Woods, C., & Tussey, C. (2009). Rater (dis)agreement on risk assessment measures in sexually violent predator proceedings: Evidence of adversarial allegiance in forensic evaluation? *Psychology, Public Policy, and Law, 15*(1), 19–53.

Neal, T. M. S., & Brodsky, S. L. (2016). Forensic psychologists' perceptions of bias and potential correction strategies in forensic mental health evaluations. *Psychology, Public Policy, and Law, 22*(1), 58–76.

Neal, T. M. S., & Grisso, T. (2014). The cognitive underpinnings of bias in forensic mental health evaluations. *Psychology, Public Policy, and Law, 20*(2), 200–211.

Neimark, G., Hurford, M. O., & DiGiacomo, J. (2006). The Internet as collateral informant. *American Journal of Psychiatry, 163*, 1842.

Otto, R. (2015). *Ethical challenges in forensic psychology.* American Psychology-Law Society Annual Conference, San Diego, CA.

Otto, R. K., Goldstein, A. M., & Heilbrun, K. (2017). *Ethics in forensic psychology practice.* Wiley.

Pew Research Center. (2021, April 7). Social media fact sheet. https://www.pewresearch.org/internet/fact-sheet/social-media/?menuItem=d102dcb7-e8a1-42cd-a04e-ee442f81505a

Pinals, D. A., Appelbaum, P. S., Bonnie, R., Fisher, C. E., Gold, L. H., & Lee, L. (2015). American Psychiatric Association: Position statement on firearm access, acts of violence and the relationship to mental illness and mental health services. *Behavioral Sciences & the Law, 33*(2–3), 195–198.

Pirelli, G., Beattey, R. A., & Zapf, P. A. (Eds.). (2017). *The ethical practice of forensic psychology: A casebook.* Oxford University Press. https://doi-org/10.1093/acprof:oso/9780190258542.001.0001

Pirelli, G., & Gold, L. (2019). Leaving Lake Wobegon: Firearm-related education and training for medical and mental health professionals is an essential competence. *Journal of Aggression, Conflict and Peace Research, 11*(2), 78–87.

Pirelli, G., Hartigan, S., & Zapf, P. A. (2018). Using the Internet for collateral information in forensic mental health evaluations. *Behavioral Sciences and the Law, Special Issue: The Internet, Cybertechnology and the Law, 36*(2), 157–169.

Pirelli, G., Otto, R. K., & Estoup, A. (2016). Using Internet and social media data as a collateral source in forensic evaluations. *Professional Psychology: Research and Practice, 47*(1), 12–17.

Pirelli, G., Wechsler, H., & Cramer, R. J. (2019). *The behavioral science of firearms: A mental health perspective on guns, suicide, and violence.* Oxford University Press.

Recupero, P. R. (2008). Forensic evaluation of problematic Internet use. *Journal of the American Academy of Psychiatry and the Law, 36,* 505–514.

Recupero, P. R. (2010). The mental status examination in the age of the Internet. *Journal of the American Academy of Psychiatry and the Law, 38,* 15–26.

Scurich, N., Krauss, D. A., Reiser, L., Garcia, R. J., & Deer, L. (2015). Venire jurors' perceptions of adversarial allegiance. *Psychology, Public Policy, and Law, 21*(2), 161–168.

Thibodaux, L. K., Breiger, D., Bledsoe, J., Sato, J., Hilsman, R., & Paolozzi, A. (2021). Teleneuropsychology: A model for clinical practice. *Practice Innovations, 6*(3), 189–198. https://doi.org/10.1037/pri0000150

Wells, M., Mitchell, K. J., Finkelhor, D., & Becker-Blease, K. A. (2007). Online mental health treatment: Concerns and considerations. *Cyberpsychology and Behavior, 10,* 453–459.

Zapf, P. A., Kukucka, J., Kassin, S. M., & Dror, I. E. (2018). Cognitive bias in forensic mental health assessment: Evaluator beliefs about its nature and scope. *Psychology, Public Policy, and Law, 24*(1), 1–10.

Zappala, M., Reed, A. L., Beltrani, A., Zapf, P. A., & Otto, R. K. (2018). Anything you can do, I can do better: Bias awareness in forensic evaluators. *Journal of Forensic Psychology Research and Practice, 18*(1), 45–56.

Zur, O., Williams, M. H., Lehavot, K., & Knapp, S. (2009). Psychotherapist self-disclosure and transparency in the Internet age. *Professional Psychology: Research and Practice, 40,* 22–30. https://doi.org/10.1037/a0014f7

Zusman, J., & Simon, J. (1983). Differences in repeated psychiatric examinations of litigants to a lawsuit. *American Journal of Psychiatry, 140*(10), 1300–1304.

INDEX

For the benefit of digital users, indexed terms that span two pages (e.g., 52–53) may, on occasion, appear on only one of those pages.

Tables, figures, and boxes are indicated by t, f, and b following the page number

239